Practical Evaluation and Management of the Shoulder

FREDERICK A. MATSEN III, M.D.
STEVEN B. LIPPITT, M.D.
JOHN A. SIDLES, M.D.
DOUGLAS T. HARRYMAN II, M.D.

University of Washington
Shoulder Team
Department of Orthopaedics
University of Washington School of Medicine
Seattle, Washington

Practical Evaluation and Management of the Shoulder

W.B. SAUNDERS COMPANY
A Division of Harcourt Brace & Company
Philadelphia London Toronto Montreal Sydney Tokyo

W.B. SAUNDERS COMPANY
A Division of
Harcourt Brace & Company

The Curtis Center
Independence Square West
Philadelphia, Pennsylvania 19106

Library of Congress Cataloging-in-Publication Data

Practical evaluation and management of the shoulder /
Frederick Matsen III . . . [et al.].

p. cm.

Includes bibliographical references and index.

ISBN 0–7216–4819–3

1. Shoulder—Diseases.   2. Shoulder joint—Diseases.
3. Shoulder—Abnormalities.   4. Shoulder joint—
Abnormalities.   5. Shoulder—Wounds and injuries.
6. Shoulder joint—Wounds and injuries.   7. Shoulder
joint—Mechanical properties.   I. Matsen, Frederick
A.   [DNLM: 1. Shoulder—physiopathology.
2. Shoulder Joint—physiopathology.   WE 810 P8945
1994]

RD557.5.P72 1994   617.5′72—dc20

DNLM/DLC   93–41664

PRACTICAL EVALUATION AND MANAGEMENT OF THE SHOULDER   ISBN 0–7216–4819–3

Printed in the United States of America.

Last digit is the print number: 9   8   7   6   5   4   3   2   1

I'm a shoulder-making man,
a shoulder-making man.
I try to stop shoulder-making,
hard as I can, but
I'm a shoulder-making man.

LAURA JANE MEGAN MATSEN
(age 4)

Proceeds from this book will be donated to the E. A. Codman Shoulder Research
Endowment at the University of Washington Department of Orthopaedics

Preface

This book presents a cost-effective approach for optimizing the function of compromised shoulders using simple exercises and appropriate surgery. It presents an integrated, practical method based on the following five precepts:

- Normal shoulder function depends on four basic mechanical characteristics: motion, stability, strength, and smoothness.
- To be surgically treatable, a disorder must be defined in terms of disturbed mechanics. Therefore, the clinician must determine both the patient's functional deficits and the mechanical reasons for these deficiencies.
- These determinations can usually be made economically, using only the history, physical examination, and plain radiographs.
- The goal of treatment is the restoration of the patient's shoulder function. Thus, the success of treatment must be measured in terms of functional improvement.

- The results of surgery are dependent both on the procedure and the surgeon performing it. Therefore, each surgeon is responsible for knowing the results of his or her own operations.

This book is directed at the type of practice we see evolving for the coming decades, when resources will not be as plentiful and increasing premiums will be placed on economy and effectiveness. In this spirit, we emphasize what can be accomplished with the basics: the clinical history, the physical examination, a few plain radiographs, simple patient-conducted rehabilitation programs, and well-characterized open surgical procedures. It is written for orthopaedic surgeons and all other investigators, physicians, therapists, coaches, and trainers who seek to understand mechanical problems of the shoulder. It is intended to be practical, informative, and, we hope, enjoyable.

Happy shouldering!

FREDERICK A. MATSEN III, M.D.
STEVEN B. LIPPITT, M.D.
JOHN A. SIDLES, Ph.D.
DOUGLAS T. HARRYMAN II, M.D.

Foreword

With the ever increasing number of volumes being written about afflictions of the shoulder, one might ask, "Do we really need another book on the shoulder?" Before reading this text, the answer might well be "No." However, after careful perusal of this bold and somewhat unconventional initiative, I believe our original response would prove to be mistaken. The salient features of this publication that distinguish it from those that have gone before are that

1. It attempts to provide a practical, common sense, basic approach to evaluating and managing the most important clinical shoulder problems.
2. The physical examination and management recommendations are solidly founded in basic science investigation.

The challenge of this text is that it attempts to wed a practical approach to evaluating shoulder problems to sophisticated laboratory investigations. If this task is accomplished successfully, readers have a tremendous asset at their disposal for management of this difficult anatomic region. The authors have been able to embody the integration of clinical and research data and, in so doing, have met this challenge ably.

The authors' program, which starts with the initial clinical evaluation and describes the spectrum of shoulder pathology in terms of the broad categories comprising motion, strength, stability, and roughness, will appeal to experienced orthopaedic surgeons as well as to those still in training. An additional unique feature is the detailed presentation of material designed to be shared with patients to enhance their understanding of the disease processes and management options.

It should be noted that this text does not portend to be a comprehensive text reference on the shoulder. Rather, the authors have achieved a practical and useful guide to basic evaluation and management.

BERNARD F. MORREY, M.D.
President
American Academy of Orthopaedic Surgeons

Professor and Chairman
Department of Orthopaedics
Mayo Clinic
Rochester, Minnesota

Special Acknowledgments

to the University of Washington Shoulder Team

Craig Arntz
Franz Ballmer
William Barrett
John Clark
David Collins
Elizabeth Crouch
Susan DeBartolo
Jonathan Franklin
Thurman Gillespy
Juan Carlos Gonzalez
Scott Harris
Sarah Jackins
Mark Lazarus
Laurence Mack
Michael Pearl
Yong-Girl Rhee
Michael Richardson
Anthony Romeo
Jet Tenley
Steven Thomas
Jim Vahey
Eric Vanderhooft
Joseph Zuckerman

Contents

1
Evaluating the Shoulder 1

2
Shoulder Motion 19

3
Stability 59

4
Strength 111

5
Smoothness 151

6
Synthesis: Practice
Guidelines 221

Bibliography 231

Appendix 233

Index 235

CHAPTER

1

Evaluating the Shoulder

The clinician faces the challenge of identifying the best management approach for each patient. If the patient's shoulder problem can be understood in mechanical terms, effective treatment options can usually be identified. Conversely, if a mechanical problem cannot be defined, surgical treatment will be unreliable.

Each patient presenting with a shoulder problem deserves a carefully conducted clinical history, a good physical examination, and, if appropriate, a selected series of plain radiographs; this basic evaluation cannot be replaced by MRI, arthroscopy, or examination under anesthesia. Using only the history, physical examination, and plain radiographs, the clinician can place most shoulder problems in one of three groups: (1) treatable, (2) diagnosable but untreatable, or (3) undiagnosable.

THE TREATABLE SHOULDER

There exists a group of conditions related to the shoulder for which the underlying process can be established and for which dependable treatment is available. To enable effective communication concerning the prevalence and management of these shoulder problems, we must establish the *necessary* and *sufficient* conditions for each of them. In this context, "necessary" means that the diagnosis cannot be made without meeting these criteria. "Sufficient" means that if these criteria are met, no other information or tests are required to establish the diagnosis. Table 1–1 sets forth the necessary and sufficient conditions for establishing the diagnoses of some of the important treatable conditions of the shoulder. It is significant that most of these treatable disorders can be diagnosed from the basic evaluation: the clinical history, the physical examination, and plain radiographs.

THE DIAGNOSABLE BUT UNTREATABLE SHOULDER

A second group of shoulder problems exists that are diagnosable but are not amenable to definitive surgical treatment. Examples include diagnoses such as brachial neuritis, habitual dislocations, mid-substance muscle tears, anterior sternoclavicular subluxation, generalized ligamentous laxity, instability from movement disorders, and massive rotator cuff tears in persons with paraplegia. In these situations we must inform the patient of the limitations of existing treatment methods. We can then direct the available resources to provide patient education, exercise instruction, and vocational rehabilitation.

THE UNDIAGNOSABLE SHOULDER

Some shoulder complaints are not diagnosable, no matter how many tests we order. We can spend an unlimited amount of time and money in vain pursuit of a treatable cause for vague shoulder problems or in investigating shoulder pain as a presentation of job dissatisfaction. A risk in ordering diagnostic tests when the basic evaluation suggests no shoulder pathology is that these tests may yield "findings" that do not relate to the patient's complaint. Findings of "labral fraying" on arthroscopic examination, "abnormal signals in the cuff tendons" on MRI, or "laxity" on examination under anesthesia do not help in the evaluation or management of non-specific shoulder complaints. From the standpoint of resource allocation, we must try to define which shoulder problems do *not* need expensive diagnostic evaluations on the first encounter. Our guideline is that when the basic evaluation (a careful history and physical examination along with appropriate plain radiographs) does not suggest the existence of a definable problem, we do not proceed to advanced imaging, electrodiagnostics, arthroscopy, or examination under anesthesia because the yield is so low in these circumstances. If there is nothing in the basic evaluation to suggest pathology, we are likely to tell the patient, "After a good history, physical examination, and x-rays, we do not know what your problem is; however, we doubt that further tests will change the treatment we recommend to you at this time." Repeat clinical examination after several months

TABLE 1–1. Necessary and Sufficient Diagnostic Criteria for Major Chronic Conditions of the Shoulder

Problems of Motion
I. Frozen Shoulder
  A. History
    1. Functionally significant restriction of shoulder motion
    2. Absence of history of previous major shoulder injury or surgery
  B. Physical Examination
    1. Limited glenohumeral motion in all directions
  C. Radiographs
    1. No changes in cartilaginous joint space
    2. Absence of pathologic changes other than osteopenia
II. Post-Traumatic or Post-Surgical Stiff Shoulder
  A. History
    1. Functionally significant restriction of shoulder motion
    2. History of significant shoulder injury or surgery
  B. Physical Examination
    1. Limited glenohumeral motion
  C. Radiographs
    1. No changes in cartilaginous joint space

Problems of Stability
I. Traumatic Anterior Glenohumeral Instability
  A. History
    1. Mechanism of injury appropriate to cause tearing of the anterior glenohumeral ligaments, such as a major external rotation torque applied when the arm is elevated near the coronal plane
    2. Functionally significant recurrent episodes of apprehension (fear of uncontrollable glenohumeral translations) or instability (inability to keep the humeral head centered in the glenoid fossa) when the arm is elevated near the coronal plane and externally rotated or extended
  B. Physical Examination
    1. Apprehension or instability when the arm is elevated near the coronal plane and externally rotated or extended
    2. Diagnosis is supported by grinding with translation on anterior drawer test
  C. Radiographs
    1. Diagnosis is supported by radiographs documenting a previous anterior glenohumeral dislocation
    2. Diagnosis is supported by radiographs showing a characteristic posterior lateral humeral head defect and/or anterior inferior glenoid lip defect or calcification
II. Atraumatic Instability
  A. History
    1. Functionally significant inability to keep the humeral head centered in the glenoid fossa, especially in positions not at the extremes of motion
    2. Absence of mechanism of injury likely to tear glenohumeral ligaments or capsule
    3. Spontaneous reduction of translations
  B. Physical Examination
    1. Demonstration that certain glenohumeral translations duplicate the symptoms of concern to the patient
    2. Diminished resistance to translation in multiple directions as compared with a normal glenohumeral joint
  C. Radiographs
    1. Absence of traumatic lesions

Problems of Strength
I. Full Thickness Rotator Cuff Tear
  A. History
    1. Functionally significant weakness of glenohumeral elevation and/or rotation
    2. Age over 30 years, usually over 40 years
    3. Diagnosis is supported by a history of sudden, unexpected loading of the arm followed by shoulder weakness
  B. Physical Examination
    1. Weakness on elevation and/or rotation
    2. Diagnosis is supported by supraspinatus and/or infraspinatus atrophy, subacromial crepitance, and/or palpable defect in rotator cuff
  C. Radiographs
    1. Diagnosis is supported by upward displacement of humeral head in relation to the acromion and by acromial spurring
  D. Definite identification of a full thickness cuff defect by an expert observer using one of the following: ultrasonography, arthrography, MRI, arthroscopy, or open surgery
II. Incomplete Thickness Cuff Lesion
  A. History
    1. Compromise of shoulder function in activities requiring rotator cuff function
    2. Mechanism for damaging the rotator cuff, such as unanticipated eccentric load applied to the elevated arm
  B. Physical Examination
    1. Pain and weakness on tests of rotator cuff function, such as resisted elevation and resisted external rotation
    2. Diagnosis is supported by subacromial crepitance

Table continued on following page

TABLE 1–1. Necessary and Sufficient Diagnostic Criteria for Major Chronic Conditions of the Shoulder *Continued*

C. Radiographs
   1. Diagnosis is supported by upward displacement of humeral head in relation to the acromion and by acromial spurring
D. Definite identification of an incomplete thickness cuff lesion by an expert observer using one of the following: arthrography, arthroscopy, or open surgery

Problems of Smoothness
I. Subacromial Abrasion
   A. History
      1. Limited function with the arm in intermediate positions of elevation
   B. Physical Examination
      1. Subacromial crepitance that reproduces the function-limiting symptoms, particularly on rotation of the humerus with the arm in intermediate positions of elevation
   C. Radiographs
      1. Diagnosis is supported by primary or secondary changes on the undersurface of the coracoacromial arch, such as acromial sclerosis or a traction spur in the coracoacromial ligament
      2. Diagnosis is supported by the coexistence of incomplete thickness cuff lesion or full thickness rotator cuff tear
II. Degenerative Joint Disease (primary)
   A. History
      1. Absence of major joint trauma, previous surgery, or other known causes of secondary degenerative joint disease
      2. Age over 30 years, usually over 40 years
      3. Limited motion and function
   B. Physical Examination
      1. Limited glenohumeral motion
      2. Diagnosis is supported by bone on bone crepitance
   C. Radiographs
      1. Joint space narrowing
      2. Periarticular sclerosis
      3. Periarticular osteophytes
      4. Absence of other pathology
      5. Diagnosis is supported by posterior glenoid erosion with posterior subluxation of humeral head
III. Secondary Degenerative Joint Disease
   A. History
      1. Evidence of major joint trauma or other known causes of secondary degenerative joint disease
      2. Limited motion and function
   B. Physical Examination
      1. Limited glenohumeral motion
      2. Diagnosis is supported by bone-on-bone crepitance
   C. Radiographs
      1. Joint space narrowing
      2. Periarticular sclerosis
      3. Periarticular osteophytes
      4. Diagnosis is supported by radiographic evidence of previous trauma or other known causes of secondary degenerative joint disease
IV. Rheumatoid Arthritis
   A. History
      1. American Rheumatological Association criteria for rheumatoid arthritis
      2. Limited motion and function
   B. Physical Examination
      1. Limited glenohumeral motion
      2. Diagnosis is supported by findings of muscle atrophy and weakness and/or bone-on-bone crepitance
   C. Radiographs
      1. Joint space narrowing
      2. Periarticular osteopenia
      3. Diagnosis is supported by the absence of osteophytes and sclerosis
      4. Diagnosis is supported by the presence of periarticular erosions and medial erosion of glenoid
V. Avascular Necrosis (Atraumatic)
   A. History
      1. Limited shoulder function
      2. Diagnosis is supported by the presence of risk factors, such as steroid use
   B. Physical Examination
      1. Diagnosis is supported by glenohumeral crepitance
   C. Radiographs
      1. Sclerosis within head of humerus
      2. Collapse of subchondral bone of humeral head
      3. Absence of other pathologic changes (e.g., tumor, cuff tear arthropathy)

TABLE 1–1. Necessary and Sufficient Diagnostic Criteria for Major Chronic Conditions of the Shoulder *Continued*

VI. Capsulorrhaphy Arthropathy
  A. History
    1. Functionally significant restricted glenohumeral motion
    2. History of previous repair for glenohumeral instability
  B. Physical Examination
    1. Limited motion and function (especially external rotation)
    2. Diagnosis is supported by bone-on-bone crepitance
  C. Radiographs
    1. Joint space narrowing
    2. Periarticular sclerosis
    3. Periarticular osteophytes
    4. Diagnosis is supported by posterior glenoid erosion with posterior subluxation of the humeral head
VII. Cuff Tear Arthropathy
  A. History
    1. Limited motion and function
    2. Weakness in elevation and rotation
    3. Diagnosis is supported by previously confirmed cuff tear
  B. Physical Examination
    1. Limited glenohumeral motion
    2. Evidence of large cuff defect, such as
      a. Supraspinatus and infraspinatus atrophy
      b. Weakness of external rotation and elevation
      c. Superior position of humeral head relative to the scapula
      d. Palpable rotator cuff defect
    3. Bone-on-bone crepitance
  C. Radiographs
    1. Superior displacement of the humeral head relative to the glenoid leading to contact with the coracoacromial arch
    2. Secondary degenerative changes of the glenohumeral joint
    3. Diagnosis is supported by erosion of the greater tuberosity ("femoralization" of the proximal humerus)
    4. Diagnosis is supported by a contoured coracoacromial arch and upper glenoid to produce a socket for the proximal humerus ("acetabularization")
    5. Diagnosis is supported by the collapse of the superior subchondral bone of the humeral head

often provides additional insight into the nature of the problem. The diagnosis for "shoulder pain without identified pathology" should be just that. Assigning a label with minimal therapeutic significance, such as fibromyalgia, myofasciitis, and trigger points, does not help us determine a curative treatment. Usually, we can best serve these patients by shifting the expenditure of resources from evaluation to a program of physical, vocational, and social support.

AGE AT PRESENTATION AS AN AID IN DIAGNOSIS

Certain conditions are strongly age related; thus, the patient's age is a practical guide to the diagnostic probabilities. To explore these relationships, we recorded the ages of a consecutive series of new patients at the time of presentation to the University of Washington Shoulder Team for treatment of one of nine diagnoses that can be rigorously confirmed: degenerative joint disease, rheumatoid arthritis, capsulorrhaphy arthropathy (arthritis after previous instability repair), avascular necrosis, incomplete thickness cuff lesions (including what is referred to by some as the "impingement syndrome"), full thickness cuff tears, frozen shoulder, traumatic anterior instability, and atraumatic instability. Table 1–2 and Figures 1–1 and 1–2 show the distribution of these diagnoses by age at presentation to our service. Although the numbers in some groups are small, and the data reflect the particular nature of the practice of the University of Washington Shoulder Team, several observations are significant. Diagnoses other than instability were rare in patients younger than 30 years of age. No patient under 30 years of age had a complete cuff tear. With advancing age, incomplete thickness cuff lesions became less common as full thickness cuff lesions became more common. Degen-

TABLE 1–2. Age at Presentation to University of Washington Shoulder Team for Patients with Nine Major Shoulder Diagnoses

Diagnosis	Mean Age in Years ± SD (range)	Number
Atraumatic instability	23 ±7 (13–43)	51
Traumatic anterior instability	30 ± 10 (16–62)	32
Avascular necrosis	39 ± 12 (27–58)	8
Capsulorrhaphy arthropathy	40 ± 7 (30–48)	7
Incomplete thickness cuff lesion	41 ± 11 (30–72)	18
Rheumatoid arthritis	56 ± 18 (26–77)	13
Frozen shoulder	53 ± 10 (35–71)	39
Degenerative joint disease	64 ± 10 (39–83)	46
Full thickness rotator cuff tear	62 ± 12 (31–80)	58

erative joint disease, cuff tears, and frozen shoulder were the most common diagnoses in patients older than 45 years of age.

Patients presenting with chronic, diagnosable shoulder problems fell into three age groups (Fig. 1–3). The *Young* group, aged 13 to 30 years, was dominated by problems of traumatic anterior instability and atraumatic instability. The *Middle* group, aged 31 to 45 years, included representation of all the major diagnoses. Finally, the *Older* group, with age at presentation over 45 years, was dominated by degenerative joint disease, cuff tears, and frozen shoulders.

PRACTICAL CLINICAL EVALUATION OF SHOULDER FUNCTION: THE SIMPLE SHOULDER TEST

It is evident that each of the conditions potentially afflicting the shoulder may vary substantially in severity. The diagnoses of instability, cuff disease, arthritis, or frozen shoulder do not, in themselves, indicate the need for treatment. The need for treatment arises from the effect of the condition on the patient's function. Furthermore, the success of the treatment is best measured in terms of its ability to restore function. We conclude that a practical method for documenting the patient's shoulder function is essential to planning and evaluating treatment.

The clinical course of a shoulder problem before and after treatment can be mapped by its effect on shoulder function. The most important and practical assessment of a shoulder's function is the patient's view of it. Figure 1–4 charts the course of a shoulder problem. From the clinical onset of the disease, the patient's function deteriorates. The physician makes the diagnosis and institutes a conservative course of treatment that results in a temporary improvement in shoulder function. The physician then performs an operation that is followed by a progressive improvement, maximizing after a recovery period. The incremental changes in function resulting from treatment represent the effectiveness of the treatment.

To facilitate and standardize the patient's reporting of the functional status of his or her problematic shoulder, we have developed a brief questionnaire called the *Simple Shoulder Test,* or SST. The SST consists of a minimal data set of twelve "yes" or "no" questions derived from the common complaints of patients presenting to the Shoulder Team for evaluation. These twelve questions are the following:

1. Is your shoulder comfortable with your arm at rest by your side?
2. Does your shoulder allow you to sleep comfortably?
3. Can you reach the small of your back to tuck in your shirt with your hand?
4. Can you place your hand behind your head with the elbow straight out to the side?
5. Can you place a coin on a shelf at the level of your shoulder without bending your elbow?

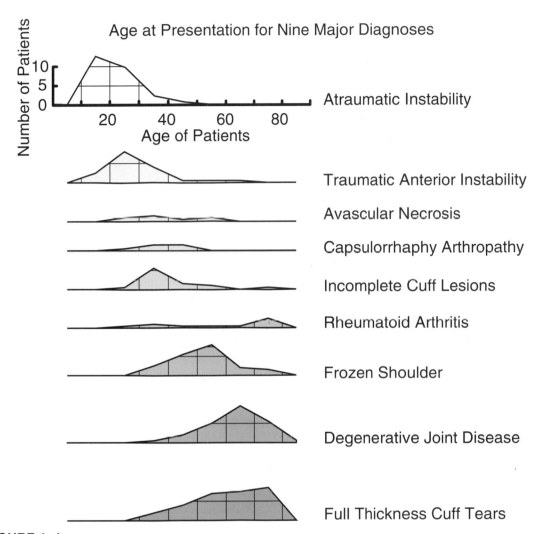

FIGURE 1–1.

Distribution of ages at presentation for 272 consecutive patients with nine major diagnoses. The abscissa indicates age in years. The ordinate indicates the number of patients in each decade; each ordinate mark indicates five patients. The total numbers of patients with each diagnosis were atraumatic instability, 51; traumatic anterior instability, 32; avascular necrosis, 8; capsulorrhaphy arthropathy, 7; incomplete cuff lesions, 18; rheumatoid arthritis, 13; frozen shoulder, 39; degenerative joint disease, 46; and full thickness cuff tears, 58.

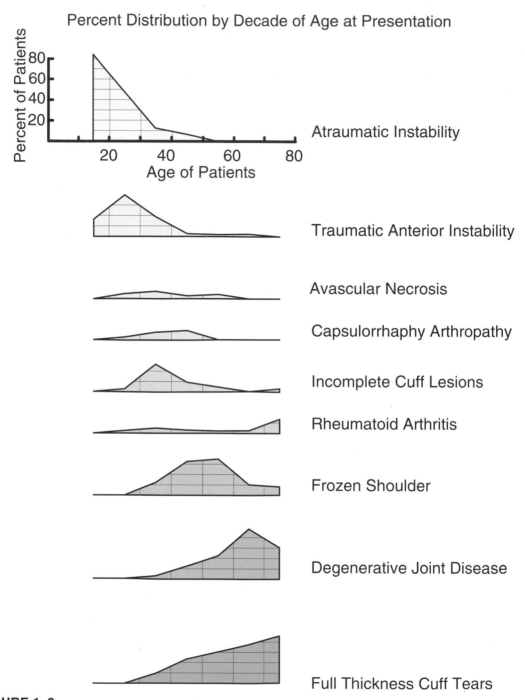

FIGURE 1–2.

Percent distribution by decade of age at presentation for 272 consecutive patients with nine major diagnoses. The abscissa indicates age in years. The ordinate indicates the percentage of patients in each decade with each of the diagnoses. Each ordinate mark indicates 5 percent of the patients in the indicated decade with the indicated diagnosis.

Diagnoses Presenting in Three Age Groups

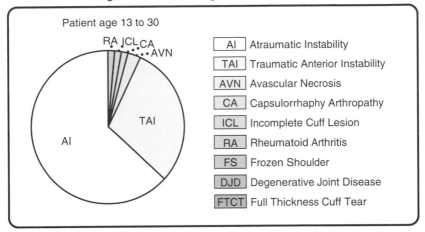

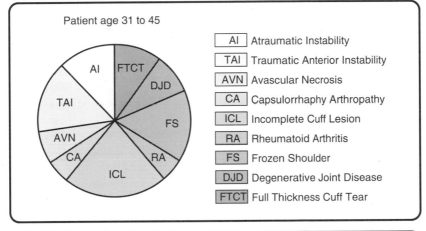

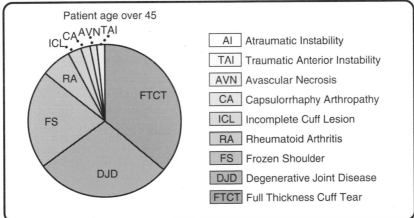

FIGURE 1–3.

Diagnoses presenting in the age groups 13 to 30, 31 to 45, and over 45. In the age group 13 to 30, the predominant diagnoses were atraumatic instability and traumatic anterior instability. In the age group 31 to 45, all nine diagnoses were substantially represented. In the age group over 45, the predominant diagnoses were cuff tear, frozen shoulder, and degenerative joint disease.

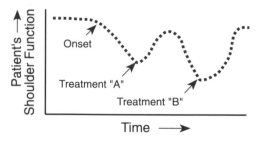

FIGURE 1–4.

Hypothetical clinical course of a shoulder problem, charted according to its effect on the patient's view of his or her shoulder function. Treatment "A" led to a temporary increment in function. Treatment "B" led to a greater improvement in function.

6. Can you lift 1 lb (a full pint container) to the level of your shoulder without bending your elbow?
7. Can you lift 8 lb (a full gallon container) to the level of the top of your head without bending your elbow?
8. Can you carry 20 lb at your side with the affected extremity?
9. Do you think you can toss a softball underhand 10 yards with the affected extremity?
10. Do you think you can throw a softball overhand 20 yards with the affected extremity?
11. Can you wash the back of your opposite shoulder with the affected extremity?
12. Would your shoulder allow you to work full-time at your usual job?

It is important that the patient answer these questions without assistance: it is the patient's own evaluation of his or her shoulder function that is wanted. Because the patient is the consistent evaluator of the shoulder, concern about interobserver variability is eliminated. The SST reflects the status of the shoulder in functional terms rather than in degrees of motion, appearance of radiographs, or isokinetic torque measurements. If the situation requires, we can add questions to the original twelve, keeping the minimal data set intact. For example, in studying high-performance athletes, we add to the basic SST questions such as, "Does your shoulder allow you to pitch (or serve) with your usual speed and control?" "Does

your shoulder allow you to swim your normal workout?" "Does your shoulder allow you to compete at the varsity level in your sport?"

Prior to the clinical introduction of the SST, we verified that almost all normal patients aged 60 to 70 years were able to perform the twelve basic functions (Fig. 1–5). Subsequently, we have used the SST on thousands of clinical occasions.

The SST has demonstrated a high degree of reproducibility. In normal subjects, the reproducibility is essentially 100 percent, with almost all subjects answering "yes" to all twelve questions. As a more stringent test, we tested 70 patients with *abnormal* SSTs and then retested them 5 to 30 days later (average 14 days) (Figs. 1–6 and 1–7). Sixty-three percent of the patients had identical responses on retesting. Ninety percent of the patients answered no more than one question differently on retest. More than 96 percent made no more than two different responses on retest. This lack of absolute reproducibility is not a deficiency of the SST; instead it reflects an actual day-to-day variation in some patients' view of their shoulder function.

The SST provides a practical method for determining the pretreatment shoulder function as well as the shoulder function at various intervals after the treatment (Fig. 1–8). Sequential SSTs indicate the length of time required to achieve maximum functional benefit after treatment. The difference between the shoulder function before treatment and after the recovery period is a measure of the effectiveness of the treatment.

The simplicity of the SST facilitates the communication of results to patients. Prospective surgical candidates are able to compare their own pretreatment status with the typical pretreatment status of others having the same diagnosis. This information enables them to answer questions such as, "How bad is my arthritis in comparison with other people who have had a total shoulder replacement?" Similarly, by reviewing the functional results of a given treatment for their diagnosis, patients can answer the questions, "What are the chances that I will be able to do these activities after the treat-

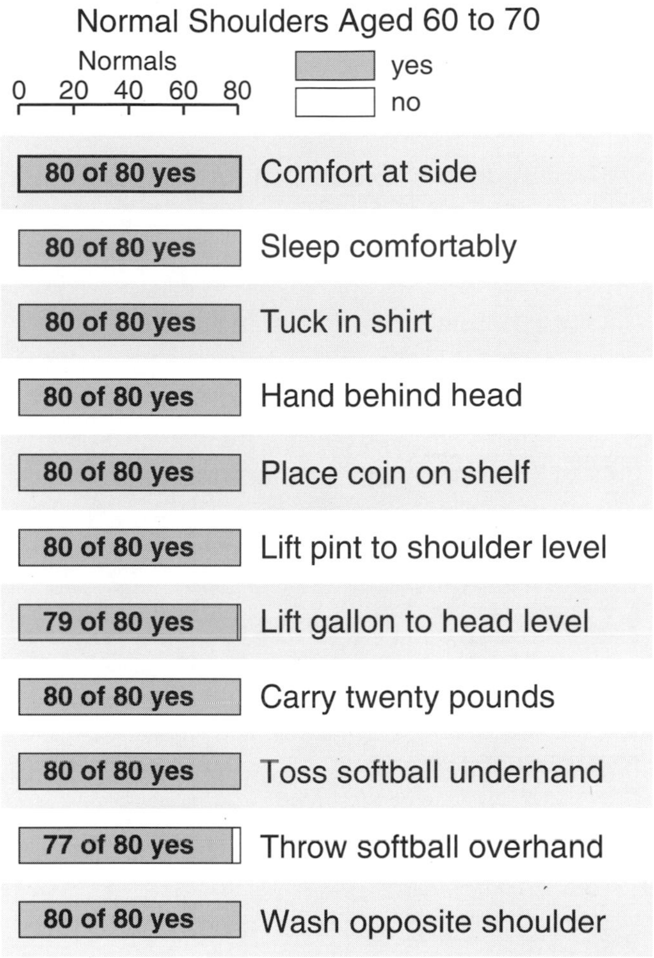

Normal Shoulders Aged 60 to 70

Normals
0 20 40 60 80

yes
no

80 of 80 yes	Comfort at side
80 of 80 yes	Sleep comfortably
80 of 80 yes	Tuck in shirt
80 of 80 yes	Hand behind head
80 of 80 yes	Place coin on shelf
80 of 80 yes	Lift pint to shoulder level
79 of 80 yes	Lift gallon to head level
80 of 80 yes	Carry twenty pounds
80 of 80 yes	Toss softball underhand
77 of 80 yes	Throw softball overhand
80 of 80 yes	Wash opposite shoulder

FIGURE 1–5.

The Simple Shoulder Test—normal shoulders. Responses from 80 subjects aged 60 to 70 years with shoulders that were normal by history, physical examination, and expert shoulder ultrasound examination to exclude cuff tear. The male/female distribution was essentially equal. Only one shoulder per subject is included. Essentially all these subjects answered "yes" to each of the test questions.

ment?" and "How long will it take before I see improvement?"

A meaningful study of a treatment outcome for a specified condition needs to capture essentially *all* of the patients meeting the necessary conditions for a given diagnosis who are treated by the individual surgeon with a specified technique. Because the patient can complete the questionnaire unassisted at home, the SST facilitates the inclusion of a maximal number of patients in the outcome analysis without the uncontrollable bias imposed by selecting only those patients who return for followup.

It is critical for the physician to have a pretreatment determination of the patient's shoulder function. For this reason, we include the SST as an integral part of our new patient information form (Patient Information 1–1). This form also gives the patient

an opportunity to supply the clinician with a wealth of other information concerning his or her shoulder problem and general health. Finally, it establishes the precedent that diagnosis and treatment require a partnership between the patient and the physician.

The outcomes for different surgeons using apparently identical procedures are often not the same. The surgeon is the critical determinant of the procedure and its outcome: "The surgeon *is* the method." It is important, therefore, for each surgeon to document the functional outcomes for his or her own surgical procedures rather than to assume that the results will be the same as another surgeon's. This personal quality control facilitates the identification of problems and suggests areas of needed improvement for the individual surgeon. Outcome measurement must not be prohibitively expensive.

Text continued on page 17

Test-retest Reproducibility of the SST

Patients
0 20 40 60

☐ same answer
☐ different answer

67 of 70 same	Comfort at side
67 of 70 same	Sleep comfortably
65 of 70 same	Tuck in shirt
63 of 70 same	Hand behind head
65 of 70 same	Place coin on shelf
62 of 70 same	Lift pint to shoulder level
64 of 70 same	Lift gallon to head level
63 of 70 same	Carry twenty pounds
64 of 70 same	Toss softball underhand
65 of 70 same	Throw softball overhand
67 of 70 same	Wash opposite shoulder
66 of 70 same	Work full-time regular job

FIGURE 1–6.

Test-retest reproducibility of each of the Simple Shoulder Test (SST) questions in 70 patients with functionally abnormal shoulders. Retests were obtained 5 to 30 days (mean 14 days) after the first test. The chart shows the number of patients providing the same answer to each of the twelve SST questions.

FIGURE 1–7.

Test-retest reproducibility of the overall Simple Shoulder Test (SST) in 70 patients with functionally abnormal shoulders. The chart shows that 63 percent of patients answered all SST questions the same on the retest. Twenty-seven percent answered all but one SST question the same; 6 percent answered all but two SST questions the same; 3 percent answered all but three questions the same.

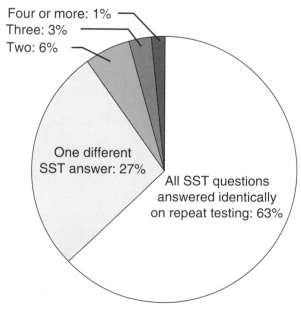

Test-retest Reproducibility of the SST in 70 Patients with Abnormal Shoulders

Four or more: 1%
Three: 3%
Two: 6%
One different SST answer: 27%
All SST questions answered identically on repeat testing: 63%

12

FIGURE 1–8.

Simple Shoulder Test data before surgery and sequentially after surgery for shoulders with degenerative joint disease having shoulder arthroplasty. For a specific surgeon, data such as these indicate (1) the typical preoperative state of patients having shoulder arthroplasty for this diagnosis, (2) the likelihood of regaining a given function after surgery, and (3) the recovery time for each function.

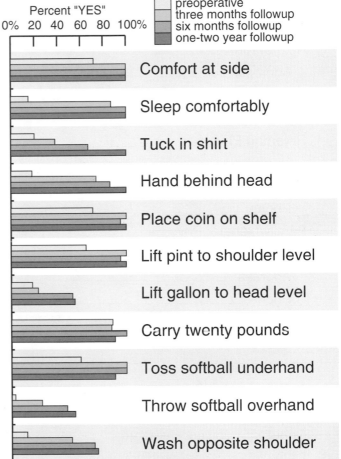

SST Data Before Surgery and Sequentially Following Total Shoulder Arthroplasty

preoperative
three months followup
six months followup
one-two year followup

Percent "YES"
0% 20 40 60 80 100%

Comfort at side
Sleep comfortably
Tuck in shirt
Hand behind head
Place coin on shelf
Lift pint to shoulder level
Lift gallon to head level
Carry twenty pounds
Toss softball underhand
Throw softball overhand
Wash opposite shoulder

PATIENT INFORMATION 1–1

UNIVERSITY OF WASHINGTON SHOULDER INFORMATION FORM
We would appreciate your volunteering some information about you and your shoulder to help us in its evaluation and treatment. Your complete answers to the information below will be helpful; however, you should feel free not to respond to any of the questions that you find objectionable. Please use the back sides of the pages as necessary.

Your Name: _____

    Address: _____

    Phone: _____

Next of Kin: _____

    Address: _____

    Phone: _____

Date of Birth: _____ Today's Date: _____

Referring Physician

    Name: _____

    Address: _____

    Phone: _____

Family/General Physician

    Name: _____

    Address: _____

    Phone: _____

Occupation: _____

    Date last worked: _____

Usual recreation: _____

Date last able to do this recreation: _____

Right-Handed: _____ Left-Handed: _____

Shoulder Involved: Right _____ Left _____

Date your shoulder problem began: _____

Were you hurt on the job? _____

Does your shoulder problem involve a legal case? _____

Please describe your current shoulder problem in your own words:

If you had an injury, please describe it in detail:

Do you currently have problems with any of the below? If so, please describe them.

    shoulder stiffness: _____

    shoulder weakness: _____

    shoulder instability: _____

PATIENT INFORMATION 1–1

UNIVERSITY OF WASHINGTON SHOULDER INFORMATION FORM *Continued*

SIMPLE SHOULDER TEST

Please answer these questions about your shoulder.   Date:_____

	YES	NO
1. Is your shoulder comfortable with your arm at rest by your side?	☐	☒
2. Does your shoulder allow you to sleep comfortably?	☐	☐
3. Can you reach the small of your back to tuck in your shirt with your hand?	☐	☐
4. Can you place your hand behind your head with the elbow straight out to the side?	☐	☐
5. Can you place a coin on a shelf at the level of your shoulder without bending your elbow?	☐	☐
6. Can you lift 1 pound (a full pint container) to the level of your shoulder without bending your elbow?	☐	☐
7. Can you lift 8 pounds (a full gallon container) to the level of the top of your head without bending your elbow?	☐	☐
8. Can you carry 20 pounds (a bag of potatoes) at your side with the affected extremity?	☐	☐
9. Do you think you can toss a softball underhand 10 yards with the affected extremity?	☐	☐
10. Do you think you can throw a softball overhand 20 yards with the affected extremity?	☐	☐
11. Can you wash the back of your opposite shoulder with the affected extremity?	☐	☐
12. Would your shoulder allow you to work full-time at your regular job?	☐	☐

Are there other important things you cannot do as a result of your shoulder problem?

Previous doctors you have seen about your shoulder problem:

Previous tests you have had concerning your shoulder problem:

Previous nonmedical treatment you have had for your shoulder problem:

How many cortisone, steroid, or other types of injections have you had in your shoulder?

Previous shoulder surgeries (please list which shoulder, procedure, and date):

Are there any other aspects of your shoulder problems that we should know about?

Any family history of shoulder problems?

PATIENT INFORMATION 1–1

UNIVERSITY OF WASHINGTON SHOULDER INFORMATION FORM *Continued*

The following information will help us understand your overall health and how it may relate to your shoulder problem.

Do you have any problems with joints other than the shoulder discussed above? _____
    If so please describe them.

Any surgeries other than those listed above? _____
    Please list:

Have you had infections, bleeding, or any other complications from previous surgeries? _____
    Please explain:

Family history of other health problems? _____
    Please explain:

Smoker? _____ Packs per day: _____ Years of smoking: _____

Alcohol consumption per average day: _____

Have you ever used recreational drugs? _____

Allergies: _____

Current medications
(including aspirin, antacids, pain medicines; heart, lung, or kidney medicines)

Do you have any of the health concerns listed below? If yes, please describe:
    Heart
    Lungs
    Seizures
    Kidneys, bladder
    Depression
    Bleeding tendencies
    Tendencies for infection
    Exposure to hepatitis
    Exposure to HIV infection (AIDS)
    Exposure to TB infection

	YES	NO
Do you have a lot of bodily pain?	☐	☐
Do you feel good most of the time?	☐	☐
Do you get depressed sometimes?	☐	☐
Do you feel your health is likely to get better?	☐	☐
Do you have as much energy as others?	☐	☐

Are there any other health-related factors we should know about you?

Your signature _____

The SST provides each practitioner with a practical, consistent tool for documenting the pretreatment and post-treatment status of each patient.

CONCLUSION

The ability of the shoulder to perform its functions depends on four basic mechanical characteristics: motion, stability, strength, and smoothness. Most of the clinically important shoulder disorders can be described in terms of abnormalities of one or more of these parameters. Thus, a frozen shoulder is primarily a problem with shoulder motion. Recurrent dislocation is primarily a problem of glenohumeral stability. Rotator cuff tears manifest themselves in terms of diminished strength. Glenohumeral arthritis produces abnormalities of both smoothness and motion. The criteria necessary for making these diagnoses can usually be established using only the history, physical examination, and plain radiographs.

Shoulder pathology that can be defined in mechanical terms has a good chance of being treatable. Treatment is determined not only by the underlying process but also by the severity of its impact on shoulder function. The Simple Shoulder Test provides an economical method for documenting a shoulder's functional status. Comparing the functional status of the shoulder before and sequentially after an operation indicates the procedure's effectiveness. The Simple Shoulder Test provides a practical tool by which surgeons can determine the outcomes for procedures in their own hands.

CHAPTER

2

Shoulder Motion

One of the special attributes of the shoulder is its ability to place the arm in a vast range of positions with respect to the thorax. In this chapter we focus on the range of positions through which the shoulder can move, how these positions are characterized in the clinic and the laboratory, and how the patient with a stiff shoulder can be managed.

SIMPLE ASSESSMENT OF SHOULDER RANGE OF MOTION

A patient's range of motion can be described in terms of the following four simple parameters:

1. The maximal angle of humeral elevation in relation to the thorax as viewed from the side (Fig. 2–1).
2. The maximal angle of external rotation with the arm at the side (zero degrees being the position in which the forearm of the flexed elbow points straight ahead in the sagittal plane) (Fig. 2–2).
3. Maximal internal rotation as indicated by the highest segment of posterior midline anatomy that can be reached by the thumb (Fig. 2–3).
4. Maximal cross-body adduction as indicated by the minimal distance between the antecubital fossa and the contralateral anterior acromion (Fig. 2–4).

The values for these parameters in a population of 81 normal subjects aged 60 to 70 years are shown in Table 2–1.

Although these four parameters provide a rapid overview of the range of motion, proper study of the shoulder requires a more specific description of the positional relationships of the humerus, the scapula, and the thorax. In the following sections we present a simple system for describing the relative positions of the humerus, the scapula, and the thorax based on simple anatomic reference lines and planes.

HUMEROTHORACIC POSITIONS

The natural reference lines for describing humerothoracic positions are the long axis of the humeral shaft and the longitudinal axis of the thorax. The angle between these lines is the angle of humerothoracic elevation.

The plane containing these two lines is the plane of humerothoracic elevation (Fig. 2–5). The plane of elevation is identified in relation to a reference plane, the coronal plane of the thorax. For example, abduction is elevation in the zero degree plane, flexion is elevation in the plus 90 degree plane, and

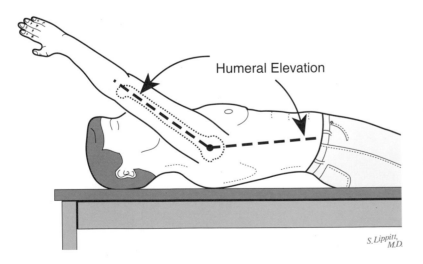

Humeral Elevation

S. Lippitt, M.D.

FIGURE 2–1.

Maximal elevation is measured with the patient supine and with the opposite arm assisting in elevation, if necessary, to gain maximal range.

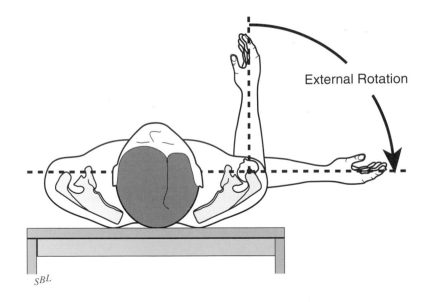

FIGURE 2–2.

Maximal external rotation is measured with the arm at the side (zero degrees being the position in which the forearm of the flexed elbow points straight ahead). We prefer to make this measurement with the patient supine to help fix the thorax.

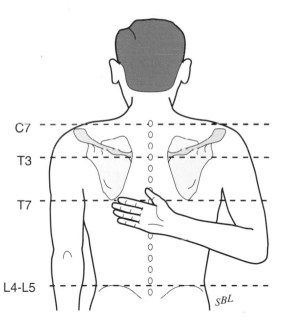

FIGURE 2–3.

Maximal internal rotation is measured by the highest segment of posterior anatomy reached with the thumb, for example, L4–L5, T7, T3, or C7.

FIGURE 2–4.

Maximal cross-body adduction is measured as the minimal distance from the antecubital fossa to the contralateral acromion when the arm is adducted horizontally across the body.

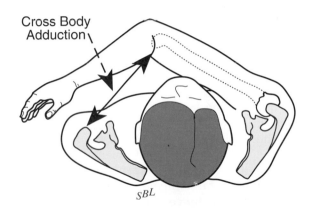

TABLE 2–1. Values for the Four Simple Parameters of Shoulder Motion in 81 Normal Subjects Aged 60 to 70 Years

	Males	Females
Maximal elevation (degrees)	160 ± 8	167 ± 7
Maximal external rotation (degrees)	72 ± 13	78 ± 15
Maximal internal rotation (segments)	T6 ± 2	T5 ± 2
Maximal cross-body adduction (cm)	15 ± 3	14 ± 3

elevation in a plane half way between is elevation in the 45 degree plane (Fig. 2–6).

Using this simple method, we can define any position of the humerus in reference to the thorax with only two numbers: the angle and the plane of humerothoracic elevation.

ACTIVITY

Position your arm to wash the back of the opposite shoulder. Describe this humerothoracic position in terms of the plane and angle of humerothoracic elevation. Do the same with your arm positioned to tuck in a shirt in back. See whether a colleague observing these positions independently arrives at the same values.

Normal Values for Ranges of Humerothoracic Positions

The ranges of humerothoracic positions in eight normal subjects were measured using electromagnetic sensors pinned to the humerus to avoid artifacts from soft tissue movement. Table 2–2 lists the average humerothoracic positions for eight common functional positions. The data demonstrate that the humerus functions in a wide range of thoracic planes from minus 88 to plus 124 degrees. Maximal humerothoracic elevation averaged 148 degrees in the plus 55 degree thoracic plane.

More detailed measurements were made of the positions attainable by a single subject, again using an electromagnetic sensor pinned to the humerus. Table 2–3 displays the maximal humeral elevation that this subject could achieve in different thoracic planes. These data define the envelope of humerothoracic positions available to this individual shoulder.

This same instrumented subject performed six of the functions of the Simple Shoulder Test (SST). The planes and angles of elevation for these activities are shown in Table 2–4. Note that the SST requires the humerus to function in a wide range of positions.

Humerothoracic Global Diagram

The global diagram (Fig. 2–7) is an effective method of displaying the range of shoulder positions because it allows presentation of both the planes of elevation ("longitudes") and the angles of elevation ("latitudes"). The "South Pole" of the globe represents zero degrees of elevation.

Figure 2–8 is a pictorial representation of the data from Tables 2–3 and 2–4. Note that

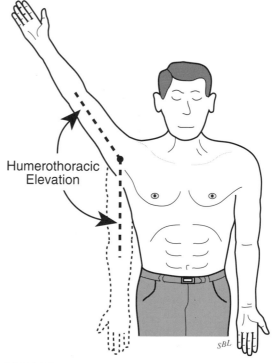

FIGURE 2–5.

Humerothoracic elevation. The angle of elevation is the angle between the humeral shaft axis and the thoracic axis. The angle is measured in the plane that contains these two axes, that is, the plane of humerothoracic elevation.

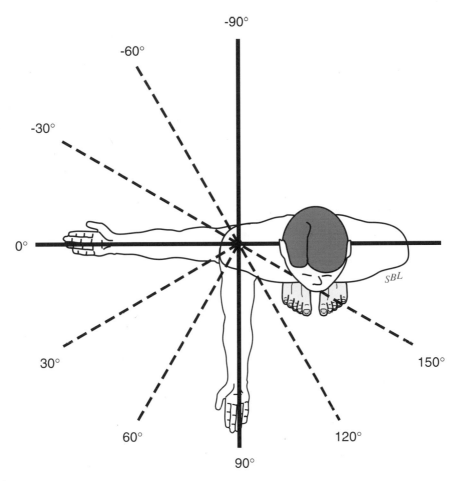

FIGURE 2–6.

The plane of humerothoracic elevation can be easily defined in relation to the zero degree thoracic plane (the coronal plane).

TABLE 2–2. Functional Humerothoracic Positions in Eight Normal Subjects*

	Plane of Elevation (degrees)	Angle of Elevation (degrees)
Cross-body adduction	124 ± 7	90 ± 1
Washing axilla	104 ± 12	52 ± 14
Eating	87 ± 29	52 ± 8
Maximal elevation	55 ± 17	148 ± 11
Combing hair	54 ± 27	112 ± 10
Maximal reach up back	-69 ± 11	56 ± 13
Reaching perineum	-86 ± 13	38 ± 10
Maximal extension	-88 ± 1	55 ± 9

*Values are mean $\pm$ SD.

TABLE 2–3. Maximal Humerothoracic Elevation in Specific Planes Observed in a Selected Subject

Humerothoracic Plane of Elevation (degrees)	Maximal Humerothoracic Angle of Elevation (degrees)
−87	73
−59	81
−30	92
0	116
31	131
60	136
90	129
118	90

the maximal elevation in the different planes defines the envelope of humerothoracic motion available to this shoulder. The positions used for the SST functions lie within this envelope.

In addition to its ability to indicate any humerothoracic position, the global diagram also provides a method of indicating unambiguously the rotational orientation of the arm. For this purpose, an arrow indicates the orientation of the anterior aspect of the humerus (which is the direction that the forearm would point if the elbow were flexed to 90 degrees).

In Figure 2–9, the rotational orientations of the humerus in the positions of maximal elevation are shown with arrows.

The rotational orientations for the functions of the SST are seen in Figure 2–10.

The details of simple and complex motions of the humerus can be indicated on a global diagram as a series of points and arrows (Fig. 2–11).

The global diagram is particularly useful because it can indicate not only the position but also the rotational orientation of the humerus in any humerothoracic position. No simple *numerical* system can describe these orientations in all possible positions of the arm. For example, a numerical system for defining zero degrees of rotation with the arm at the side becomes ambiguous when the arm is elevated 90 degrees in the 45 degree thoracic plane. The problem is familiar in navigation as well: orientations such as "north" and "west" work fine at the middle latitudes but poorly at the poles. The confusion is evident in the literature on arthrodesis positions, in describing throwing positions, and in discussions of Codman's paradox. The following activity demonstrates the value of the global system for describing humeral rotation.

ACTIVITY

CODMAN'S PARADOX

Codman proposed that the completely elevated humerus could be shown to be in either extreme external rotation or extreme internal rotation by lowering it in either the coronal or the sagittal plane, respectively, without allowing rotation about the humeral shaft axis. We can use the global diagram to examine Codman's paradox.

Part 1. Carry out the movement sequence described as follows without allowing rotation about the humeral shaft axis:

TABLE 2–4. Humerothoracic Positions Used for Simple Shoulder Test Functions by a Selected Subject

		Humerothoracic Plane of Elevation (degrees)	Humerothoracic Angle of Elevation (degrees)
SST Q3	Tuck in shirt	−54	57
SST Q1	Comfort at side	0	0
SST Q4	Hand behind head	13	118
SST Q7	Lift gallon to head level	66	93
SST Q5	Place coin on shelf	76	73
SST Q6	Lift pint to shoulder level	86	78
SST Q11	Wash opposite shoulder	128	71

SST Q = Simple Shoulder Test question no. See Patient Information 1–1.

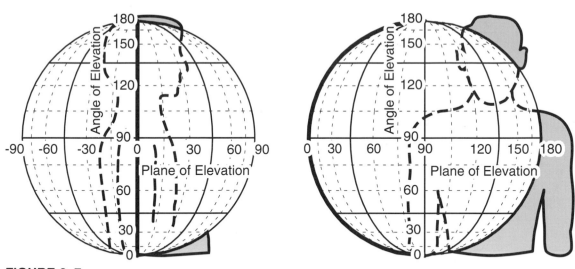

FIGURE 2–7.

Global diagrams allow the simultaneous presentation of the plane and the angle of humerothoracic elevation. Our standard format is to include both the lateral and frontal views. Zero degrees of elevation is at the "South Pole." The zero degree plane of elevation, indicated with a broad line, is the coronal plane.

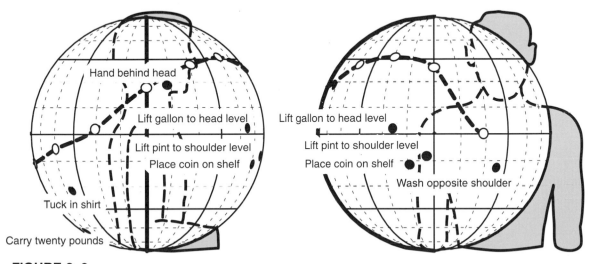

FIGURE 2–8.

Global diagram for one specific subject showing the maximal humerothoracic elevation in various thoracic planes *(unlabeled white dots)*. The labeled black dots indicate the humerothoracic positions that this subject used to perform some of the functions from the Simple Shoulder Test.

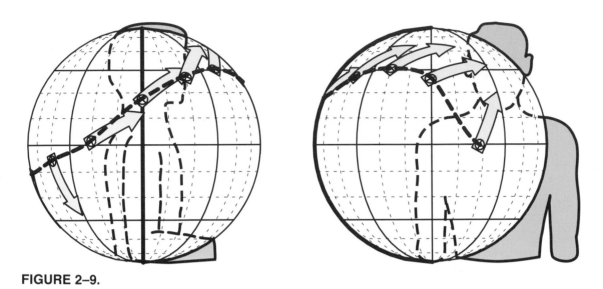

FIGURE 2–9.

The arrows indicate the rotational orientation of the forearm in positions of maximal humerothoracic elevation for the selected subject.

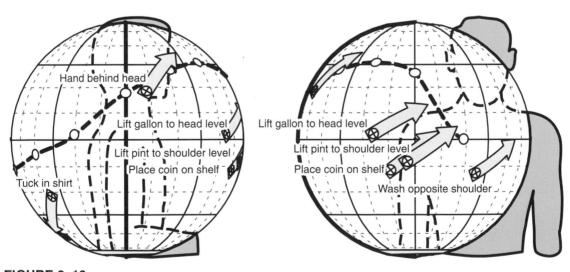

FIGURE 2–10.

The arrows indicate the rotational orientation of the arm in humerothoracic positions used by the subject to perform the activities of the Simple Shoulder Test.

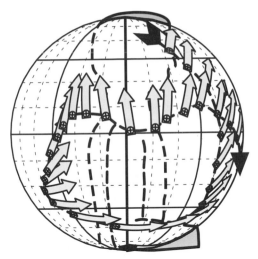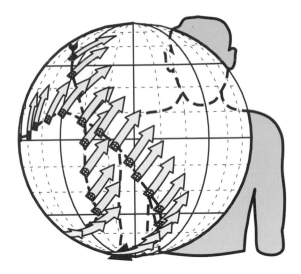

FIGURE 2–11.

The path of motion for a throw displayed as a series of points and orientations on a global diagram.

1. Place the arm at the side with the forearm internally rotated across the stomach.
2. Elevate the arm 180 degrees in the plus 90 degree thoracic (sagittal) plane.
3. Lower the arm 180 degrees to the side in the zero degree (coronal) plane.

Note that the forearm now points 180 degrees from its original position. Draw this entire motion on a global diagram (Fig. 2–12). Determine the fraction of the surface area of the sphere that is enclosed by this path of motion (answer: 1/4).

This result demonstrates the relationship between enclosed area and rotation. The area of a unit sphere is 4π. One fourth of this is π; 360 degrees of rotation is equal to 2π; thus π is equal to 180 degrees of rotation. We see that a humeral path without rotation about the humeral shaft axis circumscribing one fourth of a sphere results in an induced rotation of 180 degrees.

Part 2. To further examine this relationship, we can try another movement sequence, as follows:

1. Place the arm at the side with the forearm pointing straight ahead.
2. Elevate the arm 90 degrees in the plus 90 degree (anterior sagittal) plane (in this position the humerus is horizontal and the forearm points up).

3. Keeping the forearm pointing up, move the arm to a position of 90 degrees of elevation in the zero degree plane (arm still horizontal, forearm still pointing up).
4. Lower the arm 90 degrees to the unelevated position.

Note that the forearm now points 90 degrees from its original position. Draw this entire motion on a global diagram (Fig. 2–13). Determine the fraction of the surface area of the sphere enclosed by this path of motion (answer: 1/8). The area of one eighth of a sphere is $\pi/2$, which is equivalent to 90 degrees of induced rotation.

This relationship between area and induced rotation holds true for any sequence of motions in a closed path in which there is no rotation about the humeral shaft axis. From this relationship, we can see that the apparent paradox of induced rotations on Codman's motions is a property of motion on the surface of a sphere and not a paradox at all!

Factors Limiting Humerothoracic Positions

The range of humerothoracic positions may be limited by contact of the arm with

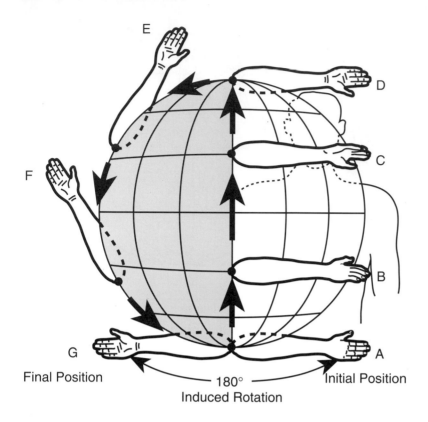

Final Position ⟵ 180° ⟶ Initial Position

Induced Rotation

FIGURE 2–12.

Codman's paradox: induced rotation of 180 degrees. If the unelevated arm is placed in maximal internal rotation across the stomach (A), then elevated 180 degrees in the sagittal plane without rotation about the humeral shaft axis (B through D), and then lowered in the coronal plane without rotation about the humeral shaft axis (E through G), it acquires a rotation of 180 degrees. In this motion, it encloses a path of a quarter of a sphere. Because a unit sphere has a total area of 4π, the enclosed area is π. Because a unit circle has a circumference of 2π, π corresponds to a hemicircle, or 180 degrees.

FIGURE 2–13.

Codman's paradox: induced rotation of 90 degrees. If the forearm of the unelevated arm is pointed straight ahead (A), then the arm is elevated 90 degrees in the sagittal plane without rotation about the humeral shaft axis (B), and then moved without rotation about the humeral shaft axis to the coronal plane (C), and lowered in that plane (D), it acquires a rotation of 90 degrees. In this motion, the arm encloses a path of one eighth of a sphere. Because a unit sphere has a total area of 4π, the enclosed area is $\pi/2$. Because a unit circle has a circumference of 2π, $\pi/2$ corresponds to one fourth of a circle, or 90 degrees.

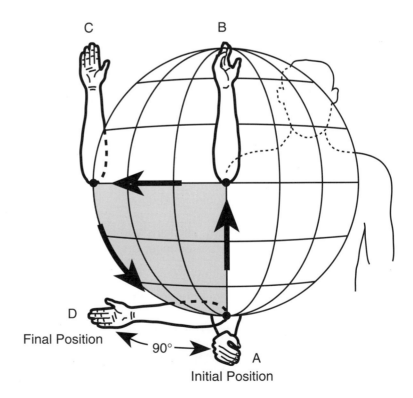

Final Position ⟵ 90° ⟶

Initial Position

the thorax or by factors limiting either of the component motions: that between the humerus and the scapula (humeroscapular) and that between the scapula and thorax (scapulothoracic).

HUMEROSCAPULAR POSITIONS

Most clinical shoulder problems involve the articulation between the humerus and scapula; thus, evaluation of clinical shoulder problems requires the specific determination of humeroscapular positions and motions. As with humerothoracic positions, humeroscapular positions are characterized in terms of the angle and the plane of elevation. The scapular references are defined in terms of the following clinically palpable landmarks (Figs. 2–14 through 2–16):

1. The inferior pole of the scapula.
2. The medial extent of the spine of the scapula.
3. The posterior angle of the acromion.
4. The tip of the coracoid process.

The angle of humeroscapular elevation is the angle between the humeral shaft axis and a parallel to the line connecting scapular reference points 1 and 2.

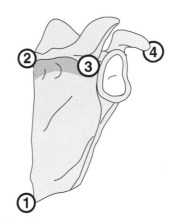

FIGURE 2–14.

Four clinically palpable scapular landmarks: (1) the inferior pole of the scapula, (2) the medial extent of the spine of the scapula, (3) the posterior angle of the acromion, and (4) the tip of the coracoid process.

The plane of humeroscapular elevation is that containing the humeral shaft axis and the reference line connecting points 1 and 2 on the medial border of the scapula. The plane of humeroscapular elevation is referenced to the plane of the scapula. The *plane of the scapula* is defined as the plane containing the scapular reference line (the line connecting points 1 and 2 on the medial scapula) and passing half-way between points 3 and 4 (see Fig. 2–16). Elevation of

FIGURE 2–15.

The four scapular reference points (see Fig. 2–14) can be easily palpated in clinical practice.

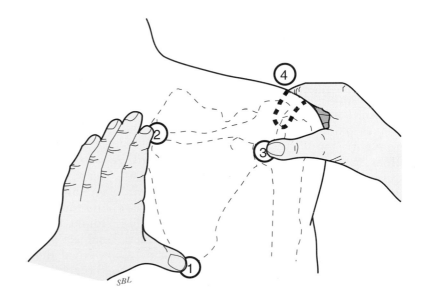

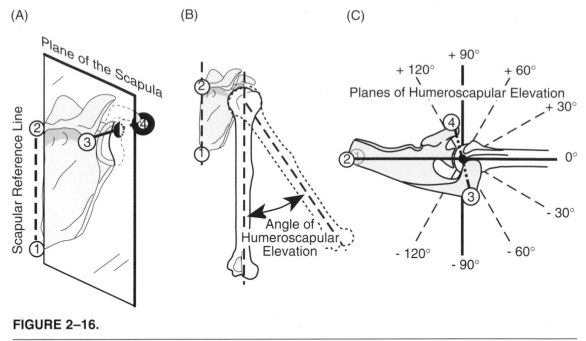

FIGURE 2–16.

A, The scapular reference line is the line connecting points 1 and 2 on the medial scapula. The plane of the scapula contains points 1 and 2 and passes midway between points 3 and 4 on the scapula. *B*, The angle of humeroscapular elevation is defined as the angle between a line parallel to the scapular reference line and the humeral shaft axis in its elevated position. *C*, The plane of humeroscapular elevation is referenced to the plane of the scapula.

the humerus in this plane is elevation in the zero degree scapular plane. Elevation anteriorly at right angles to this plane is elevation in the plus 90 degree scapular plane.

Using these four clinically accessible scapular reference points, we can define any position of the humeral shaft relative to the scapula.

Detailed measurements were made of the humeroscapular positions attained by a subject instrumented with electromagnetic sensors pinned to the humerus and the scapula. The maximal humeral elevation that this subject could achieve in different scapular planes is displayed in Table 2–5, along with the corresponding humerothoracic positions. It is critical to remember that humeroscapular elevation is defined in relation to a line connecting the two reference points on the medial scapular border and not in relation to an arbitrary "initial" position with the arm at the side. An anatomic scapular reference is necessary because patients may use a variety of combinations of humeroscapular and scapulothoracic positions to achieve a given humerothoracic position.

Thus, the only way to communicate humeroscapular positions unambiguously is by using anatomic scapular references.

The humeroscapular planes and angles noted in this subject during performance of the SST are shown in Table 2–6, along with the corresponding humerothoracic planes and angles of elevation. Note that these functions were performed between the 70 degree anterior and the 70 degree posterior planes and required less than 90 degrees of humeroscapular elevation. When the arm was at the side (humerothoracic elevation equals zero), humeroscapular elevation was not zero but rather 21 degrees in the plus 45 degree scapular plane.

In a series of 15 normal subjects, humeroscapular positions were measured using a goniometer. Clinical measurements using the four anatomic scapular landmarks were found to be quite reproducible among this subject population. When the subjects' arms were at the side in zero degrees of humerothoracic elevation, the humeroscapular position averaged 25 plus or minus 12 degrees of elevation in the 62 plus or minus 15 de-

TABLE 2–5. Maximal Humeroscapular Elevations in Various Scapular Planes by a Selected Subject*

Humeroscapular Plane of Elevation (degrees)	Humeroscapular Angle of Elevation (degrees)	Humerothoracic Plane of Elevation (degrees)	Humerothoracic Angle of Elevation (degrees)
−121	30	−87	73
−81	46	−59	81
−49	61	−30	92
−29	73	0	116
−5	87	31	131
8	94	60	136
21	96	90	129
43	78	118	90

*Shown with the corresponding humerothoracic planes and angles of elevation.

gree scapular plane. These results again emphasize that zero degrees of humerothoracic elevation does not correspond to zero degrees of humeroscapular elevation because humeroscapular elevation is defined in terms of the scapular landmarks. Maximal humerothoracic elevation averaged 140 plus or minus 7 and was accomplished with an average humeroscapular elevation of 90 plus or minus 7 degrees in the minus 4 plus or minus 7 degree scapular plane.

Humeroscapular Global Diagram

The global diagram is also useful for representing humeroscapular positions (Fig. 2–17). Figure 2–18 shows the envelope of motion available at the humeroscapular joint of the test subject measured with the electro-

magnetic sensing system and the humeroscapular positions used for the SST functions.

Arrows have been added to Figures 2–19 and 2–20 to indicate the rotational orientation of the humerus in the different humeroscapular positions.

ACTIVITY

Practice determining the four cardinal points on the scapula on a friend. Use them (1) to estimate the maximal angle of elevation in the zero degree scapular plane, (2) to determine the maximal angle of elevation in the plus 45 degree and minus 45 degree scapular planes, and (3) to determine the maximal anterior plane that can allow 45 degrees of humero-

TABLE 2–6. Humeroscapular Planes and Angles of Elevation Used by a Selected Subject to Perform Activities of the Simple Shoulder Test*

	Humeroscapular Plane of Elevation (degrees)	Humeroscapular Angle of Elevation (degrees)	Humerothoracic Plane of Elevation (degrees)	Humerothoracic Angle of Elevation (degrees)
SST Q3 Tuck in shirt	−63	27	−54	57
SST Q4 Hand behind head	−13	83	13	118
SST Q7 Lift gallon to head level	11	77	66	93
SST Q5 Place coin on shelf	18	76	76	73
SST Q6 Lift pint to shoulder level	22	80	86	78
SST Q1 Comfort at side	45	21	0	0
SST Q11 Wash opposite shoulder	60	69	128	71

*Corresponding humerothoracic positions are shown for comparison.
SST Q = Simple Shoulder Test question no. See Patient Information 1–1.

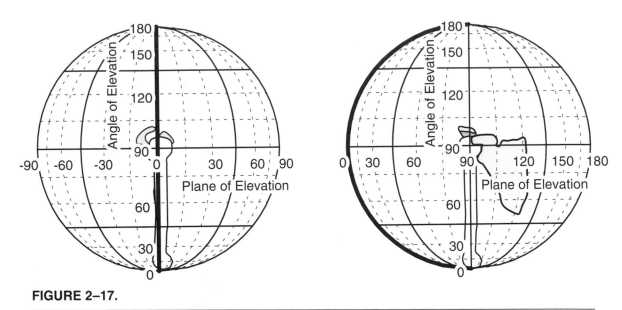

FIGURE 2–17.

The humeroscapular global diagram. Compare with the humerothoracic global diagram (see Fig. 2–7).

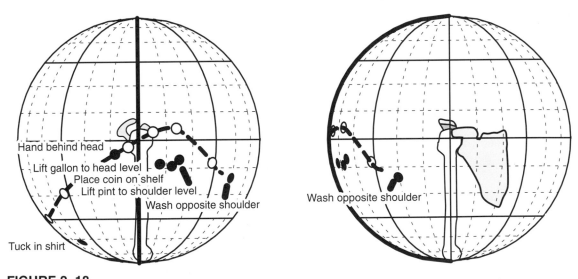

FIGURE 2–18.

Global diagram showing the envelope of humeroscapular motion for a selected subject *(white dots)*. Maximal humeroscapular elevation of nearly 100 degrees was achieved in planes just anterior to the plane of the scapula. Black dots indicate positions used by subject to perform some of the functions of the Simple Shoulder Test. Compare with Figure 2–8, which shows humerothoracic positions for these same activities.

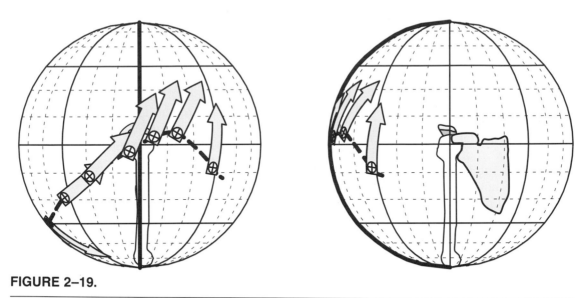

FIGURE 2–19.

The arrows indicate the rotational orientation of the arm in positions of maximal humeroscapular elevation in different planes for the selected subject. Compare with Figure 2–9, which shows humerothoracic positions for these same activities.

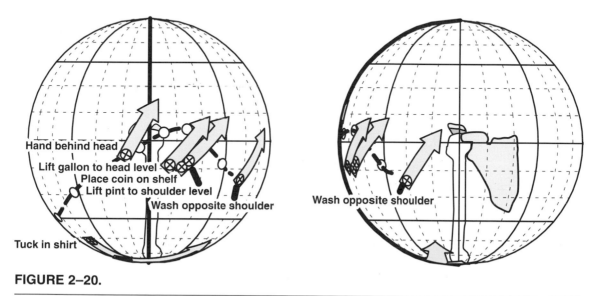

FIGURE 2–20.

The arrows indicate the rotational orientation of the arm in humeroscapular positions used by the subject to perform some of the activities of the Simple Shoulder Test. Compare with Figure 2–10, which shows humerothoracic positions for these same activities.

scapular elevation. Indicate these positions on a humeroscapular global diagram. Use a global diagram with points and arrows to indicate the humeroscapular position of touching the back of the opposite shoulder.

Humeroscapular Motion Interface

Humeroscapular motion takes place at the diarthrodial glenohumeral joint and at a large non-articular surface we call the *humeroscapular motion interface.* This largely bursa-lined interface lies between a deep group of structures (proximal humerus, rotator cuff, and biceps tendon sheath) and a superficial group of structures (deltoid, acromion, coracoacromial ligament, coracoid process, and tendons attaching to the coracoid process) (Fig. 2–21). Unrestricted motion at this interface is essential to humeroscapular motion.

The amount of relative motion occurring at this interface varies with the site of the interface being observed and the humeroscapular motion carried out. Using MRI, we measured the relative positions of the scapula, the inner surface of the deltoid, and the external surface of the rotator cuff and humerus in the shoulders of five normal living subjects (Fig. 2–22). From a position of maximal external rotation to one of maximal internal rotation about the humeral shaft axis with the arm at the side, the relative motion was determined among these structures at four different levels along the humeral shaft (the levels of the coracoid tip, the center of the head, the distal humeral head, and the deltoid insertion).

The average interfacial motion taking place at each of the four levels in the five subjects is shown in Figure 2–23. Different excursions would be expected for different motions, such as elevation in various humeroscapular planes.

Factors Limiting Humeroscapular Motion

A number of different anatomic factors limit normal humeroscapular motion, including capsuloligamentous check reins, abutment of the cuff and capsular insertions against the margin of the glenoid, and humeroscapular bony contact.

Capsule and Ligaments

Tension in the glenohumeral capsule and ligaments limits rotation of the humeral

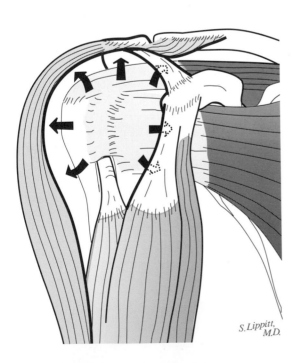

FIGURE 2–21.

The humeroscapular motion interface is an important location of motion between the humerus and the scapula. The deltoid, acromion, coracoacromial ligament, coracoid process, and tendons attaching to the coracoid lie on the superficial side of this interface, whereas the proximal humerus, rotator cuff, and biceps tendon sheath lie on its deep side.

Maximum External Rotation
(showing bone and tissue fiducial marks)

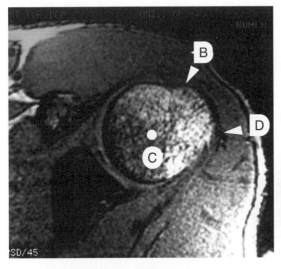

Maximum Internal Rotation
(showing same bone and tissue fiducial marks)

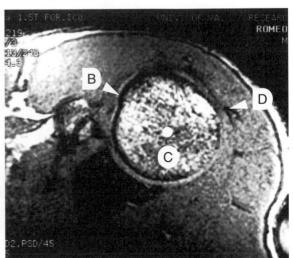

Maximum External Rotation
(with radial lines drawn between landmarks)

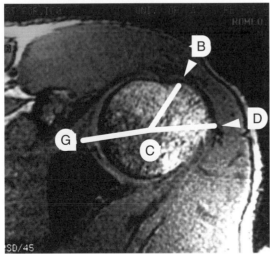

Maximum Internal Rotation
(arrow indicates sliding motion at interface)

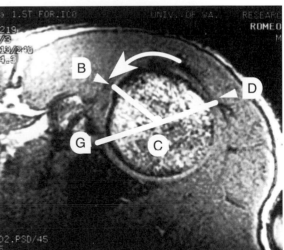

FIGURE 2–22.

MRI axial view of the shoulder *in vivo* with the arm at the subject's side in maximal active external rotation. Bone and tissue fiducial marks are used to track motion at the humeroscapular interface. *Upper left,* The fiducial marks used are the subscapularis insertion "B," a prominent deltoid raphe "D," and the center of the humeral head "C." *Upper right,* The same fiducial marks when the humerus is in maximal active internal rotation. *Lower left,* The same external rotation view as in upper left, with radial lines drawn from the center of the head "C" to the deltoid raphe "D," subscapularis insertion "B," and anterior lip of the glenoid "G." *Lower right,* The same view as in upper right, with the arrow showing the substantial sliding motion that occurs at the humeroscapular motion interface between the deltoid and the subscapularis insertion.

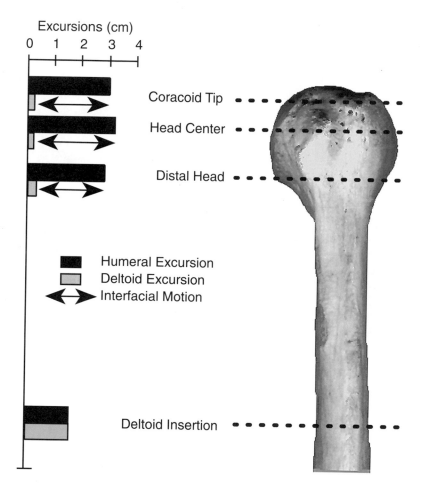

Excursions (cm)

Coracoid Tip

Head Center

Distal Head

Humeral Excursion
Deltoid Excursion
Interfacial Motion

Deltoid Insertion

FIGURE 2–23.

Mean interfacial motion from five normal subjects. The humerus at right shows the levels at which the motions were measured. The excursion (in centimeters) of the humerus (black) and deltoid (gray) from maximal internal to maximal external rotation are indicated by the horizontal bars. The magnitudes of motion at the interface between the deltoid and the humerus are indicated by the double-headed arrows. The mean excursions at the humerothoracic motion interface were between approximately 3 cm proximally and essentially 0 cm at the deltoid insertion.

head. Tension in the inferior capsule, for example, restricts elevation. Tension in the anterior and posterior portions of the capsule restricts external and internal rotation, respectively.

In eight cadaver shoulders, we investigated the kinematic effects of the rotator interval capsule–coracohumeral ligament, a particularly important aspect of the glenohumeral capsular complex, which lies between the coracoid process, the bicipital groove, the subscapularis tendon, and the supraspinatus tendon (Fig. 2–24).

We found that this area of the capsule limited humeroscapular elevation in the plus 90 degree and minus 90 degree scapular planes

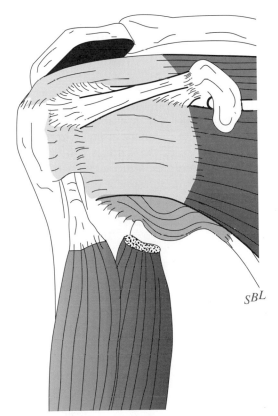

FIGURE 2–24.

The rotator interval capsule–coracohumeral ligament complex lies between the coracoid process, the bicipital groove, the subscapularis tendon, and the supraspinatus tendon. This is not a separate structure but rather a particular area of the glenohumeral capsule. Tightness of this structure can limit external rotation, adduction, and humeral elevation in anterior and posterior scapular planes.

but not in the zero degree scapular plane. Tightness of this specialized portion of the capsule also restricted adduction and external rotation, but not internal rotation of the humerus, as shown in Table 2–7.

Insertional Abutment Against Glenoid

At the extremes of humeroscapular rotation, the margins of the articular surfaces of the humeral head and the glenoid come into contact. The humeral attachments of the capsule and the rotator cuff border the articular surface of the humeral head. The labrum borders the articular surface of the glenoid. When these two groups of structures come into contact, motion is limited unless the cuff insertions slide past the labrum and into the joint. The relationships of the cuff insertion and the labrum in maximal humeral elevation are demonstrated by MRI in Figures 2–25 and 2–26.

Bony Contact

Bony factors can limit the range of humeroscapular motion. In abduction, the proximal humeral shaft can contact the acromion. In cross-body movement the humerus can contact the coracoid. In internal rotation the lesser tuberosity can contact the glenoid.

SCAPULOTHORACIC POSITIONS

The scapula moves across the thorax, gliding on the scapulothoracic motion interface. The deep surface of this interface consists of the ribs and their covering musculature. The superficial surface of the interface consists of the scapular border along with the serratus muscles. There are no generally accepted conventions for describing the position of the scapula on the thorax. Terms such as *protraction, retraction,* and *winging* are useful in describing types of movement but do not lend themselves to the definition of positions. A method of describing scapulothoracic positions and motions is needed to help us understand how the scapula functions in motions such as swinging a golf club or pushing a heavy load.

Some insight into scapulothoracic motion was gained by studying eleven patients with glenohumeral arthrodeses. Each patient had electromagnetic sensors attached to his or

TABLE 2–7. Effects of Surgical Release and Surgical Tightening of the Rotator Interval Capsule/Coracohumeral Ligament on the Range of Motion of Cadaver Shoulders

	RIC/CHL Released (degrees)	RIC/CHL Normal (degrees)	RIC/CHL Tightened (degrees)
Adduction	27	25	17
Elevation in plus 90 degree plane	82	76	68
Elevation in zero degree plane	74	76	77
Elevation in minus 90 degree plane	71	64	46
External rotation, zero degree elevation	75	70	32
External rotation, 60 degree elevation in the plus 90 degree plane	38	27	9
Internal rotation, zero degree elevation	59	59	57
Internal rotation, 60 degree elevation in the plus 90 degree plane	46	43	38

RIC/CHL = rotator interval capsule/coracohumeral ligament.

her thorax and humerus. Because all had solid glenohumeral fusions, their humerothoracic and scapulothoracic motions were equal. Starting from a position where the scapula was flat against the chest wall, these subjects averaged 47 degrees of scapular elevation in the plus 90 degree thoracic plane and 22 degrees of scapular elevation in the minus 90 degree thoracic plane. The total arc of scapular rotation about its medial reference line was 55 degrees. It is apparent that the scapulothoracic joint is able to make major contributions to shoulder motion.

Factors Limiting Scapulothoracic Motion

Movement of the scapula on the chest wall is limited by the motion allowed at the sternoclavicular and acromioclavicular joints, by the coracoclavicular ligaments, by the compliance of the scapula's musculotendinous attachments, and by the geometry of the scapulothoracic motion interface.

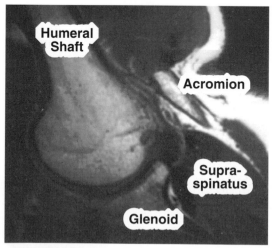

FIGURE 2–25.

This MRI view of the glenohumeral joint at maximal elevation shows abutment of the acromion against the humerus, which limits elevation. Note, however, that the supraspinatus tendon has cleared the acromion, so that contact occurs distal to the cuff insertion.

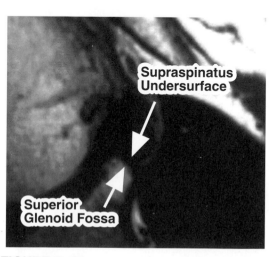

FIGURE 2–26.

In the same shoulder as shown in Figure 2–25, abutment of the undersurface of the supraspinatus tendon against the superior glenoid fossa serves to limit elevation.

PATHOLOGICALLY LIMITED SHOULDER MOTION

Humerothoracic motion is a major determinant of shoulder function. Pathologic processes affecting either humeroscapular or scapulothoracic motion may limit the effective range of humerothoracic motion. Humeroscapular motion can be limited by capsular contracture, arthritis, avascular necrosis, infection, fracture, dislocation, or interruption in the smooth functioning of the humeroscapular motion interface. Scapulothoracic range of motion can be limited by factors such as sternoclavicular arthritis, acromioclavicular arthritis, contracture, rib or scapular fracture, post-traumatic scarring, tumor, dislocation, or others disrupting the scapulothoracic motion interface.

Soft Tissue Causes of Limited Humeroscapular Motion

Shoulder stiffness resulting from disruption of the glenohumeral joint surface is discussed in a later section. Here we consider stiffness in the presence of normal glenohumeral joint surfaces, that is, stiffness resulting from problems of the humeroscapular soft tissues. Two variations of soft tissue restriction of humeroscapular motion are recognized. The term *frozen shoulder* refers to an idiopathic limitation of humeroscapular motion from contracture and loss of compliance of the glenohumeral joint capsule. By contrast, in a *post-traumatic* or *post-surgical stiff shoulder,* adhesions, scarring, and capsular contracture result from previous injuries or surgery to the soft tissues around the glenohumeral joint and non-articular humeroscapular motion interface.

Contracture of the glenohumeral capsule may be generalized or localized. Localized capsular contractures produce predictable limitations of shoulder motion, as indicated in Table 2–8.

Important effects of capsular tightness occur in addition to limited range of motion. One of these effects is the phenomenon of *obligate translation.* When rotational torque is applied to the humerus in a direction that

TABLE 2–8. Effect of Localized Capsular Tightness on Shoulder Motion

Location of Capsular Tightness	Motion(s) Limited
Posteroinferior	Elevation in anterior planes Internal rotation of the elevated arm Cross-body adduction
Posterosuperior Anterosuperior Anteroinferior	Reach up the back External rotation at the side External rotation of the elevated arm

tightens one aspect of the capsule, the head of the humerus may be forced in the opposite direction. Therefore, we would expect that when the capsule is tight anteriorly and an external rotation torque is applied, the humeral head is forced posteriorly (Fig. 2–27). This phenomenon may link anterior

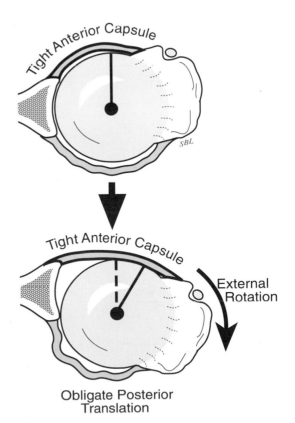

FIGURE 2–27.

Obligate posterior translation. When the anterior capsule is tight, external rotation against the tight capsule produces a posteriorly directed force that can push the humeral head in a posterior direction.

capsular tightness and posterior humeral subluxation with posterior glenoid wear seen commonly in glenohumeral osteoarthritis. It is furthermore consistent with the posterior glenohumeral subluxation and posterior glenoid erosion in shoulders with excessively tight anterior capsular repairs—a condition we refer to as *capsulorrhaphy arthropathy.*

Similarly, tightness of the posterior capsule may produce obligate anterior-superior translation with shoulder flexion (Fig. 2–28). In a series of experiments using cadaver shoulders, we found that humeral elevation in the plus 90 degree scapular plane with a torque of three Newton-meters produced anterior translation of 5 mm and superior translation of 0.5 mm. When the posterior capsule was shortened surgically, the anterior translation on forward elevation increased to over 7 mm and the superior translation to over 2 mm. These translations are

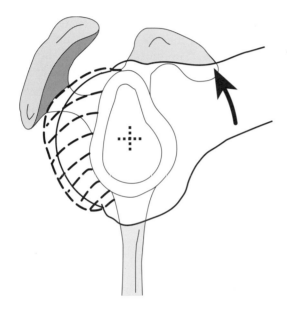

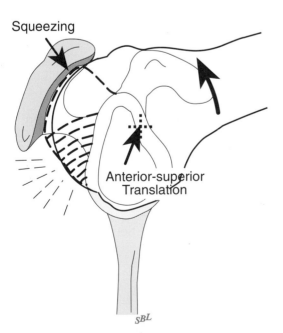

FIGURE 2–28.

Normal capsular laxity allows the humeral head to remain centered during elevation. Tightness of the posterior capsule can create obligate anterior-superior translation with anterior humeroscapular elevation. This may cause squeezing between the humerus and the undersurface of the acromion.

sufficient to press the humeral head and cuff against the coracoacromial arch, producing "subacromial impingement." These data suggest that "impingement signs" (either in maximal flexion or in abduction internal rotation) are likely to be positive in the presence of a tight posterior capsule.

The phenomenon of obligate translation suggests that caution should be exercised in applying large rotational torques to shoulders with tight capsules because of the risk of forcing obligate translation and increasing joint contact pressures.

EVALUATION OF THE PATIENT WITH LIMITED SHOULDER MOTION

Clinical evaluation of the patient presenting with a complaint of shoulder stiffness includes a good history, physical examination, and appropriate plain radiographs. The two principal soft tissue causes of a stiff shoulder are idiopathic frozen shoulder and post-traumatic stiff shoulder. The necessary and sufficient criteria for these conditions are listed in Table 2–9. The clinician must remember that a stiff shoulder may accompany or even mask other conditions, including cervical radiculopathy, cuff disease, or a neoplasm.

History

In evaluating stiff shoulders, it is essential to establish the circumstances surrounding the onset of stiffness, the duration of the condition, any tendency toward worsening or improvement, and the possible existence of risk factors, such as a period of immobilization, metabolic disease (such as diabetes), or referred pain from the neck, chest, or abdomen. In post-traumatic stiff shoulders the relationship of loss of motion to previous surgery or injury becomes evident from the history.

The age of patients with idiopathic frozen shoulders presenting to our service is typically between 43 and 63 years (Fig. 2–29).

Patients with frozen shoulders may have substantial functional losses. Figure 2–30 shows the SST results for patients meeting the strict criteria for idiopathic frozen shoulder. Patients with frozen shoulders had greatest difficulty sleeping comfortably on the affected side, putting their hands behind their heads with the elbow out to the side, lifting 8 pounds to the level of the top of their head without bending their elbow, and throwing overhand.

Physical Examination

As described at the beginning of this chapter, a simple assessment of shoulder motion can be obtained by examining the maximal ranges of elevation, external rotation, internal rotation and cross-body adduction. Then the humeroscapular range can be determined by stabilizing the scapula with one hand and putting the humerus through a passive range of motion with the other. The patient should remain relaxed during this examination to assure that muscle contraction is not limiting motion. Specific ranges of humeroscapular elevation and rotation can be measured by determining the positions that the humerus can attain in relation to the four palpable scapular reference points. Humeroscapular elevation of less

TABLE 2–9. Necessary and Sufficient Criteria for Frozen Shoulders and Post-Traumatic Stiff Shoulders

I. Frozen Shoulder
 A. History
  1. Functionally significant restriction of shoulder motion
  2. Absence of previous major shoulder injury or surgery
 B. Physical Examination
  1. Limited glenohumeral motion in all directions
 C. Radiographs
  1. No changes in cartilaginous joint space
  2. Absence of pathologic changes other than osteopenia
II. Post-Traumatic and Post-Surgical Stiff Shoulder
 A. History
  1. Functionally significant restriction of shoulder motion
  2. History of significant shoulder injury or surgery
 B. Physical Examination
  1. Limited glenohumeral motion
 C. Radiographs
  1. No changes in cartilaginous joint space

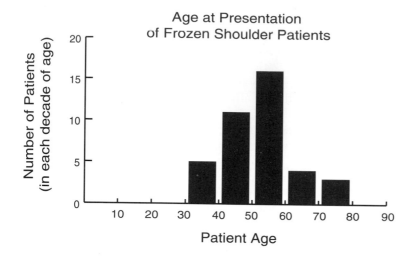

Age at Presentation of Frozen Shoulder Patients

(Chart: Number of Patients (in each decade of age) vs Patient Age)

FIGURE 2–29.

The distribution of age at presentation of 41 patients meeting the strict criteria for the diagnosis of frozen shoulder (see Table 2–9).

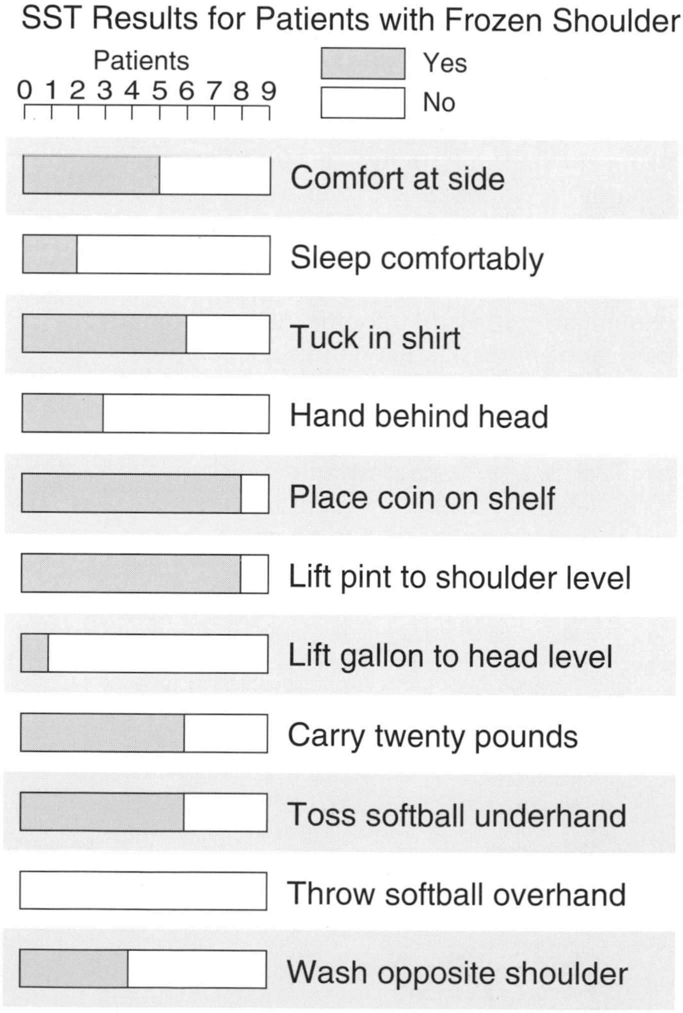

SST Results for Patients with Frozen Shoulder

Patients
0 1 2 3 4 5 6 7 8 9

Yes / No

- Comfort at side
- Sleep comfortably
- Tuck in shirt
- Hand behind head
- Place coin on shelf
- Lift pint to shoulder level
- Lift gallon to head level
- Carry twenty pounds
- Toss softball underhand
- Throw softball overhand
- Wash opposite shoulder

FIGURE 2–30.

The Simple Shoulder Test responses of nine patients meeting the criteria for idiopathic frozen shoulder. As a group, these patients had particular problems sleeping comfortably, putting their hands behind their heads, lifting eight pounds to the level of their heads, and throwing.

than 90 degrees indicates stiffness, especially if it is less than the contralateral normal shoulder.

Localized areas of capsular tightness or adhesions are identified by the pattern of motion restriction. For example, a shoulder with limited humeral elevation in anterior scapular planes, limited cross-body adduction, and limited internal rotation is likely to have tightness of the posterior capsule. A postoperative shoulder with isolated limitation of external rotation with the arm at the side is likely to have some combination of the following problems: scarring at the humeroscapular motion interface between the coracoid muscles and the subscapularis, excessive tightness of the subscapularis and anterior capsule, or contracture of the rotator interval capsule. Finally, a shoulder with limited elevation after a previous acromioplasty is likely to have scarring at the humeroscapular motion interface between the acromion, deltoid, and rotator cuff.

Radiographs

The definition of a frozen shoulder requires a normal joint space and normal joint relationships. Thus, in the evaluation of a shoulder with restricted humeroscapular motion, an axillary view and an anteroposterior radiograph in the plane of the scapula should be ordered to exclude the presence of narrowing of the radiographic joint space, glenohumeral dislocation, or joint surface fracture (Fig. 2–31A to D).

When scapulothoracic range is limited, a tangential (lateral) radiographic view of the scapula and a chest film are included to seek displaced fractures of the ribs or scapula, scapulothoracic dislocation, or an osteochondroma on the anterior aspect of the scapula.

NON-OPERATIVE MANAGEMENT

Shoulder stiffness tends to be a chronic condition. In this light, the patient must play a major role in its treatment. We use a patient-conducted rehabilitation program with two major elements: (1) gentle shoulder stretching exercises, and (2) an aerobic fitness program (Patient Information 2–1). These frequent, gentle exercises are performed at least three times a day, in a manner similar to what an athlete would use to develop more flexibility. Forceful passive stretching is avoided because of the risk of creating repeated capsular tears, which then go on to heal with additional tight scar tissue. Vigorous passive stretching also carries the risk of damage to the articular cartilage and labrum by causing obligate translation, which forces the humeral head away from the center of the joint.

If Exercises Are Not Successful

In the rare situation in which a well-motivated patient continues to have major functional limitations after 6 months of a first-rate effort at the home exercise program, a more aggressive approach is considered. For a classic frozen shoulder refractory to this program, examination is performed under anesthesia with gentle manipulation (unless there is significant osteopenia). Manipulation is not used in post-traumatic or post-surgical stiff shoulders because the scar tissue may be stronger than the cuff or the bone. Before proceeding, it is important that the surgeon and patient agree on a plan if freedom of motion is not achieved with manipulation. One option is to return to the exercise program; another is to proceed to a surgical release while the patient is still under the same anesthetic. Manipulation is performed under a brachial plexus block or under general anesthesia with total muscle relaxation. The brachial plexus block is preferable because the prolonged analgesia greatly facilitates the patient's ability to continue the range of motion program during the critical 12 hours after the procedure. Low levels of torque are applied in elevation, cross-body adduction, internal rotation, and external rotation. Sometimes, a gentle examination may produce lysis of essentially all the restrictions to motion. At other times, the examination may reveal firm blocks to motion that do not yield with the

Text continued on page 50

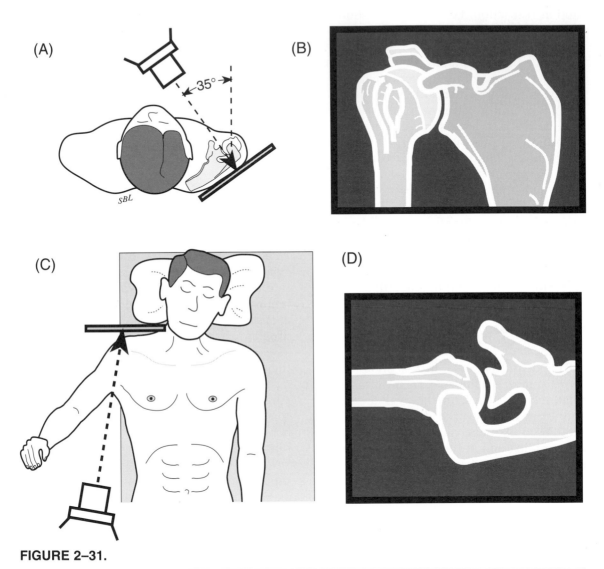

FIGURE 2–31.

Radiographic series for a stiff shoulder. *A,* The anteroposterior view in the plane of the scapula is obtained by orienting the beam perpendicular to the plane of the scapula and centering it on the coracoid tip while the film is parallel to the plane of the scapula. *B,* The resulting radiograph should clearly reveal the radiographic joint space between the humeral head and the glenoid. *C,* The axillary view is obtained by centering the beam between the coracoid tip and the posterior angle of the acromion. *D,* The resulting radiograph should project the glenoid midway between the coracoid and acromion, providing a clear view of the joint space.

PATIENT INFORMATION 2–1

UNIVERSITY OF WASHINGTON SHOULDER AND ELBOW SERVICE

Home Exercise Program for the Stiff Shoulder

Shoulders can become stiff for a wide variety of reasons. In many situations, the stiffness is related to tightness of the soft tissues around the joint. Normally, these tissues are flexible, allowing the shoulder to maintain its usually large range of motion. When these tissues become thickened or scarred, they lose their normal resilience and suppleness. Sometimes this stiffness develops after an injury or surgery. On many occasions, however, shoulder stiffness occurs for no apparent reason.

After a medical examination has excluded such conditions as arthritis, which may require a different kind of treatment, most stiff shoulders are treated effectively by a simple program that you can do at home. This program is the safest of all treatments for frozen shoulders. Although months of these specific exercises may be required, persistence almost always pays off.

There are two components to the home program for stiff shoulders. The first is a series of stretching exercises, and the second relates to regular participation in a fitness program.

THE STRETCHING PROGRAM. Your opposite arm is a great therapist for your stiff shoulder. Your "therapist arm" is always available to apply a gentle stretch in any direction of tightness. Each of these gentle stretches needs to be held up to a count of 100. The basic program includes the following four directions of stretching:

1. Overhead reach.
2. External rotation.
3. Internal rotation.
4. Cross-body reach.

If other directions of stiffness are identified, they can be stretched with a similar approach. An important principle of the stretching exercises is to allow your muscles to relax so that the stretch can be applied to the soft tissues without muscle interference. Tissues of a tight shoulder do not like to be stretched suddenly, roughly, or with a lot of force. Thus, the strategy is to apply a stretch sufficiently gentle that only minimal soreness results. Any soreness should go away within 15 minutes after you conclude the exercises.

Overhead reach is lifting your stiff arm up as high as it will go. To stretch your overhead reach, lie flat on your back, relax, and grasp the wrist of the tight shoulder with your opposite hand. Using the power in your opposite arm, bring the stiff arm up as far as it is comfortable. Start holding it for 10 seconds, and then work up to where you can hold it for a count of 100. Breathe slowly and deeply while the arm is moved. Repeat this stretch three times, trying to help the arm up a little higher each time (Fig. 2–32).

An alternative method of stretching to overhead reach is to use the "progressive forward lean." In this method you sit beside a table, shelf, armchair back, or other fixed object with your arm in a comfortable amount of elevation in overhead reach. Then, by leaning forward, allow the fixed object to apply a gentle, upward-directed force on the arm for a count of 100. The advantage of this method is that it does not require the help of the other arm, and

45

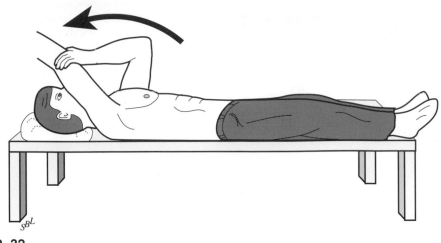

FIGURE 2–32.

Stretching in overhead reach using the opposite arm as the "therapist."

it can be sustained for a longer period (Fig. 2–33).

External rotation is turning the arm out to the side while your elbow stays close to your body. External rotation is best stretched while you are lying on your back. Hold a cane, yardstick, broom handle, or dowel in both hands. Bend both elbows to a right angle. Use steady, gentle force from your normal arm to rotate

the hand of the stiff shoulder out away from your body. Continue the rotation as far as it will go comfortably. Work up to holding it there for a count of 100. Repeat this exercise three times (Fig. 2–34).

An alternative method of stretching in external rotation is to hold onto a fixed object and gently turn your body away while keeping your elbow at the side. The advantage of this method is that it does

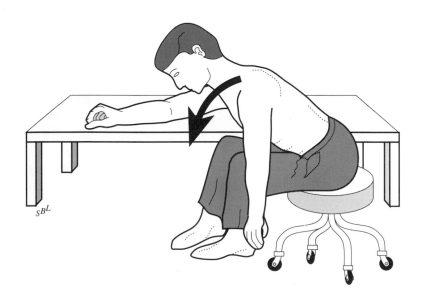

FIGURE 2–33.

Stretching in overhead reach using the progressive forward lean to apply a gentle elevating force to the arm.

46

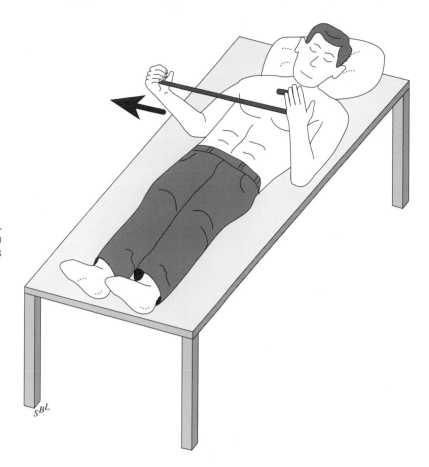

FIGURE 2–34.

Stretching in external rotation using the opposite hand as the "therapist."

not require the help of the other arm, and it can be sustained for a longer period (Fig. 2–35).

Internal rotation is the motion of reaching up the back. Grasp a towel behind your back in both hands. Gently pull the hand of the stiff shoulder up your back. Work up to holding the maximum comfortable stretch for a count of 100. Repeat the exercise three times (Fig. 2–36).

An alternative method of stretching in internal rotation is to hold onto a fixed object behind you with your hand as high up your back as it will easily reach. Then, by bending your knees, a gentle stretching force can be applied and sustained for a count of 100.

Cross-body reach is reaching across your chest so that your elbow approaches your opposite shoulder. Grasp the elbow of the stiff shoulder in your opposite hand and pull it toward the opposite shoulder.

Work up to holding the maximum comfortable stretch for 100 seconds. Repeat the exercise three times (Fig. 2–37).

You should carry out this shoulder stretching sequence three times a day. As much as possible, these sessions should be performed after the shoulder has been relaxed by a hot shower, bath, or aerobic exercise. For each stretch, make a note of the maximum range obtained with each session. Try to establish a new "bench mark" each time you do them, so that you can see your progress.

The beauty of this exercise program is that *you* are in control. You can adjust the vigor of the stretching to do what is most easily tolerated by your shoulder. The exercise program is totally portable and can be performed in your home, office, car, the bus, the airplane, or wherever you happen to be. This is important because consistency in this exercise program pays

47

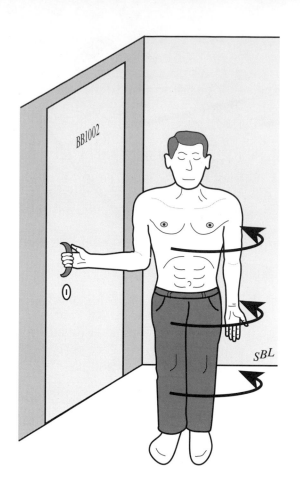

FIGURE 2–35.

Stretching in external rotation by turning the body away from a fixed object to apply a gentle stretching force.

FIGURE 2–36.

Stretching in internal rotation using a towel to apply a gentle stretching force.

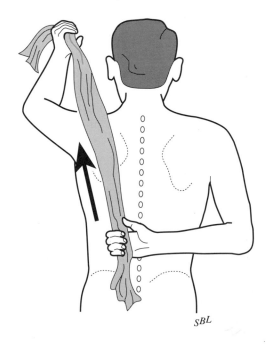

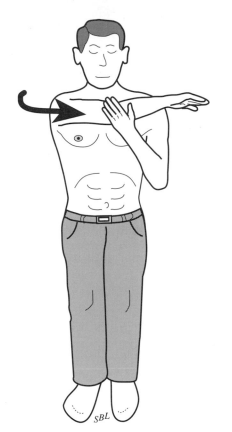

FIGURE 2–37.

Stretching in cross-body reach using the opposite arm as the "therapist."

off. If pain results from the exercise program, do not stop or change the frequency of your exercise sessions—just reduce the vigor of the stretches.

FITNESS. Regular fitness exercise helps keep your joints supple. This "lubricating" effect is optimized if you perform a half-hour of aerobic exercise each day. This exercise may take a variety of forms, including brisk walking, jogging, riding a stationary or mobile bicycle, rowing, climbing stairs, or using a cross-country skiing simulator. If you have concerns about your ability to carry out such an exercise program, you should consult your general physician. It is not important that these exercises be carried out vigorously; it is only important that in addition to the stretching program, a half-hour of your day be devoted to some form of aerobic exercise. A guideline for someone with a healthy heart, lungs, and blood pressure is to work up to 30 minutes of exercise at a target of two thirds of his or her maximum heart rate. The maximum heart rate is estimated by subtracting your age from 220. If you are older than 35 and have not been exercising much, or if you are not sure of your health, you should consult your doctor before starting this aspect of the program.

Many patients are reluctant to try this stretching and aerobic program because they have already "had therapy." Our repeated observation is that many patients who have not responded to formal therapy sessions can improve their shoulder function using this home program. Remember that your shoulder stiffness has been present for quite a while. Improvement in your range of motion and comfort may not begin until 6 weeks of persistence with the program. You should not stop these exercises until your shoulder has regained normal motion and comfort.

We have found that medication is not very helpful in managing stiff shoulders. Mild analgesics (such as aspirin, ibuprofen, and acetaminophen) may be used in conjunction with this program if desired. Narcotic medications, "muscle relaxants," and sleeping pills have not proved helpful to our patients.

We encourage you to use your shoulder actively within the range of comfort. For example, if you can do some water exercises or swimming without aggravating the shoulder, please do so. On the other hand, activities that produce shoulder pain should be avoided.

We hope this program is easy for you to understand and carry out. If you have any questions, please let us know.

application of low torques; if so, this is time to stop and go to "plan B." If freedom of motion is achieved by manipulation, continuous passive motion is instituted in the recovery room (Fig. 2–38).

The immediate institution of continuous motion has two important benefits: (1) it influences the early phases of the healing process in a direction that encourages motion and discourages adhesions, and (2) it enables the patient to wake up from the anesthetic seeing the shoulder in motion. As soon as possible after the procedure, the patient reinstitutes the same stretching program used before the procedure.

If Manipulation Is Not Successful

Open surgical release is considered for informed, consenting patients if the manipulation is not successful in reestablishing motion in a stiff shoulder. The patient's role in the recovery process is emphasized (Patient Information 2–2).

The type of stiffness dictates the surgical approach to the refractory stiff shoulder. We usually approach a post-surgical stiff shoulder through an incision that provides access to the previous surgical site. This is because the densest adhesions and scars are usually located beneath the surgical incision. The idiopathic frozen shoulder is reached through a deltopectoral approach, which allows access to the rotator interval, the motion interface, the subscapularis, and the glenohumeral joint capsule. The surgical release is analogous in many ways to the subscapularis and capsule release performed during glenohumeral arthroplasty.

We proceed sequentially through a series of distinct stages of shoulder release, reassessing the range of motion after each stage.

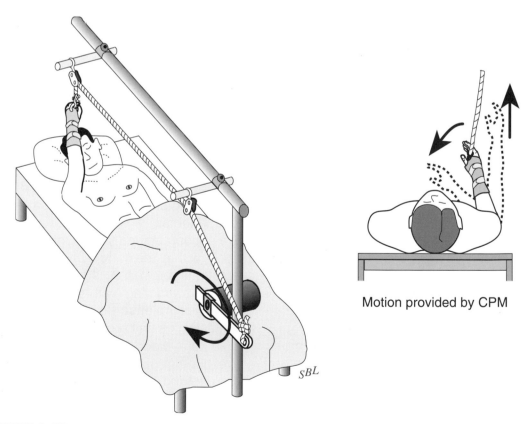

Motion provided by CPM

FIGURE 2–38.

Continuous passive motion (CPM) is helpful for the first 24 to 48 hours after a procedure to mobilize the shoulder. Elevation to 90 degrees is easily achieved using a simple pulley system with a motor-driven eccentric cam.

PATIENT INFORMATION 2–2

UNIVERSITY OF WASHINGTON SHOULDER AND ELBOW SERVICE

Open Release for Refractory Stiff Shoulders

Most patients with stiff shoulders can improve their comfort and function with a home exercise program. We consider an open surgical release for the few stiff shoulders that do not improve with a persistent effort at the exercises. The purpose of the surgical release is to cut through the adhesions, scar tissue, and other structures that may be interfering with the motion of your shoulder. This procedure is purely elective. The alternatives are to continue with the exercises or to accept the current range of motion.

Because this is a surgical operation, it carries some risks. These include the risk of anesthesia, infection, nerve injury, blood vessel injury, excessive looseness and instability of the shoulder, persistent or increased shoulder stiffness, fracture, increased pain, or the need for repeat surgery.

After surgery, it is essential that you resume your shoulder stretching program so that adhesions will not have an opportunity to reform. Although we can loosen the shoulder at surgery, you are the only person who can maintain the motion during the healing period. These exercises will need to be continued for as long as a year after your surgery. If you have concerns about your ability to carry out this important aspect of your treatment, please discuss this with us before you undertake surgery. We will keep you in the hospital until your exercise program is well launched. At the time of discharge, we will encourage you to be physically active and to avoid narcotic and sleeping medications. You will be unable to drive for at least 2 weeks after this procedure, so you should make appropriate provisions for getting around during this time.

We hope this information is helpful. If you have questions, please ask us at any time.

51

We continue through these stages until the desired motion is obtained.

Stage 1: Reestablishment of the Humero-scapular Motion Interface. Our *in vivo* MRI studies demonstrated that there is normally a substantial excursion at the humeroscapular motion interface. In post-surgical and post-traumatic stiff shoulders, adhesions, or "spot welds," are common between the deltoid, acromion, coracoacromial ligament, coracoid, and coracoid muscles on the one hand and the rotator cuff and humerus on the other. These spot welds can virtually eliminate motion at the interface. Thus, each area of the interface needs to be smooth and free of adhesions for the shoulder to achieve its normal range. At times the motion interface can be obscured and difficult to identify. In the "totally stuck shoulder," we start under the acromion, knowing that it is part of the outer aspect of the motion interface. Dissecting beneath the acromion and coracoacromial ligament with a knife, we can free the subjacent cuff tissue. By rotating the humerus internally and externally during this step of the dissection, we continue the dissection under the coracoacromial arch to the coracoid. The sharp dissection proceeds beneath the coracoid and coracoid muscles, freeing the subjacent subscapularis muscle. Adhesions between the coracoid muscles and the subscapularis cause a major limitation of external rotation owing to the magnitude of interfacial motion here. It must be remembered that the brachial plexus, especially the musculocutaneous and axillary nerves, are close by and vulnerable. Thus, we stay lateral to the coracoid muscles (the "safe side"), dissecting on the surface of the subscapularis as it is externally rotated rather than diving medial to the coracoid muscles (the "suicide").

In a similar manner, sharp dissection continues laterally from the acromion to reestablish the motion interface between the deltoid and the rotator cuff. Again, the nerve supply, in this instance the branches of the axillary nerve, lie in the motion interface. We avoid them by keeping our sharp dissection on the superficial aspect of the rotator cuff and proximal humerus. If the dissection enters the deltoid muscle, its nerve supply is at risk (Fig. 2–39).

Stage 2: Opening the Rotator Interval. As our cadaver research has demonstrated, tightness at the rotator interval can substantially restrict the range of glenohumeral motion. We release the rotator interval by sharply dissecting the subscapularis and supraspinatus tendons free from their moorings to the base of the coracoid. We verify the completeness of this release by passing a blunt elevator between the tendons on both sides of the coracoid process.

Stage 3: Reestablishment of Subscapularis Length and Excursion. The subscapularis and the anterior capsule may be contracted and scarred, particularly after previous anterior shoulder injury or surgery (Fig. 2–40*A*). We perform a coronal plane Z-lengthening of the subscapularis tendon and capsule using a step cut. We cut the superficial lateral aspect of the tendon at the lesser tuberosity near the long head of the biceps. We then split the tendon medially in the coronal plane. Finally, we complete the medial aspect of the cut by transecting the remaining tendon and capsule adjacent to the glenoid

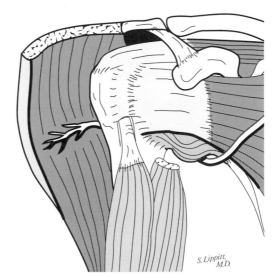

FIGURE 2–39.

The axillary nerve lies in the motion interface. It is thus at risk in the release of a tight shoulder.

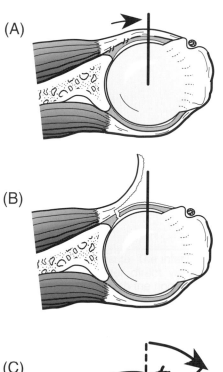

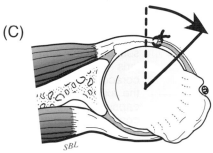

FIGURE 2–40.

A, Contracted subscapularis and anterior capsule, limiting external rotation. *B,* Subscapularis is incised from the lesser tuberosity laterally. The capsule is incised from the labrum medially. *C,* At the conclusion of the procedure, the lateral end of the subscapularis tendon is sutured to the medial end of the capsule, resulting in a substantial lengthening of these structures. As a rule of thumb, each centimeter of length gained by this procedure increases external rotation by approximately 20 degrees.

labrum (Fig. 2–40*B*). At the conclusion of the procedure, we suture the lateral end of the superficial flap to the medial end of the deep flap. Each centimeter of length gained by the step cut increases external rotation by approximately 20 degrees (Fig. 2–40*C*). Prior to the closure, we perform a "360 degree"

release of the subscapularis tendon from the coracoid muscles anteriorly, the axillary nerve below, the capsule and scapular neck posteriorly and the coracoid above. This release should reestablish the normal "bounce" and excursion of the subscapularis (Fig. 2–41).

Stage 4: Release of the Capsule. Capsular tightness is the major component of an idiopathic frozen shoulder, but it may also be a major component of post-traumatic and post-surgical stiff shoulders. In the surgical release, we section the tight capsular tissue just lateral to the glenoid labrum. The capsule can be released selectively or circumferentially according to the pattern of stiffness. A circumferential capsular release can be started anterosuperiorly, then carried down the anterior glenoid. We release the inferior capsule sharply while a finger protects the axillary nerve (Fig. 2–42). We expose the origin of the triceps from the infraglenoid tubercle with this release. We insert a humeral head retractor into the joint and twist it slightly to tension the posterior inferior capsule so that it can be safely sectioned. By twisting the retractor a little more with each bit of posterior capsular release (Fig. 2–43), we can safely release the posterior capsule up to the origin of the biceps tendon at the supraglenoid tubercle.

The lengthened subscapularis tendon is then sutured to the capsule attached to the lesser tuberosity (see Fig. 2–40*C*).

The hallmarks of an adequate release are (1) translation of the humeral head on the posterior drawer test of at least 1.5 cm; (2) a "scarecrow" test demonstrating almost 90 degrees of internal rotation of the arm elevated 90 degrees in the zero degree thoracic plane; (3) at least 45 degrees external rotation with the arm at the side; and (4) total elevation of the arm to at least 140 degrees.

As soon as the procedure is completed, we place the arm in continuous passive motion (see Fig. 2–38). Early motion achieves several goals. It prevents formation of adhesions or scarring during the critical early healing period. It also demonstrates to the patient that the shoulder can and should be moved immediately. Finally, early movement seems to increase the comfort, speed, and com-

Text continued on page 58

Progress Chart

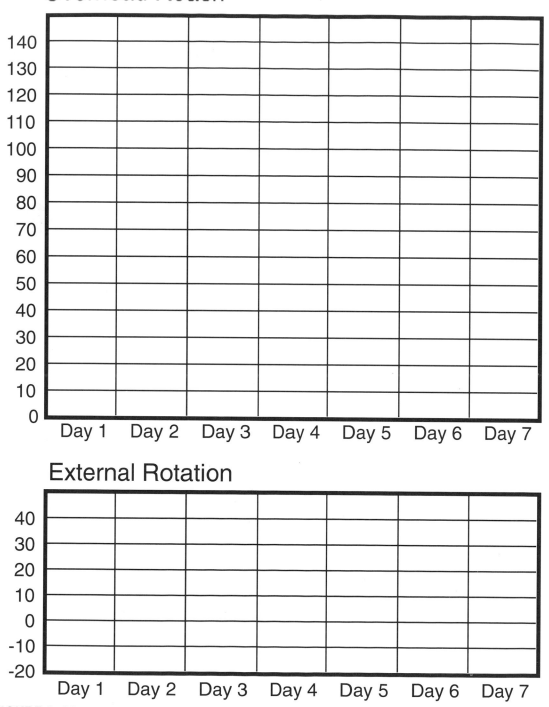

FIGURE 2–44.

A, Wall charts are used to display the patient's overhead reach *(top)* and external rotation *(bottom)*. These charts are posted in the patient's room to provide positive feedback to the patient. Using a colored marker, the physical therapist, nurse, or physician charts the range of motion achieved each day.

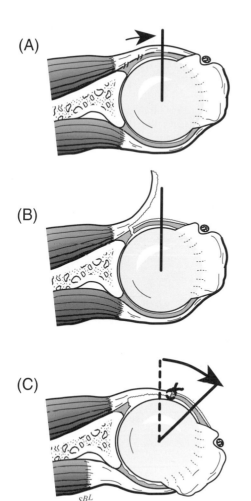

(A)

(B)

(C)

SBL

FIGURE 2–40.

A, Contracted subscapularis and anterior capsule, limiting external rotation. *B,* Subscapularis is incised from the lesser tuberosity laterally. The capsule is incised from the labrum medially. *C,* At the conclusion of the procedure, the lateral end of the subscapularis tendon is sutured to the medial end of the capsule, resulting in a substantial lengthening of these structures. As a rule of thumb, each centimeter of length gained by this procedure increases external rotation by approximately 20 degrees.

labrum (Fig. 2–40B). At the conclusion of the procedure, we suture the lateral end of the superficial flap to the medial end of the deep flap. Each centimeter of length gained by the step cut increases external rotation by approximately 20 degrees (Fig. 2–40C). Prior to the closure, we perform a "360 degree"

release of the subscapularis tendon from the coracoid muscles anteriorly, the axillary nerve below, the capsule and scapular neck posteriorly and the coracoid above. This release should reestablish the normal "bounce" and excursion of the subscapularis (Fig. 2–41).

Stage 4: Release of the Capsule. Capsular tightness is the major component of an idiopathic frozen shoulder, but it may also be a major component of post-traumatic and post-surgical stiff shoulders. In the surgical release, we section the tight capsular tissue just lateral to the glenoid labrum. The capsule can be released selectively or circumferentially according to the pattern of stiffness. A circumferential capsular release can be started anterosuperiorly, then carried down the anterior glenoid. We release the inferior capsule sharply while a finger protects the axillary nerve (Fig. 2–42). We expose the origin of the triceps from the infraglenoid tubercle with this release. We insert a humeral head retractor into the joint and twist it slightly to tension the posterior inferior capsule so that it can be safely sectioned. By twisting the retractor a little more with each bit of posterior capsular release (Fig. 2–43), we can safely release the posterior capsule up to the origin of the biceps tendon at the supraglenoid tubercle.

The lengthened subscapularis tendon is then sutured to the capsule attached to the lesser tuberosity (see Fig. 2–40C).

The hallmarks of an adequate release are (1) translation of the humeral head on the posterior drawer test of at least 1.5 cm; (2) a "scarecrow" test demonstrating almost 90 degrees of internal rotation of the arm elevated 90 degrees in the zero degree thoracic plane; (3) at least 45 degrees external rotation with the arm at the side; and (4) total elevation of the arm to at least 140 degrees.

As soon as the procedure is completed, we place the arm in continuous passive motion (see Fig. 2–38). Early motion achieves several goals. It prevents formation of adhesions or scarring during the critical early healing period. It also demonstrates to the patient that the shoulder can and should be moved immediately. Finally, early movement seems to increase the comfort, speed, and com-

Text continued on page 58

(A)

(B)

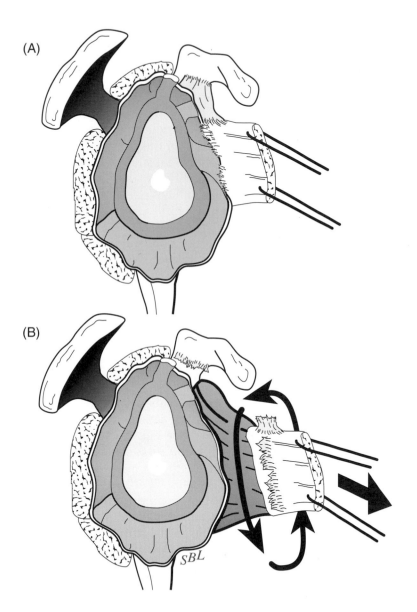

FIGURE 2–41.

A, 360-degree release of the subscapularis. The subscapularis must be freed from the coracoid muscles anteriorly, the axillary nerve inferiorly, the capsule posteriorly, and the coracoid superiorly. *B,* Once this release is complete, traction on the subscapularis should produce a normal "bounce."

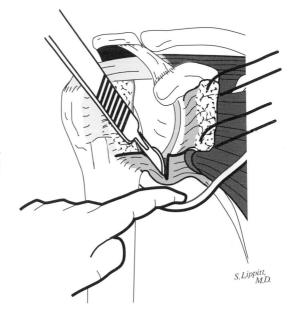

FIGURE 2–42.

Release of the inferior capsule. The inferior capsule is released sharply and under direct vision while the axillary nerve is protected with the finger.

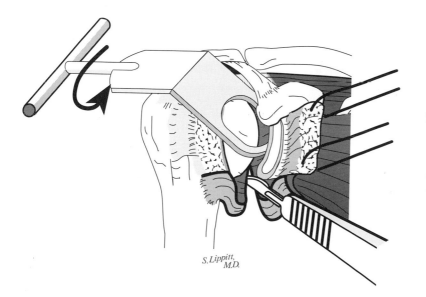

FIGURE 2–43.

The posterior capsule is released from the glenoid labrum under direct vision. It is exposed by progressively twisting the humeral head retractor.

Progress Chart

Overhead Reach

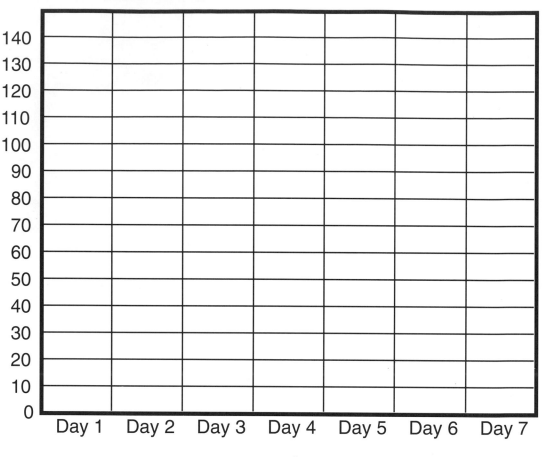

External Rotation

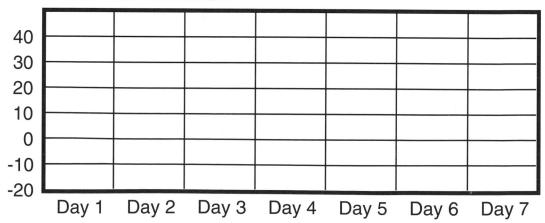

FIGURE 2–44.

A, Wall charts are used to display the patient's overhead reach *(top)* and external rotation *(bottom)*. These charts are posted in the patient's room to provide positive feedback to the patient. Using a colored marker, the physical therapist, nurse, or physician charts the range of motion achieved each day.

Progress Chart

Overhead Reach

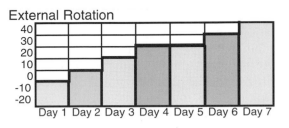

FIGURE 2–44. *Continued*

B, Typical wall charts showing the improvement in overhead reach and external rotation after an open release.

External Rotation

(A) Increment in Elevation after Open Release

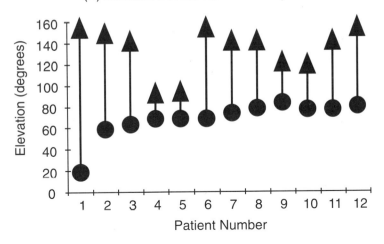

FIGURE 2–45.

A, Increment in humerothoracic elevation after open release. *B*, Increment in external rotation after open release.

(B) Increment in External Rotation after Open Release

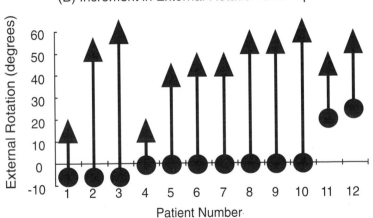

pleteness of motion recovery. The use of the continuous passive motion after surgery is greatly facilitated by a brachial plexus block for the surgical procedure. This type of anesthesia can give 12 to 18 hours of postoperative analgesia, allowing the awake patient the opportunity to observe the increase in motion gained by the procedure without experiencing early postoperative pain.

On the first day after surgery, the patient resumes the range of motion exercise program (see Patient Information 2–1). Each day the patient is in the hospital, we plot the range of elevation (overhead reach) and rotation on charts posted in the patient's hospital room (Fig. 2–44A). These charts provide positive reinforcement for the patient's progress (Fig. 2–44B). Ideally, before discharge the patient can demonstrate comfortable assisted motion to 140 degrees of elevation, 40 degrees of external rotation, internal rotation until able to reach T12 with the thumb, and cross-body adduction comparable with the normal side. The wall charts reflect these discharge goals. With this program, the patient becomes the center of the treatment team and is motivated to continue the exercises after discharge. Two-year followup data for twelve patients having open surgical release for refractory frozen shoulders are seen in Figure 2-45A and B.

CONCLUSION

The evaluation and management of shoulder stiffness require localizing the site of involvement and quantifying the severity of each limited motion. We are most often successful in the management of an idiopathic frozen shoulder with a patient-conducted home exercise and fitness program. For the rare case of idiopathic frozen shoulder refractory to non-operative management and for symptomatic post-traumatic or postoperative stiff shoulders, we consider more aggressive treatment. This next step may include sequential surgical release, immediate postoperative motion, and aggressive resumption of the patient-conducted home exercise program.

CHAPTER

3

Stability

For the upper extremity to carry out its many and varied functions, the shoulder must provide a stable link between the humerus and the thorax. This chapter concentrates on the most important aspect of this linkage: the stability of the glenohumeral joint. Some precise definitions help resolve some of the imprecision and ambiguity that have surrounded this topic.

The *glenoid center line* is the line perpendicular to the surface of the glenoid fossa at its midpoint (Fig. 3–1).

The *net humeral joint reaction force* is the vector sum of all forces acting on the humeral head relative to the glenoid fossa (Fig. 3–2). It is this force that needs to be stabilized at the glenohumeral joint. This force includes component forces applied to the humerus by muscles, capsule, and ligaments as well as by external factors such as gravity, contact with objects, and inertia.

Glenohumeral translation is movement of the center of the humeral head with respect to the face of the glenoid (Fig. 3–3).

Glenohumeral translational laxity is the translation observed on examination of the joint. A substantial amount of laxity is characteristic of normal glenohumeral joints.

Glenohumeral stability is the ability to maintain the humeral head centered in the glenoid fossa.

Glenohumeral instability is the inability to maintain the humeral head centered in the glenoid fossa.

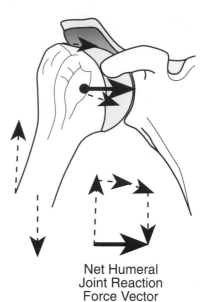

Net Humeral
Joint Reaction
Force Vector

FIGURE 3–2.

The *net humeral joint reaction force* is the vector sum of all forces acting on the head of the humerus relative to the glenoid fossa.

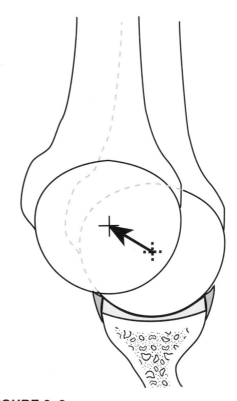

FIGURE 3–3.

Glenohumeral translation is the movement of the center of the humeral head with respect to the face of the glenoid.

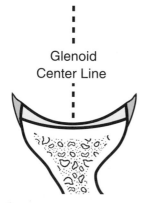

Glenoid
Center Line

FIGURE 3–1.

The *glenoid center line* is a line perpendicular to the surface of the glenoid fossa at its midpoint.

Glenohumeral apprehension is the sense of impending instability in certain glenohumeral positions.

Traumatic instability is instability that arises from an injury of sufficient magnitude to tear the glenohumeral capsule, labrum, ligaments, or rotator cuff or to produce a fracture of the humerus or glenoid.

Atraumatic instability is instability that arises in the absence of significant trauma.

STABILIZING MECHANISMS

In comparison with the hip joint, the glenohumeral joint is not centered by an intrinsically stable ball-and-deep-socket articulation. In the hip, the cup of the acetabulum surrounds much of the head of the femur, providing substantial resistance to dislocation. By contrast, in the shoulder the small arc of the glenoid captures relatively little of the head of the humerus (Fig. 3–4).

As opposed to other joints with shallow sockets, such as the knee, interphalangeal joints, elbow, and ankle, the shoulder is not stabilized by isometric articular ligaments. For such ligaments to be effective stabilizers throughout the range of motion, a joint is required to move around an axis of ligament isometry, so that the ligaments remain stretched out to full length in all positions. If the ligaments of the glenohumeral joint

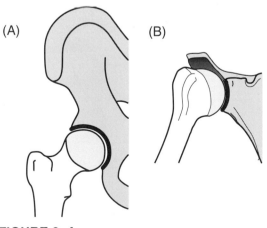

FIGURE 3–4.

In contrast with the situation in the hip *(A)*, the shallow glenoid captures relatively little of the articulating ball *(B)*.

were all stretched out to length in a given position, the joint would be unable to move from that position. To allow ample movement, the capsule and ligaments of a ball-and-socket joint are slack in most of the joint's positions (Fig. 3–5).

The glenohumeral joint must therefore achieve stability by mechanisms other than a deep socket or ligaments that are isometric about a single axis of motion. The following sections describe some of these mechanisms. Particular emphasis is placed on mechanisms that can contribute to glenohumeral stability in midrange positions, in which most of the daily activities of the joint take place.

Balance

Glenohumeral balance is a stabilizing mechanism in which the glenoid is positioned so that the net humeral joint reaction force passes through the glenoid fossa (Fig. 3–6). No other stabilizing mechanism is necessary as long as the humeroscapular position is such that the glenoid supports the net humeral joint reaction force. When the joint is in balance, its stability is independent of the *magnitude* of net humeral joint reaction force. However, balance is sensitive to the *direction* of the net humeral joint reaction force vector with respect to the glenoid fossa. The larger the arc subtended by glenoid concavity, the larger the range of directions of the net humeral joint reaction force vector that will be stabilized by it. This range of directions can be estimated from simple geometric calculations. A radian is the central angle of a circle that subtends an arc equal in length to the radius of the circle. There are 2π radians in a circle; thus, one radian equals 360 degrees divided by 2π, or almost 60 degrees. The arc of stability from glenohumeral balance can be predicted by dividing the length of the glenoid arc by the radius of the humeral head and multiplying the quotient by 360 degrees/2π (Fig. 3–7). As an example, if the anteroposterior arc length of the glenoid were equal to the radius of the humeral head, the glenoid would balance net humeral joint reaction force vec-

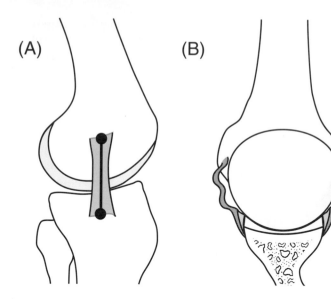

(A)

(B)

FIGURE 3–5.

In contrast with the knee, where the ligaments remain isometric during joint motion *(A)*, the glenohumeral ligaments must be slack in most of the joint's positions *(B)*.

tors through a range of directions of approximately 60 degrees (from about 30 degrees anterior to 30 degrees posterior to the glenoid center line). Hypoplasia, erosion, or fracture of the glenoid rim can diminish the arc available for balance stability (Fig. 3–8).

range of directions of the ball's gravitational force vector that would be stabilized on the tee by dividing the length of the tee arc by the ball radius and multiplying the quotient by 360 degrees/2π. Check your estimate by performing the experiment. Start with the ball on the

ACTIVITY

Measure the radius of a golf ball. Measure the length of the arc of a golf tee. Estimate the

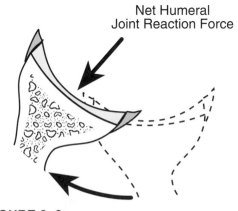

Net Humeral
Joint Reaction Force

FIGURE 3–6.

Glenohumeral balance is a stabilizing mechanism in which the glenoid is positioned so that the net humeral joint reaction force passes through the glenoid fossa.

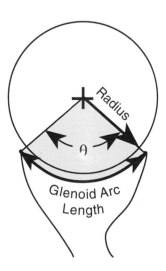

Radius

θ

Glenoid Arc
Length

$$\text{Angular Range of Stability} = \frac{\text{Glenoid Arc Length}}{\text{Radius}} \times \frac{360°}{2\pi}$$

FIGURE 3–7.

The angular range of stability from glenohumeral balance can be predicted by dividing the length of the glenoid arc by the radius of the humeral head and multiplying the quotient by 360 degrees divided by 2π.

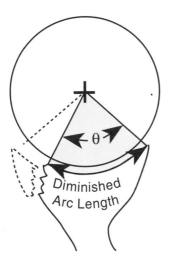

FIGURE 3–8.

A glenoid rim fracture, or Bankart lesion, diminishes the glenoid arc length and therefore reduces the angular range of glenohumeral stability.

tee held in the usual vertical orientation. Then, slowly tip the tee and determine the maximal angulation with the vertical that can be achieved before the ball falls off the tee. Multiply this angle by 2 to obtain the total angle of balance stability, and compare with your prediction. Would the stability angle be different for a heavier golf ball of the same size? Next, chip the edge of the golf tee and repeat the experiment. Does this provide insight into a possible mechanism for the instability seen with glenoid rim fractures and labral avulsions from the glenoid?

In an experiment with a series of cadaver shoulders, we demonstrated this balancing effect in a manner similar to the golf ball and tee demonstration. After removing the muscles and capsule, we positioned the humeral shaft vertically (head down) in a stand

through which it was free to slide. In this situation, the weight of the humerus provided the net joint reaction force. We designed a frame that positioned the scapula under the humeral head, with the glenoid center line pointing vertically upward. We then slowly tipped the scapula anteriorly, increasing the angle between the glenoid center line and the joint reaction force applied by the humerus, until the head of the humerus slipped over the glenoid lip. We defined the *balance stability angle* as the maximal angle between the net joint reaction force and the glenoid center line before dislocation occurred. We carried out three trials and calculated the average maximal angle of tip before dislocation. In a similar way, we determined the balance stability angle for tipping in the superior, inferior, and posterior directions. Finally, we repeated the anterior tipping after we had created a 3-mm defect in the anterior glenoid lip. Table 3–1 shows the results of these experiments. Balance stabilized the net humeral joint reaction force vector through a wide range of angles. The combined anteroposterior balance stability angle averaged 36 degrees and that for the superoinferior directions averaged 57 degrees. In these cadaver shoulders, balance stability was relatively symmetrical around the glenoid center line (the anterior and posterior stability angles were approximately equal, as were the superior and inferior angles). Owing to the increased vertical extent of the glenoid, the superoinferior stability angle was greater than the anteroposterior stability angle. The anterior stability angle was reduced by an average of more than 25 percent by the presence of a relatively small glenoid rim defect.

The large number of component forces operating on the humerus makes it difficult to calculate the exact direction of the net hu-

TABLE 3–1. Angles of Balance Stability

Superior	Inferior	Posterior	Anterior	Anterior (3-mm anterior lip defect)
24	31	17	19	16
31	21	24	15	10
21	32	17	18	13
28	41	15	20	13

*Data are in degrees; each row represents one of four cadaver shoulders.

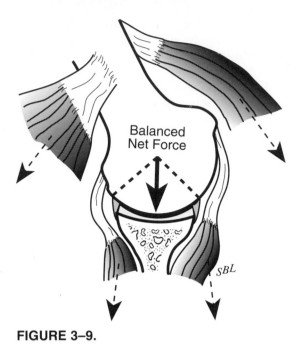

FIGURE 3–9.

The vector sum of the deltoid and cuff muscle forces lies close to the axis of the humerus in many functional positions of the shoulder.

meral joint reaction force vector *in vivo.* A rough approximation is that in midrange humeroscapular positions, the vector sum of the deltoid and cuff muscle forces lies close to the axis of the humerus (Fig. 3–9). In many vigorous shoulder activities, the scapula is positioned so that the glenoid center line is closely aligned with the humerus. During the critical moments of the boxer's knockout punch, the bench press, or the tennis stroke, for example, the humeroscapular position appears to be such that the glenoid center line and the humerus are aligned. Under these circumstances the glenohumeral joint is stabilized by balance so that muscle energy is preserved for power. This observation emphasizes two special features of balance stability: (1) as long as the net humeral joint reaction force vector is relatively aligned with the glenoid center line, the resulting stability is unaffected by increasing the magnitude of this force; and (2) the only muscular effort required to achieve balance is that for positioning the glenoid in relation to the net humeral joint reaction force.

Stability from balance is of particular interest because of its relationship to humeroscapular position. It is apparent that essentially identical *humerothoracic* positions

can be achieved using different *humeroscapular* positions. Some of these positions favor glenohumeral balance, whereas others do not. Consider the arm elevated 90 degrees in the plus 90 degree thoracic plane. If the scapula is protracted, the humerus is closely aligned with the glenoid center line. Alternatively, if the scapula is retracted, the humerus is almost at right angles to the glenoid center line (Fig. 3–10). The essential point is

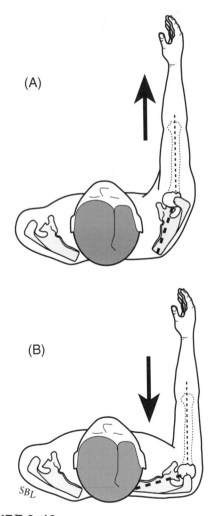

FIGURE 3–10.

Essentially identical humerothoracic positions can be achieved using different humeroscapular positions, which, in turn, have different implications for the balance mechanism. *A,* The humerus is elevated so that it is closely aligned with the glenoid center line. This should be the most stable position. *B,* The same humerothoracic position is achieved with the humerus almost perpendicular to the glenoid center line, challenging the balance stability of the joint.

FIGURE 3–11.

A, Stability is compromised by muscle imbalance. In this example, the humerus is aligned with the glenoid center line, but the net humeral joint reaction force is misaligned owing to weakness of the posterior cuff musculature. *B,* Balance stability is compromised with abnormal glenoid version. In this example, the humerus is aligned with the plane of the scapula, but severe glenoid retroversion results in a posteriorly directed glenoid center line that is divergent from the net humeral joint reaction force.

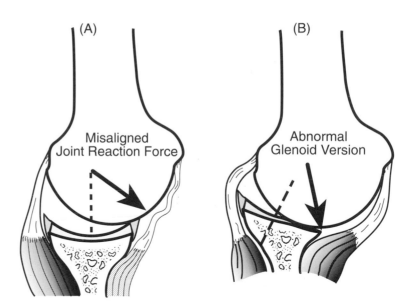

that balance at the glenohumeral joint is determined by humeroscapular position rather than the more easily observed humerothoracic position. Which humeroscapular position is used to achieve a given humerothoracic position is a question of neuromuscular control, habit, and training. In analyzing patients with glenohumeral instability, it is important to document the humeroscapular positions in which the instability occurs. Neuromuscular retraining may help the patient regain stabilizing balance.

The precision of neuromuscular control required for balance is inversely related to the size of the glenoid fossa. The angle through which the balancing mechanism can function is less in the anterior and posterior directions, where the glenoid arc is relatively small, than in the superior and inferior directions, where it is larger. The balance stability angle is diminished in glenoid hypoplasia, fracture, or degenerative erosion. In prosthetic shoulder arthroplasty, components with a large articular surface offer a greater balance stability angle.

The balance stability mechanism may fail in cases of severe muscle imbalance in which the net humeral joint reaction force is not aligned with the glenoid, even though the humerus is close to the glenoid center line (Fig. 3–11*A*). The balance stability mechanism may fail in the presence of abnormal glenoid version where the glenoid center line deviates substantially from the plane of the scapula and from the net humeral joint reaction force (Fig. 3–11*B*).

Concavity Compression

Concavity compression is a stabilizing mechanism in which compression of the convex humeral head into the concave glenoid fossa stabilizes it against translating forces. The stability is related to the depth of the concavity and the magnitude of the compressive force.

ACTIVITY

Take a smooth ball, such as a marble or a billiard ball. First, press it down on a hard, smooth surface while a partner applies a translating force parallel to the surface. Note how little force your partner needs to exert before the ball begins to translate. No matter how hard you push down, stability against translation is minimal in the absence of a concavity in the hard surface. Next, create a small concavity in the hard surface and repeat the experiment, this time pressing the ball into the concavity. Note that it is much harder for your partner to make the ball slide for the same amount of downward push. Make an even greater concavity and note that stability for the same downward push is still greater. Finally, note that for a given size concavity, pressing down harder gives even greater stability.

ACTIVITY

The importance of concavity compression as a stabilizing mechanism for the glenohumeral joint can be demonstrated in the normal person. When the subject is completely relaxed, the examiner may easily translate the humeral head anteriorly or posteriorly with respect to the glenoid. If the subject gently contracts the shoulder muscles (e.g., by slightly abducting the shoulder), this anteroposterior excursion is virtually eliminated.

The anatomy of the glenohumeral joint is well adapted to facilitate stabilization through concavity compression. The rotator cuff is ideally situated to provide a compressive load throughout the range of motion of the glenohumeral joint. The concavity in the glenoid is provided by the shape of the glenoid bone, by the increased thickness of the articular cartilage at the periphery of the glenoid fossa, and by the glenoid labrum (Fig. 3–12).

As the humeral head is translated from the center of the glenoid fossa over the glenoid lip, it must displace laterally (i.e., in a direc-

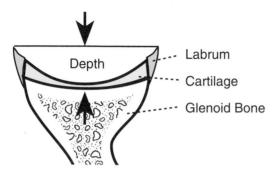

FIGURE 3–12.

The glenoid fossa. The depth of the glenoid fossa is a result of the slight concavity of the glenoid bone, the articular cartilage, which is thicker at the periphery than in the center, and the fossa-deepening effect of the glenoid labrum.

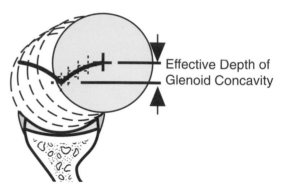

FIGURE 3–13.

The effective depth of the glenoid concavity. The gull wing–shaped line indicates the path of the center of the head as it is translated from the glenoid center to the top of the lip. The effective depth of the glenoid concavity in a specified direction of translation is equal to the lateral displacement of the humeral head at the top of the lip relative to its starting point centered in the glenoid fossa.

tion parallel to the glenoid center line). The path of the humeral head center during this ascent from the center over the lip has a particular "gull wing" shape, as shown in Figure 3–13. The narrowness of this gull wing is a major contributor to the centering of the head in the glenoid: essentially no translation is possible without the head being lifted from the depths of the glenoid fossa. The effective depth of the glenoid in a specified direction of translation is the amount of displacement in the lateral direction required for the head of the humerus to translate from the center of the glenoid to the top of the lip of the glenoid.

We conducted a series of experiments to determine the degree to which concavity compression can stabilize the humeral head against translating forces parallel to the surface of the glenoid. We used ten cadaver shoulders in which the muscles, tendons, and capsule had been resected, leaving only the glenoid bone, cartilage, and labrum to stabilize the head of the humerus. For each shoulder we measured the effective glenoid depth in each of four directions of translation. Figure 3–14 shows the data for the superior, inferior, anterior, and posterior directions in a typical shoulder.

For all ten cadaver shoulders, the average effective glenoid depth was greater superi-

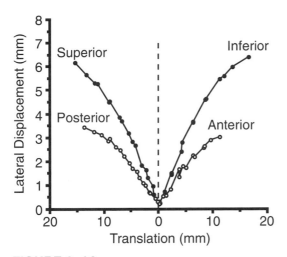

FIGURE 3–14.

Lateral displacement of the humeral head necessary for translation to the lip of the glenoid in four different directions in a typical young shoulder. The effective glenoid depth in this shoulder was 3.4 mm for translation in the posterior direction, 3.2 mm in the anterior direction, 6.2 mm in the superior direction, and 6.4 mm in the inferior direction. Note the high degree of symmetry about the glenoid center line and the deep valley when the head is exactly centered in the glenoid socket.

orly (4.8 ± 1.0 mm) and inferiorly (4.9 ± 1.1 mm) than anteriorly (2.2 ± 0.9 mm) and posteriorly (2.1 ± 0.9 mm). The greater depth for translation in the superior and inferior directions is a direct consequence of the oblong shape of the fossa and its constant radius of curvature (Fig. 3–15).

We measured the stability from concavity compression with compressive loads of 50

and 100 Newtons. Concavity compression proved to be an effective mechanism for stabilizing the humeral head against translating forces (Table 3–2). For example, a compressive load of 50 Newtons stabilized the humeral head against inferiorly directed translating forces averaging 32 Newtons. Doubling the compressive load to 100 Newtons increased the inferior force that could be stabilized to an average of 56 Newtons. The effectiveness of the concavity compression mechanism varied with different directions of translating force. For a given compressive load, the stability was greater against superiorly and inferiorly directed forces than against forces directed anteriorly and posteriorly. Doubling the compressive load from 50 to 100 Newtons did not quite double the translating force that can be stabilized. This suggests that deformability of the lip of the glenoid fossa may provide less effective glenoid depth with greater applied loads.

To facilitate the comparison of the effectiveness of concavity compression under different conditions, a "stability ratio" was calculated as:

Stability ratio (%) =
$$\frac{\text{Translation force}}{\text{Compressive load}} \times 100$$

The stability ratios for the different directions of translation are shown in Figure 3–16.

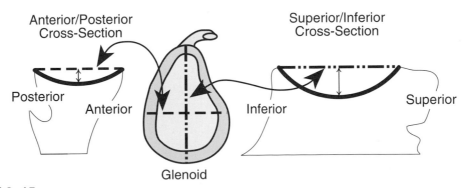

FIGURE 3–15.

The width of the glenoid in the superoinferior direction is greater than the width of the glenoid in the anteroposterior direction. For a given radius of curvature, an increase in width results in an increase in depth. Thus, the depth of the glenoid as measured along the superoinferior direction is greater than the depth measured along the anteroposterior direction.

TABLE 3–2. Concavity Compression Stability: Translating Force Resisted for Compressive Loads of 50 and 100 Newtons

Direction	Compressive Load (Newtons)	Translating Force (just before dislocation) (Newtons)
Superior	50	29 ± 7
	100	51 ± 9
Anterior	50	17 ± 6
	100	29 ± 5
Inferior	50	32 ± 4
	100	56 ± 12
Posterior	50	17 ± 6
	100	30 ± 12

After characterizing the stability ratios for the ten shoulders with the labrum intact, the labrum was excised entirely and the tests repeated. Excision of the labrum diminished the stability ratios for all directions of displacement and for both magnitudes of compressive loading (Table 3–3). In the shoulder specimens from these older cadavers with relatively atrophic labra, labral excision reduced the stability ratio by an average of 20 percent. The contribution of the labrum to stability is likely to be even greater in younger shoulders.

The stability ratios correlated with the effective depth of the glenoid concavity, both when the labrum was present and after it was excised (Table 3–4). A plot of the eight stability ratios as a function of the respective values for the effective glenoid depth reveals a consistent relationship (Fig. 3–17).

The strong relationship between depth and stability from concavity compression suggests that this stabilizing mechanism is compromised when the glenoid is developmentally small or flat or when the effective concavity of the glenoid has been lessened by injury or wear. Glenoids with flat posterior lips contribute to posterior glenohumeral subluxation and dislocation. Glenoid rim fractures involving significant loss of glenoid concavity are associated with glenohumeral instability. Avulsion of the glenoid labrum in traumatic instability lessens the effective depth of the glenoid concavity, predisposing the joint to recurrent subluxation and dislocation. Anatomic reattachment of a detached labrum and glenohumeral ligament back to the glenoid rim helps restore the effective glenoid depth and stability (Fig. 3–18).

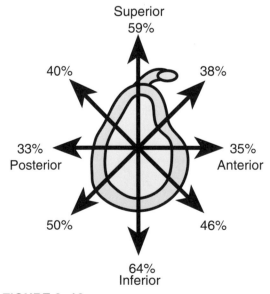

FIGURE 3–16.

Stability ratios for ten glenohumeral joints with the labrum intact and a compressive load of 50 Newtons.

Superior Stability

Concavity compression is the primary mechanism by which the head of the humerus is centered and stabilized in the glenoid fossa to resist the upward pull of the deltoid. By virtue of this stability, the head and rotator cuff are held down away from the coracoacromial arch. Previously, the rotator cuff muscles were viewed as head "depressors." However, the net force vector of

TABLE 3–3. Effect of Load and Labrum on Stability: Changes in the Stability Ratio with Different Compression Loads and with Removal of the Labrum*

Direction of Translating Force (Degree)	Stability Ratios at 50 Newtons Compressive Load			Stability Ratios at 100 Newtons Compressive Load		
	Labrum Intact	Labrum Excised	P Value	Labrum Intact	Labrum Excised	P Value
Superior (zero)	59 ± 13	47 ± 8	0.012	51 ± 9	45 ± 7	0.028
Superoanterior (45)	38 ± 11	30 ± 10	0.032			
Anterior (90)	35 ± 11	28 ± 6	0.062	29 ± 5	26 ± 5	0.021
Anteroinferior (135)	46 ± 6	39 ± 8	0.008			
Inferior (180)	64 ± 8	41 ± 13	0.0001	56 ± 12	40 ± 13	0.0002
Inferoposterior (225)	50 ± 19	30 ± 10	0.001			
Posterior (270)	33 ± 12	25 ± 11	0.017	30 ± 12	23 ± 9	0.01
Posterosuperior (315)	40 ± 16	32 ± 14	0.032			

*Values are means of ten shoulders $\pm$ SD.

TABLE 3–4. Relationship of Depth and Stability: Comparison of Effective Depth of Glenoid Concavity and Stability Ratio for Superoinferior and Anteroposterior Directions with 50 Newton Compression Loads*

	Superoinferior		Anteroposterior	
Labrum Intact				
Depth (mm)	4.8 ± 1	4.9 ± 1.1	2.2 ± 0.9	2.1 ± 0.9
Stability ratio (%)	64 ± 13	64 ± 8	35 ± 11	33 ± 12
Labrum Excised				
Depth (mm)	3.7 ± 0.8	3.0 ± 1.3	1.6 ± 0.6	1.4 ± 0.5
Stability ratio (%)	47 ± 13	41 ± 13	28 ± 6	25 ± 11

*Data reported as mean $\pm$ SD.

FIGURE 3–17.

A nearly linear relationship exists between the effective depth of the glenoid concavity and the stability ratio with a 50-Newton compressive load. These data include points representing superior, inferior, anterior, and posterior translations with and without the glenoid labrum. Linear regression by the least squares method yields the following relationship:

Stability ratio (%) = 10.3 × (glenoid ratio in mm) + 9.7

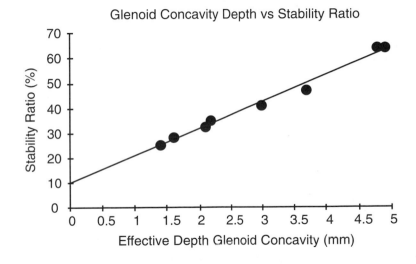

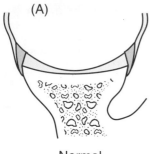

(A) Normal

(B) Bankart lesion

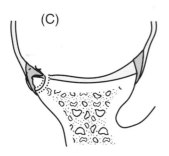

(C) Anatomic repair

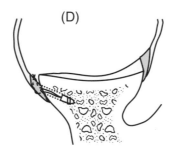

(D) Suboptimal repair

FIGURE 3–18.

Normally, the capsule and labrum deepen the effective glenoid fossa *(A)*. This effect is lost in the presence of a Bankart lesion *(B)*. Anatomic repair of the detached glenoid labrum and glenohumeral ligaments to the glenoid rim helps restore the effective depth of the glenoid concavity *(C)*. In contrast, when the labrum and capsule heal to the neck, concavity is not restored *(D)*.

the supraspinatus muscle is not oriented optimally to depress the head of the humerus against the upward pull of the deltoid (Fig. 3–19). We suggest that the cuff muscles provide stability by functioning as "compressors" of the head into the glenoid concavity.

The coracoacromial arch provides a rigid backstop to upward displacement of the humeral head relative to the glenoid. Even when a substantial supraspinatus defect is present, compression from the subscapularis and infraspinatus can hold the humeral head centered on the glenoid away from the coracoacromial arch (Fig. 3–20).

More severe cases of chronic rotator cuff

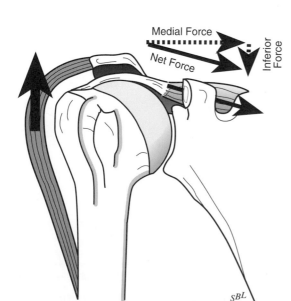

FIGURE 3–19.

The supraspinatus muscle is not optimally oriented to depress the head of the humerus against the upward pull of the deltoid, because the inferiorly directed component of the supraspinatus force is small.

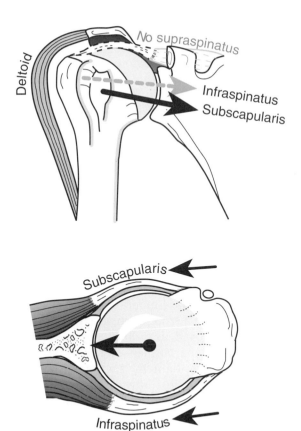

FIGURE 3–20.

Compression by the infraspinatus and subscapularis can help stabilize the humeral head in the absence of a supraspinatus, provided the glenoid concavity is intact.

deficiency, however, may be associated with superior subluxation of the head of the humerus and wear on the superior lip of the glenoid fossa. This erosive wear flattens the superior glenoid concavity and thereby reduces the effective glenoid depth in that direction. Once the effective glenoid concavity is lost, repair of the rotator cuff tendons or complex capsular reconstruction cannot completely restore the glenohumeral stability provided by compression into an intact concavity (Fig. 3–21).

Concavity compression is a versatile mechanism for stabilizing the glenohumeral joint. When an effective glenoid concavity is present, this mechanism can operate in any position in which a compressive force can be generated. Furthermore, concavity compression does not require intact capsule or glenohumeral ligaments.

Concavity compression is an important mechanism of stability in shoulder arthroplasty. In this situation, the capsule and ligaments are routinely sectioned as a part of the soft tissue release. In the design of shoulder arthroplasty components, the depth of the prosthetic glenoid fossa is a function of the radius of curvature of the joint surface and the height and width of the glenoid component. For a given radius of curvature, higher and broader glenoid components provide more depth. Oblong components have less stability anteroposteriorly than superoinferiorly. Components that narrow at the superior aspect are less stable in the anterosuperior and posterosuperior directions.

Adhesion-Cohesion

Adhesion-cohesion is a stabilizing mechanism by which joint surfaces wet with joint fluid are held together by the molecular attraction of the fluid to itself and to the joint surfaces. Fluids such as water and joint fluid demonstrate the property of cohesion; that is, they tend to hang together. Some surfaces, such as clean glass or articular cartilage, can

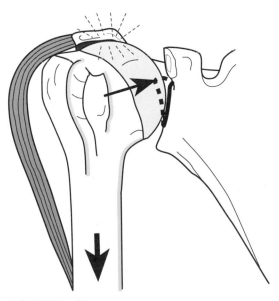

FIGURE 3–21.

Erosion of the superior glenoid concavity compromises the concavity compression stability mechanism, allowing upward translation.

be wet with water or synovial fluid, meaning that the fluid adheres to them. When two surfaces with adherent fluid are brought in contact, the adhesion of the fluid to the surfaces and the cohesion of the fluid tend to hold the two surfaces together. The amount of stability generated by adhesion-cohesion is related to the adhesive and cohesive properties of the joint fluid, the "wetability" of the joint surfaces, and the area of contact between the glenoid socket and the humerus.

ACTIVITY

Place a drop of water between two clean microscope slides. Note how it wets their surfaces. Observe the minimal resistance to their gliding on one another in the plane of the interposed water layer. Attempt to pull the surfaces apart with a force at right angles to the plane of the interposed water layer. The adhesion of water to the glass surfaces and the cohesion of water resist strongly the separation of these surfaces.

The magnitude of the stabilizing effect of adhesion-cohesion in the glenohumeral joint is unknown. The known wetability of articular cartilage and the cohesiveness of joint fluid suggest that this adhesion-cohesion mechanism may conserve energy by providing stability against low distracting loads without use of muscle action. This mecha-

nism can function in any position of the glenohumeral joint.

Stability from adhesion-cohesion is reduced by any factors that would lower either the cohesion of joint fluid (such as in inflammatory joint disease), the degree to which the joint surfaces could be wet (such as in degenerative joint disease), or the glenohumeral contact area (such as in a displaced articular surface fracture or a congenitally small glenoid).

Glenohumeral "Suction Cup"

The glenohumeral *suction cup* provides stability by virtue of the seal of the labrum and capsule to the humeral head. A suction cup adheres to a smooth surface by expressing the interposed air or fluid and then forming a seal to the surface. A rubber suction cup is noncompliant in the center but becomes more flexible toward its periphery. Like a suction cup, the glenoid surface has "feathered" edges that become increasingly flexible with increasing distance from the center (Fig. 3–22). The center of the glenoid is covered with a relatively thin layer of articular cartilage. At greater distances from the center, the articular cartilage becomes thicker, providing greater flexibility. More peripherally, the glenoid labrum and, finally, the capsule provide even more flexibility. This graduated flexibility permits the socket to conform and seal to the smooth humeral articular surface. Compression of the head into the glenoid fossa expels any intervening

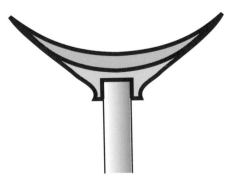 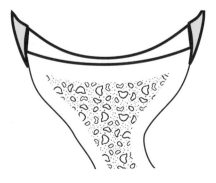

FIGURE 3–22.

In cross section, the glenoid looks much like a rubber suction cup with respect to its feathered, compliant edges and a more rigid center.

fluid so that a "suction" is produced that resists distraction.

The glenoid suction cup stabilization mechanism is easily demonstrated in young cadaver shoulders in which the articular cartilage, glenoid labrum, and joint capsule are compliant. The magnitude of this stabilizing effect has not been measured. Like stabilization from adhesion-cohesion, the glenoid suction cup centers the head of the humerus in the glenoid without muscle action and is effective in midrange positions in which the capsule and ligaments are not under tension. The suction cup mechanism is disrupted in situations where the socket cannot seal to the surface of the humeral head, such as an avulsion of the glenoid labrum and glenoid fracture.

ACTIVITY

Study the "design" of a suction cup, and compare it with a cross section of the glenoid socket with respect to the change in pliability from the center to the periphery. Press a wet rubber suction cup against a smooth ball. Get a feel for the force necessary to pull them apart. Repeat this test after trimming away one edge of the suction cup. If possible, obtain the fresh shoulder of a young cadaver, and verify the stability afforded by the suction cup mechanism.

Limited Joint Volume

Limited joint volume is a stabilizing mechanism in which the humeral head is held to the socket by the relative vacuum created when they are distracted. Although it is common to speak of the glenohumeral joint space, there is essentially no space and minimal free fluid within the confines of the articular surfaces and the joint capsule of the normal glenohumeral joint. The lack of fluid within the joint can be confirmed on MRI scans of normal joints, on inspection of normal joints, and on attempts to aspirate fluid from normal joints. The appearance of the *potential* joint volume can be demonstrated

only after instilling air, saline, or contrast materials into the joint. Osmotic action by the synovium removes free fluid, keeping a slightly negative pressure within the normal joint. This negative intraarticular pressure holds the joint together with a force proportional to the joint surface area and the magnitude of the negative intraarticular pressure. Because the normal joint is sealed, attempted distraction of the joint surfaces lowers the intraarticular pressure even more, progressively adding substantial resistance to greater displacement.

This mechanism is defined as the *limited joint volume effect.* Our cadaver experiments demonstrated that this mechanism is sufficiently strong enough to support the weight of the arm. The limited joint volume effect is reduced if the joint is vented (opened to the atmosphere) (Fig. 3–23A). These studies indicated that simply venting the capsule with an 18-gauge needle reduced the force necessary to translate the head of the humerus halfway to the edge of the glenoid by an average of 50 percent (28 to 13 Newtons anteriorly, 25 to 14 Newtons posteriorly, and 33 to 14 Newtons inferiorly). The limited joint volume effect is also compromised if the joint contains free fluid or if the capsule is very compliant.

This mechanism of glenohumeral stability is, therefore, compromised with arthrography, arthroscopy, articular effusions, hemarthrosis and in other situations in which free fluid is present within the glenohumeral joint. The limited joint volume effect is also compromised when the capsular boundaries of the joint are very compliant. Under these circumstances, attempted distraction draws the flexible capsule into the joint, producing a "sulcus" (Fig. 3–23B). This may be one of the factors that contributes to midrange glenohumeral instability in patients with generalized ligamentous laxity.

ACTIVITY

To demonstrate the stabilizing effect of limited joint volume, attempt to distract the plunger from the barrel of a plugged syringe. To demonstrate the destabilizing effect of capsular

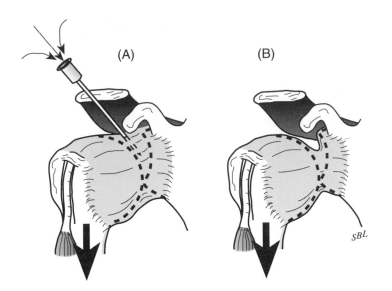

FIGURE 3–23.

The glenohumeral capsule establishes a limited joint volume so the distraction of the humeral head produces a relative vacuum within the capsule, thus resisting displacement. *A,* Venting of the capsule diminishes the stabilization from limited joint volume, allowing inferior translation. *B,* Displacement of a compliant capsule into the joint area produces a sulcus, also allowing inferior translation.

venting, distract the plunger after the hole in the end of the barrel is opened to the air. To demonstrate the destabilizing effect of compliant capsular walls, saw off the end of the syringe and replace it with a compliant material such as a rubber dam. Distract the plunger, noting that a "sulcus" is formed as the dam invaginates into the barrel (Fig. 3–24).

Taken together, balance, concavity compression, adhesion-cohesion, the glenoid

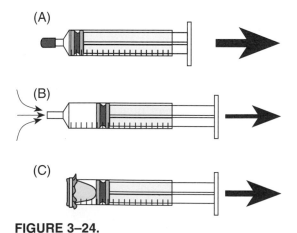

FIGURE 3–24.

Limited joint volume. Substantial force is required to pull the plunger from a plugged syringe *(A)*. This stabilizing effect is lost if the syringe is uncapped *(B)* or if the end of the syringe is covered with a compliant material *(C)*.

suction cup, and limited joint volume provide a family of stabilizing mechanisms that function throughout the range of glenohumeral motion, including the midrange where the glenohumeral ligaments and capsule are not under tension. Midrange stability is critical in that most of the activities of daily living, such as dressing, eating, working, and writing, are performed in midrange positions.

Capsuloligamentous Constraint

The capsule and ligaments of the glenohumeral joint serve as check reins to glenohumeral translation and rotation. They are not "primary stabilizers" in that they do not effectively hold the humeral head centered in the glenoid socket in most functional positions of the joint.

The capsule and its ligaments arise in continuity with the articular surface of the glenoid through the glenoid labrum, so that when they are under tension they provide a smooth continuation of the glenoid concavity. By serving as check reins at the limits of glenohumeral motion, the capsule and ligaments control the maximal humeroscapular angle that can be achieved in a given direction as well as the amount of internal and external rotation that is allowed at each humeroscapular position (Figs. 3–25 and 3–26). For example, the posterior capsule lim-

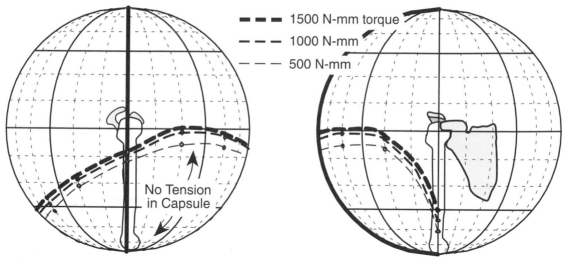

FIGURE 3–25.

Range of humeroscapular elevation with no capsular tension. This global diagram represents data from a cadaver experiment in which the humerus was elevated in a variety of scapular planes, allowing free axial rotation. Elevation was performed until the torque reached 500, 1000, and 1500 Newton/mm. The positions associated with these torque levels are indicated by the isobars. The area within the inner isobar indicates the range of positions in which there was no tension in the capsuloligamentous structures.

its how far the elevated arm can be brought across the body. Glenohumeral joints with lax posterior capsules can reach the 90 degree anterior humeroscapular plane. Shoulders with tight posterior capsules have difficulty reaching the 45 degree anterior humeroscapular plane. Similarly, the anterior capsule limits posterior motion of the elevated arm. Shoulders with anterior capsular laxity achieve significantly more posterior humeroscapular planes than shoulders with tight anterior structures. In this

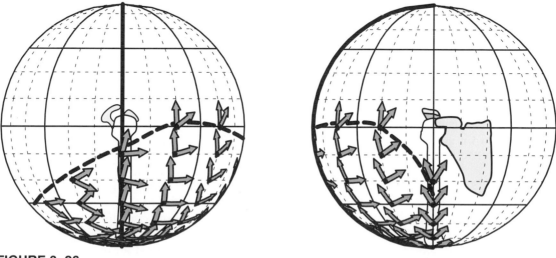

FIGURE 3–26.

Rotational laxity. Data are from the same cadaver experiment discussed in Figure 3–25. At each position, the range of internal and external rotation allowed by the capsular laxity is indicated by arrows pointing in the direction of the forearm.

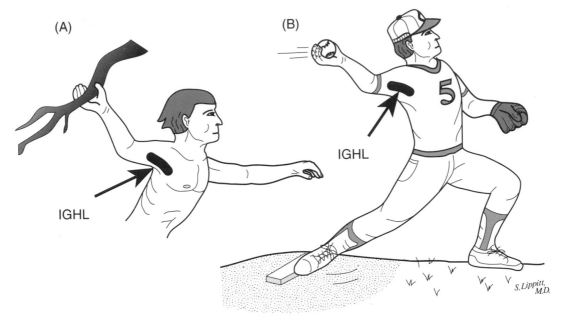

FIGURE 3–27.

The anterior band of the inferior glenohumeral ligament (IGHL) becomes tight in swinging from a branch *(A)* and in the transition between cocking and acceleration in the throw *(B).*

way, the capsule prevents the humerus from deviating far from positions of glenohumeral balance.

Certain portions of the capsular complex that serve major roles are condensed and thickened in the form of capsular ligaments. These ligaments appear to represent capsular reinforcements in directions where large torques may be encountered at the extremes of motion, as in swinging from branch to branch or in the transition between the cocking and the acceleration phases in a baseball pitch (Fig. 3–27). These motions apply major torques to the joint. The strong anterior band of the inferior glenohumeral ligament is strategically positioned to check the range of rotation of the joint when the arm is elevated and forced into external rotation.

CAPSULAR LAXITY

The capsule and its associated ligaments are lax in most of the common functional positions of the glenohumeral joint (compare Fig. 2–18 and Fig. 3–25). This laxity is necessary for the joint to achieve its large range of positions. Because of this midrange

laxity, the capsule cannot stabilize the joint in many important functional positions. In a study of eight cadaveric shoulders, we measured the anterior, posterior, and inferior translational laxity (Fig. 3–28A). These shoulders were vented using an 18-gauge needle to admit air to the capsule, thus eliminating the stabilizing effect of finite joint volume. The largest translational laxity was found in midrange positions of approximately 15 to 45 degrees of elevation, in planes of elevation from zero to 30 degrees anterior to the plane of the scapula. Typically, the amount of laxity was 1 to 2 cm for translation in any of the three directions. As the joint was brought near its limit of motion (e.g., 75 degrees of elevation in the -30 degree scapular plane), the joint laxity was substantially reduced consequent to the tightening of the capsular ligaments.

It is thus apparent that capsular ligaments alone do not hold the humeral head centered in the glenoid, at least in the midrange positions where most activities of daily living occur. Instead, centering of the humeral head in the glenoid fossa must depend on other mechanisms, such as concavity compression. Therefore, we must distinguish be-

Mean Translational Laxity in Intact Shoulders

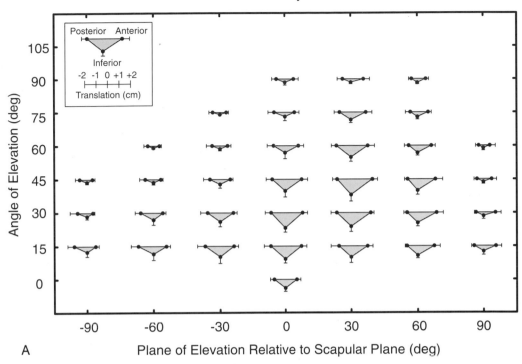

A

Plane of Elevation Relative to Scapular Plane (deg)

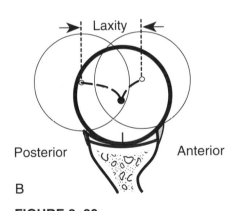

B

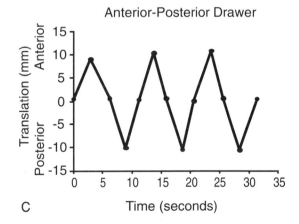

C

FIGURE 3–28.

A, Mean translational laxity as measured in eight cadaveric shoulders. The applied translational force was 30 Newtons (approximately 6 lb), and it was applied along each of the following axes: anterior, posterior, and inferior. The capsule was vented to the surrounding atmosphere. Planes of elevation are measured relative to the plane of the scapula, not the thoracic plane. Standard deviations are shown at the vertex of each triangle. *B, Laxity* is the translation allowed by the glenohumeral joint in a specified direction (anteroposterior laxity is diagrammed here). The stability of the joint is related to the shape and effective depth of the glenoidogram (indicating the path taken by the humeral head center as it translates across the glenoid face), shown as the gull wing pattern. Tight V-shaped graphs favor precise centering of the humeral head in the glenoid. Note that neither the laxity nor the glenoidogram need be symmetrical about the glenoid center. *C*, Translations on anterior and posterior drawer tests in the shoulder of a normal living subject. Note the reproducible translations of approximately 1 cm in both directions.

tween capsular laxity (which is normal and necessary to the proper function of the glenohumeral joint) and glenohumeral instability, which may be operationally defined as an inability to hold the humeral head centered in the glenohumeral joint (Fig. 3–28B).

To demonstrate the degree of laxity present in eight normal shoulders, electromagnetic sensors were pinned to the humerus and scapula to allow accurate measurement of the magnitude of translation on standard clinical tests of glenohumeral laxity: the anterior and posterior drawer tests, the sulcus test, and the push-pull test. The anterior and posterior drawer tests were performed by stabilizing the scapula and clavicle with one hand while grasping the proximal humerus with the other hand. The arm was placed in a relaxed position at the subject's side. The humeral head was pushed forward to assess maximal anterior translation and then pushed posteriorly to assess maximal posterior translation. In the sulcus test, downward traction was applied to the subject's arm while the shoulder girdle was stabilized with the other hand.

The push-pull test was performed with the subject supine and the arm elevated 90 degrees in the plus 20 degree thoracic plane. The examiner pushed down on the proximal humerus with one hand while pulling up on the subject's wrist with the other.

The shoulders were stressed to the clinical end point. Even though the force applied was not quantified, the amount of translation was highly reproducible, as shown for a typical test in Figure 3–28C. The results of these tests (Table 3–5) indicate that this group of normal shoulders demonstrated substantial translations on these clinical laxity tests. These data indicate that, in the positions tested, the capsule and ligaments were lax and were not contributing to the centering of the humeral head in the glenoid fossa. We conclude that in these midrange positions, the head is centered by stabilizing mechanisms other than the capsule and ligaments.

Because laxity is a feature of stable shoulders, it is of interest to ask whether unstable shoulders have more laxity than do stable shoulders. Of greater clinical relevance are the questions: Are laxity tests useful in discriminating stable from unstable shoulders? Do laxity tests reveal the primary pathologic changes in glenohumeral instability? As a step toward answering these questions, we measured the laxity of 16 patients requiring surgery because of symptomatic recurrent instability that was refractory to non-operative management. We then compared these results with those of normal shoulders presented earlier. Eight of these patients had classic anterior traumatic instability, and eight had classic atraumatic instability. Each patient was studied under anesthesia just prior to surgical repair, with our electromagnetic position sensors rigidly attached to the humerus and scapula. The laxity tests were carried out exactly as described earlier for the normal subjects. The magnitudes of the passive glenohumeral translations measured in the unstable shoulders were remarkably similar to those measured in the normal subjects (Fig. 3–29).

These results suggest that glenohumeral laxity is not the preponderant factor in determining the clinical stability of the shoulder. Shoulders that are quite lax may be completely stable, whereas those without major laxity may be clinically unstable. These data further serve to caution against using the magnitude of translation on these laxity tests to distinguish between clinically stable and unstable shoulders. As we will see, the diagnosis of instability must rest on a careful history and physical examination that endeavor to define the problem that is symptomatic for the patient.

In conclusion, substantial translational laxity is allowed by the normal glenohumeral joint capsule, especially in midrange positions. The wide variance in translation

TABLE 3–5. Normal Laxity *in Vivo*: Means (± SD) Translation on Clinical Laxity Tests for Eight Normal Subjects

Test	Direction	Translation (mm)
Anterior drawer	Anterior	8 ± 4
Posterior drawer	Posterior	8 ± 6
Sulcus test	Inferior	11 ± 4
Push-pull test	Posterior	9 ± 6

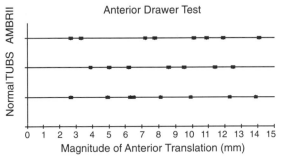

Anterior Drawer Test

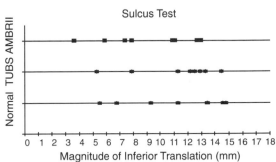

Sulcus Test

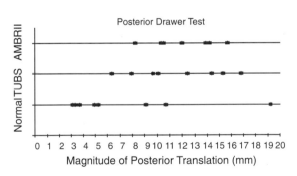

Posterior Drawer Test

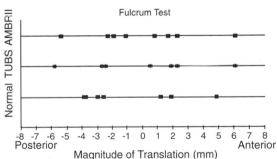

Fulcrum Test

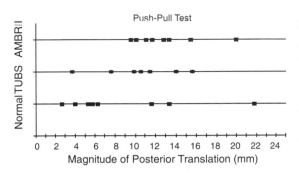

Push-Pull Test

FIGURE 3–29.

The magnitude of translation on laxity tests for three groups of shoulders *in vivo*: eight normal shoulders, eight shoulders with symptomatic atraumatic instability (AMBRII), and eight shoulders with symptomatic traumatic instability (TUBS). Each shoulder is represented by a square box. Note that for each of these laxity tests, the *range* of translations for the normal subjects is essentially the same as the range of translations for subjects with symptomatic instability requiring surgical repair.

among normal shoulders precludes the definition of a "normal" amount of translation on laxity tests. Translation on clinical laxity tests is not an indication of instability. Stability of the glenohumeral joint, especially in midrange positions, must be due to factors other than tension in the capsular structures.

GLENOHUMERAL INSTABILITY

Glenohumeral instability is the inability to maintain the humeral head articular surface centered in the glenoid fossa. Instability may arise from a traumatic episode in which an injury occurs to the bone, rotator cuff, labrum, capsule, and/or ligaments. Recurrent traumatic instability typically produces symptoms when the arm is placed in positions near that of the original injury. Conversely, instability may arise atraumatically from decompensation of the mechanisms providing midrange glenohumeral stability. The necessary and sufficient criteria for these diagnoses are listed in Table 3–6.

ATRAUMATIC INSTABILITY

Atraumatic instability is instability that arises without major trauma. In that many factors provide normal midrange stability, it is likely that atraumatic midrange instability may arise from a variety of causes. A shoulder that has been stable may become unstable after a minor injury or a period of disuse. Certain shoulders may be more susceptible to atraumatic instability. A flat or small glenoid fossa may jeopardize the balance, concavity compression, adhesion-cohesion, and glenoid suction cup mechanisms. Attenuation of the glenoid labrum may further compromise these stabilizing mechanisms. Thin, excessively compliant capsular tissue may invaginate into the joint when traction is applied, limiting the effectiveness of stabilization from limited joint volume. An extensive glenohumeral joint capsule may allow humeroscapular positions outside the range of balance stability. Weak rotator cuff muscles may provide insufficient compression for

TABLE 3–6. Necessary and Sufficient Diagnostic Criteria for Traumatic Anterior and Atraumatic Glenohumeral Instability

I. Traumatic Anterior Glenohumeral Instability
  A. History
    1. Mechanism of injury appropriate to cause tearing of the anterior glenohumeral ligaments, such as a major external rotation torque applied when the arm is elevated near the coronal plane
    2. Functionally significant recurrent episodes of apprehension (fear of uncontrollable glenohumeral translations) or instability (inability to keep the humeral head centered in the glenoid fossa) when the arm is elevated near the coronal plane and externally rotated or extended
  B. Physical Examination
    1. Apprehension or instability when the arm is elevated near the coronal plane and externally rotated or extended
    2. Diagnosis is supported by grinding with translation on anterior drawer test
  C. Radiographs
    1. Diagnosis is supported by radiographs documenting a previous anterior glenohumeral dislocation
    2. Diagnosis is supported by radiographs showing a characteristic posterior lateral humeral head defect and/or anterior inferior glenoid lip defect or calcification
II. Atraumatic Instability
  A. History
    1. Functionally significant inability to keep the humeral head centered in the glenoid fossa, especially in positions not at the extremes of motion
    2. Absence of mechanism of injury likely to tear glenohumeral ligaments or capsule
    3. Spontaneous reduction of translations
  B. Physical Examination
    1. Demonstration that certain glenohumeral translations duplicate the symptoms of concern to the patient
    2. Diminished resistance to translation in multiple directions as compared with a normal glenohumeral joint
  C. Radiographs
    1. Absence of traumatic lesions

the concavity compression stabilizing mechanism. Poor neuromuscular control may fail to position the scapula to balance the net humeral joint reaction force. Voluntary or inadvertent malpositioning of the humerus in excessive anterior or posterior scapular planes may cause the net reaction force to lie outside the confines of the glenoid fossa.

Any of these factors, individually or in combination, could contribute to instability of the glenohumeral joint. For example, posterior glenohumeral subluxation may result from the combination of a relatively flat posterior glenoid and the tendency to retract the scapula during anterior elevation of the arm,

FIGURE 3–30.

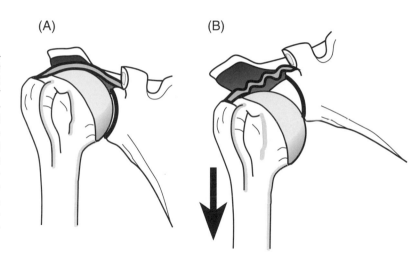

Scapular dumping. With the scapula in a normal position (A), the superior capsular mechanism is tight, supporting the head in the glenoid concavity. Drooping of the lateral scapula (B) relaxes the superior capsular structures and rotates the glenoid concavity so that it does not support the head of the humerus. Conversely, stability is enhanced by elevating the lateral aspect of the scapula.

resulting in use of the elevated humerus in anterior scapular planes. Excessively compliant capsular tissue in combination with relatively weak rotator cuff muscles could contribute to inferior subluxation on attempted lifting of objects with the arm at the side. If the lateral scapula is allowed to droop (whether voluntarily or involuntarily), the superior capsular structures are relaxed, permitting inferior translation of the humerus with respect to the glenoid (Fig. 3–30).

Because they usually result from loss of midrange stability, atraumatic instabilities are more likely to be multidirectional. Pathogenetic factors such as a flat glenoid, weak muscles, and a compliant capsule may produce instability anteriorly, inferiorly, and/or posteriorly. Although the onset of atraumatic instability may be provoked by a period of disuse or a minor injury, many of the underlying contributing factors may be developmental. As a result, the tendency for atraumatic instability is likely to be bilateral and familial as well.

It is now apparent that atraumatic instability is not a simple diagnosis but rather a syndrome that may arise from a multiplicity of factors. To help recall the various aspects of this syndrome, we use the acronym AMBRII. The instability is atraumatic, usually associated with multidirectional laxity and with bilateral findings. Treatment is predominantly by rehabilitation, directed at restoring optimal neuromuscular control. If surgery is necessary, it needs to include reconstruction of the rotator interval cap-

sule–coracohumeral ligament mechanism and tightening of the inferior capsule.

History

Figure 3–31 shows the age distribution of 51 patients presenting to our service with the atraumatic (AMBRII) instability. It appears to be a condition that presents predominantly in persons younger than 30 years of age.

AMBRII instability often begins with some minor event or series of events that lead to progressive decompensation of the glenohumeral stability mechanisms. An awkward lift, reaching over the back seat of the car, or a sneeze may be all that is necessary to launch the predisposed, but compensated, shoulder down the path toward instability. The patient notices that the shoulder has become loose and may feel it slip out and "clunk" back in with different activities. These episodes almost never require manipulative reduction. The instability may be sufficiently subtle that the patient is unaware of the humerus translating on the glenoid. The patient may be aware only of a feeling that the shoulder does something unnatural in certain positions or that certain functions cannot be performed, such as reaching out in front or lifting at the side. In contrast with the situation in traumatic instability, discomfort with activities of daily living may be a significant component of the complaint. A patient may volunteer that he or she can make the shoulder "pop out" and

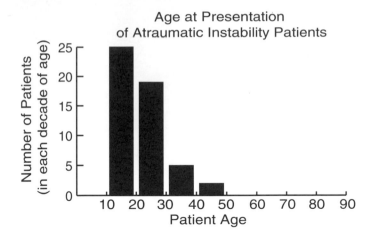

Age at Presentation of Atraumatic Instability Patients

FIGURE 3–31.

The age distribution of 51 patients with atraumatic instability.

that at times the shoulder feels as if it "needs to be popped out" on purpose. The patient should indicate each and every position in which problems with instability have been noted. Instability with the arm out in front of the body and problems lifting or reaching down are particularly suggestive of the AMBRII condition. It is important to note how frequently the problem occurs and whether the problem is "avoidable" if the patient concentrates on how the shoulder is used. Finally, we record the extent and effectiveness of previous non-operative and operative treatments and the presence or absence of instability symptoms in the opposite shoulder or other joints.

The Simple Shoulder Test provides a minimal data set for characterizing some of the functional impairment from atraumatic multidirectional glenohumeral instability (Fig. 3–32). These patients have greatest difficulty sleeping, lifting overhead, and throwing.

Particular emphasis is placed on the patient's functional goals with respect to work and sport activities. We try to determine whether these goals are realistic, considering the condition of the shoulder.

In summary, patients with atraumatic instability are usually young, perhaps with a family predisposition to "loose shoulders." The instability is most prevalent in midrange positions, those commonly used in activities of daily living such as lifting at the side and raising the arm to the front. The contralateral shoulder may also seem "loose." The patient may have difficulty defining exactly what it is about the shoulder that is bothersome. The history does not re-

veal an injury of sufficient magnitude to tear the capsule or ligaments.

Physical Examination

The physical examination of patients with AMBRII syndrome is usually started by asking them to demonstrate the positions in which the shoulder feels unstable. They may demonstrate a spontaneous jerk test by bringing the elevated arm horizontally across the chest, causing the humeral head to subluxate posteriorly. Then, by returning the elevated humerus to the coronal plane, they produce a clunk on reduction of the glenohumeral joint (much like the Ortolani and Barlow signs of the hip). Using the palpable scapular coordinates, we can estimate the scapular plane in which the shoulder subluxates and the plane in which it reduces. Patients may also demonstrate that when they attempt to lift an object or tie their shoes, the shoulder subluxates inferiorly. They may demonstrate that when they lie on the affected shoulder, it is pushed forward out of joint. Finally, they may demonstrate by elevating the arm in a posterior humerothoracic plane that they can produce anterior subluxation with spontaneous reduction on return to the coronal plane. By allowing the patient to demonstrate the symptomatic positions and motions of instability, our hands are free to define the humeroscapular positions at the moments of interest. These observations may reveal faulty patterns of scapulohumeral mechanics, such as allowing the lateral scapula to droop during lifting or retracting the

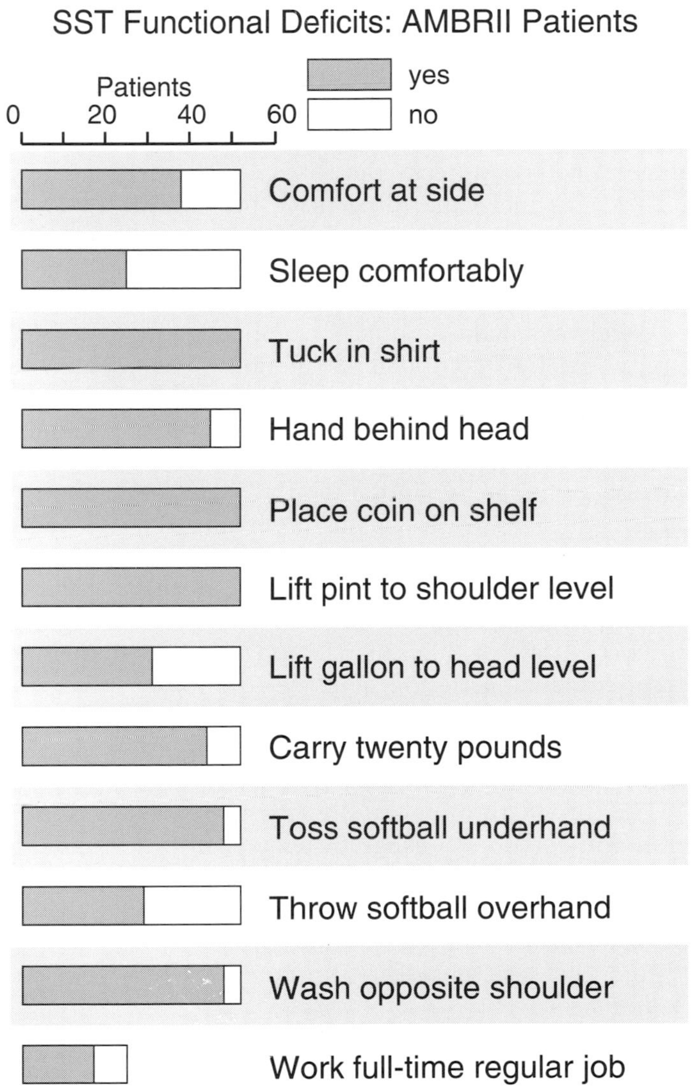

FIGURE 3–32.

The functional deficits presented by 52 patients with atraumatic instability.

SST Functional Deficits: AMBRII Patients

Patients

yes

no

0   20   40   60

Comfort at side

Sleep comfortably

Tuck in shirt

Hand behind head

Place coin on shelf

Lift pint to shoulder level

Lift gallon to head level

Carry twenty pounds

Toss softball underhand

Throw softball overhand

Wash opposite shoulder

Work full-time regular job

scapula during anterior elevation of the humerus.

We have described our investigations of classic clinical laxity tests showing that, in a small group of subjects, the *magnitude* of translation for shoulders with atraumatic instability is essentially the same as that of normal shoulders or shoulders with traumatic instability. Therefore, we pay particular attention to the patient's response during laxity testing; we are seeking to reproduce the translations that duplicate the symptoms that brought the patient in for treatment. Our best diagnostic confirmation occurs when, during a laxity test, the patient states, "That's it—that's the thing that's bothering me." We refer to this as *recognition* of the symptomatic event when it is reproduced during the examination.

We always make a point of examining the laxity of the contralateral glenohumeral joint. Occasionally, laxity tests yield different results on the symptomatic side. More often, however, examination of the contralateral shoulder is similar to the symptomatic one. This allows us the opportunity to demonstrate to the patient and the family that, although both shoulders demonstrate similar degrees of laxity, the patient is able to control one of them using good mechanics. This demonstration helps set the foundation for our discussion of the need to regain stabilizing neuromuscular control of the symptomatic shoulder.

Finally, we examine the strength of abduction and rotation to gauge the power of the muscles contributing to stability through concavity compression. We also examine the strength of the scapular protractors and elevators that are necessary to position the scapula securely.

Radiographs

In atraumatic instability, shoulder radiographs characteristically show no bony pathologic changes. Because these patients characteristically demonstrate midrange instability, radiographs may show translation of the humeral head with respect to the glenoid. The axillary view may show posterior subluxation. Occasionally, radiographs may suggest factors underlying the atraumatic instability, such as a hypoplastic, a posteriorly inclined, or an otherwise dysplastic glenoid. The bony glenoid fossa may appear quite flat; however, it is difficult to relate the apparent depth of the bony socket to the effective depth of the fossa formed by cartilage and labrum covering the bone.

We do not use stress radiographs, arthrography, MRI, or arthroscopy in the diagnosis of atraumatic instability.

Treatment

The goal of treatment of patients with atraumatic instability is the restoration of shoulder function. Many patients with AMBRII syndrome have simply become deconditioned from their normal state of dynamic glenohumeral stability. They have lost the proper neuromuscular control of humeroscapular positioning; concavity compression has become dysfunctional. Neuromuscular control cannot be restored surgically; rather, it requires prolonged adherence to a well-constructed reconditioning program. The patient may need to be convinced that training and exercises constitute a reasonable therapeutic approach. Many would prefer a surgical "cure." We have found it useful to demonstrate that the contralateral shoulder often has substantial laxity on examination yet is clinically stable. In this way we try to educate the patient and family that a loose shoulder is not necessarily clinically unstable. We emphasize that gymnasts usually have very lax, yet very stable shoulders.

There are two aspects of the non-operative management of atraumatic instability: strengthening the compressor muscles and training for humeroscapular balance. First, it is essential to optimize the strength and endurance of the muscles compressing the head of the humerus into the glenoid concavity. Weakness or poor endurance of the rotator cuff muscles can usually be managed by a regular exercise program. The second component of the exercise program emphasizes regaining stability through neuromuscular control of humeroscapular positions.

Our program is outlined in Patient Information 3–1.

PATIENT INFORMATION 3-1

UNIVERSITY OF WASHINGTON SHOULDER AND ELBOW SERVICE

Exercise Program for Atraumatic Instability

Normal shoulders are stabilized by good muscle strength and by proper technique in their use. Many shoulders, like those of gymnasts, are very loose when the muscles are relaxed but function superbly with proper training and technique. Your shoulder may have problems of instability after a minor injury or a period of disuse. You may notice that your shoulder slips or feels unstable with certain activities. In these situations, the most effective treatment is to restore the normal strength and coordination of the shoulder.

There are four parts to this reconditioning program. The first is to do all you can to avoid having your shoulder "pop out of place." Even if it feels like it "needs" to be popped, **don't do it.** Each time you let it pop, it makes it easier for it to happen the next time (just like blowing up a balloon repetitively makes it easier on each successive occasion).

The second part of the reconditioning program concerns strengthening the muscles that press the ball of the shoulder into the socket. These muscles are called the *rotator cuff muscles.* They are strengthened by working against resistance in rotation internally (toward the body) and externally (away from the body). It is important that your shoulder have both strength and endurance of internal and external rotation. This means that you need to carry out at least five exercise sessions each day, each taking only about 5 minutes. Internal rotation is strengthened by holding the elbow close to the side and trying to rotate the arm inward against resistance. This resistance

can be isometric (unmoving), such as the opposite hand, a wall, or other fixed object. You can also use dynamic exercises against rubber tubing, weights and pulleys, or free weights while you lie on your side (Fig. 3–33). External rotation is strengthened by holding the elbow at the side and trying to rotate the arm outward against either isometric or dynamic resistance (Fig. 3–34). The reason these exercises are started with your arm at the side is because that is usually a position in which your shoulder is stable. As you get stronger, you should be able to perform these rotations in other stable positions.

The third component of the reconditioning program for your shoulder is to train the muscles that balance the ball in the socket. These muscles are primarily those that power your shoulder blade or scapula. When your scapula gets lazy or weak, the shoulder tends to become malaligned and unstable. The purpose of these exercises is to strengthen the muscles and to eliminate bad habits that your shoulder may have developed. The largest and most important muscle groups are those that move your shoulder blade forward (the serratus and pectoralis) and those that lift the shoulder blade (the trapezius, levator scapulae, and rhomboids). The first group, the protractors, are strengthened by a bench press–type exercise performed supine holding the bar with the hands about a meter (yard) apart. At first, only the bar is used while you concentrate on powering the shoulder blade upward. When you lift your shoulder blade off the bed or table, we call this the *press "plus"* (Fig. 3–35). The "plus" is important for training the shoulder blade muscles. Once you can control the bar alone for 20 repetitions, add weight to the bar progressively

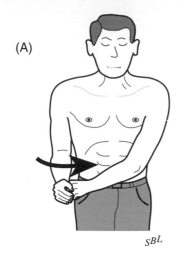

(A)

SB^L

doing a one hand press using a 1-pound weight and building up to 20 percent of your body weight. This series of exercises will restore the strength and technique necessary to use your arm stably in front of you. The second muscle group helps balance your shoulder during lifting at your side (Fig. 3–36). Start with a simple

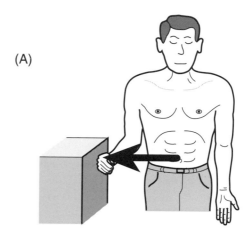

(A)

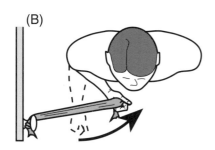

(B)

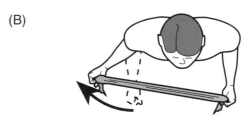

(B)

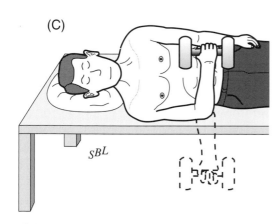

(C)

SB^L

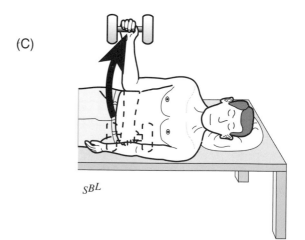

(C)

SB^L

FIGURE 3–33.

Internal rotation can be strengthened with isometrics *(A)*, rubber tubing *(B)*, or free weights *(C)*.

up to about half your body weight. Never use a weight greater than what you can control for 20 repetitions. Once you feel confident in the shoulder, you can start

FIGURE 3–34.

External rotation strengthening using isometrics *(A)*, rubber tubing *(B)*, or free weights *(C)*.

86

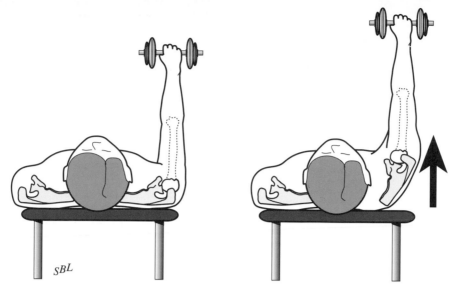

FIGURE 3–35.

In the press plus, the arm is pushed upward until the shoulder blade is lifted off the table or bed.

FIGURE 3–36.

The shoulder shrug exercise: lift the tip of the shoulder toward the ear while holding the elbow straight.

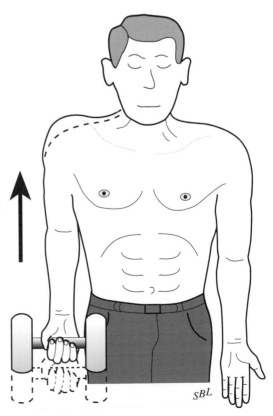

87

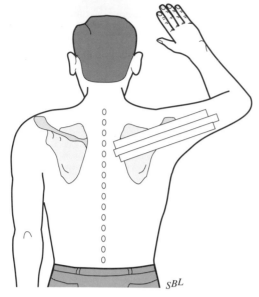

FIGURE 3–37.

Training tape applied across the back of the shoulder as a reminder to avoid unbalanced positions.

shoulder shrug, lifting the point of your shoulders as high as they will go 20 times. Once the shoulder shrug becomes easy, add weight 1 pound at a time to each hand, keeping the number of repetitions at 20. With each shrug, concentrate on lifting the tip of the shoulder.

The fourth component of the exercise program concerns performing activities with the arm away from the body. Lift your arm 90 degrees to the side holding several pounds in your hand. Notice that the shoulder is stable in that position. Rotate your hand in a small circle. Repeat this exercise with the arm in progressively more forward positions as long as your shoulder feels stable. Try to accomplish this movement with the shoulder blade and not at the shoulder joint *per se.* If you have difficulty keeping your shoulder stable while you are doing this exercise, try using the "training tape" technique. Have someone apply some tape to the back of your shoulder joint (from the shoulder

blade to the back of the arm) while you have your arm elevated straight out to the side (Fig. 3–37). This tape will tend to keep the shoulder blade and your arm lined up and stable while you bring the arm forward. Just like with training wheels on a bike, once you have learned the technique of balance, you can discard the training tape.

As you gain strength and coordination, try to carry out progressively more of your usual activities, concentrating on keeping the ball of your shoulder in the socket. Avoid activities and positions that threaten your shoulder's stability, while practicing those that you can perform with confidence. Swimming, rowing, and using cross-country skiing simulators are all good exercises for developing strength, coordination, and endurance. They also have the advantage of exercising both shoulders at the same time.

Persistent, regular sessions of these exercises are essential for success. We cannot say that "exercises don't help" unless you have adhered to a quality program for at least 6 months. Please keep a daily log of your exercise sessions so we can go over it when you return to the office.

In summary, the cornerstones of the rehabilitative program are to (1) avoid letting your shoulder pop out, (2) strengthen the rotator cuff muscles, (3) optimize the strength and endurance of the muscles that control your scapula, and (4) regain the technique and confidence in normal use of your shoulder. Remember that the shoulders of many athletes, such as gymnasts, are quite lax yet are stabilized by excellent muscle strength and learned techniques of neuromuscular control. Only exercises and training can reestablish proper use of your shoulder.

If you have any questions about your shoulder or our recommended treatment, please let us know.

Surgical Management of Atraumatic Instability

The ability of surgery alone to *cure* atraumatic instability is limited. Usually there is no single lesion that can be repaired. Most of the factors providing midrange stability cannot be enhanced by surgical reconstruction. Problems of poor neuromuscular control or relative glenoid flatness do not have surgical solutions. Even after a snug capsulorrhaphy, the midrange stabilizing mechanisms of balance and concavity compression must be optimized through muscle strengthening and kinematic training. Otherwise, excessive loads will be applied to the surgically tightened glenohumeral capsule, leading to stretching and failure of the surgical reconstruction.

In this light, the indications for surgical treatment of atraumatic instability need to be carefully considered. First, the patient must have major functional problems that are clearly related to atraumatic glenohumeral instability. Second, the patient must clearly understand that good strength and kinematic technique are the primary stabilizing factors for the shoulder rather than capsular tightness. Third, the patient must have participated in a strengthening and training program conscientiously and recognize that strength and proper technique will continue to be major stabilizing factors for the shoulder even after reconstructive surgery is performed. The patient must also recognize that capsulorrhaphy is designed to stiffen the shoulder; the surgery will compromise the range of motion in the hope of gaining stability. If attempts to regain normal range are made early, instability is likely to recur. Thus, the limitations imposed by surgical capsulorrhaphy may be incompatible with the goals of normal or supernormal range of motion. Therefore, gymnasts, dancers, and baseball pitchers may not be good candidates for this surgical procedure. Similarly, this procedure has a limited ability to hold up under the demands of heavy physical labor unless it is accompanied by a superb strength and kinematic rehabilitation program. Finally, the patient must understand that rehabilitation after this procedure is protracted. It is important that the shoulder be immobilized in a brace for a month, during which time muscles get weak and normal kinematics are lost. After this month of immobilization, many months are required for the re-establishment of good strength and shoulder kinematics. In spite of the best operative and postoperative management, the success of this procedure in reestablishing normal shoulder function is substantially less than that of procedures for traumatic instability.

The foregoing is a large amount of important information that must be understood by the patient considering the surgical procedure. The situation is further complicated by the fact that many patients who present with atraumatic midrange instability are young and may have difficulty understanding and accepting the ramifications of this information. Thus, during the preoperative discussions with young patients, it may be important that parents participate actively. We find that many families who present requesting that "the shoulder be fixed" are prepared to work more diligently on the non-operative program after this discussion. We provide the Patient Information Form 3–2 to patients and families interested in the surgical management of atraumatic multidirectional instability.

UNIVERSITY OF WASHINGTON SHOULDER AND ELBOW SERVICE

Surgery for Atraumatic Instability

Your shoulder has problems with instability even though you have not had a major traumatic injury. As a result, your shoulder slips or feels unstable with certain activities. Most often, atraumatic shoulder instability can be managed by restoring the normal strength and coordinated use of the shoulder through a reconditioning program. Rarely, the instability is so severe that surgery is considered as an adjunct to the exercise and training program. Shoulder surgery itself cannot "fix" the problem of atraumatic instability because there is no simple rip to sew up. Instead, the goal of shoulder surgery for this type of instability is to tighten the tissues around the shoulder joint, restricting its range of motion but also helping add some stability.

In this surgery, an incision is made in the skin and through the tendon of one of the shoulder muscles to gain access to the tissues surrounding the joint called the *capsule.* The operation takes some of the slack out of the capsule and then reattaches it to the bone. It also reconstructs a new stabilizing ligament for the shoulder joint. Like all surgeries, this operation carries some risk of infection, nerve injury, blood vessel injury, excessive tightness, persistent looseness and instability, pain, and the need for revision surgery. The recovery from surgery takes much longer than the recovery after a repair of the traumatic type of shoulder instability.

For a month after surgery, your shoulder will be immobilized in a brace at your side to allow for healing of the repaired capsule (Fig. 3–38). This brace complicates your hygiene and dressing—you will need some help with these activities. Following this period of immobilization, you must resume the program of shoulder strengthening and training that you worked on before surgery. Your shoulder must relearn how to function in stable positions. You must avoid efforts to regain full shoulder motion because this would defeat the purpose of the surgical procedure. It is essential that you avoid "testing" the shoulder to see if it is stable—you can defeat the operation if you work at stretching out the repair. Instead, all your

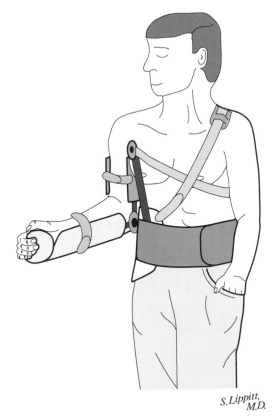

S. Lippitt, M.D.

FIGURE 3–38.

The neutral rotation brace used to immobilize the arm after a global capsular repair.

efforts must be directed toward relearning normal stable use of this joint and preventing stress on the repair. The postoperative program usually includes 1 month in the brace, during which time you carry out isometric strengthening exercises at regular intervals. The following exercises are simple:

1. External rotation isometrics: without moving your arm, push your wrist out against a fixed resistance (for example, your other hand). Hold for a count of ten. Repeat 100 times per day.
2. Abduction isometrics: without moving your arm, push your elbow out against a fixed resistance (for example, the wall). Hold for a count of ten. Repeat 100 times per day.

The next 2 months are directed at enhancing the strength of the shoulder and increasing its usage in stable positions. Again, do not test the stability of your shoulder by trying any motion that may challenge its stability.

You will not be able to lift more than 10 pounds with this shoulder for the first 6 months. You will continue to perform your isometric exercises and to use the shoulder for activities that do not challenge its stability.

At 6 months after surgery and after your shoulder has gained strength, endurance, and normal patterns of use, you can start activities such as gentle swimming. You will not be able to participate in sports until at least 1 year after this operation, and then only if you have excellent strength and dynamic control of your shoulder.

In summary, surgery for atraumatic instability cannot "fix" your shoulder. Rather, it is an operation that can help your shoulder regain stability if you couple the operation with sincere efforts to optimize your shoulder's dynamic stability after surgery. Your partnership and compliance with the postoperative management program are at least as important as the operation itself.

It is our hope that you will take time to consider this information in great detail before deciding to proceed with a surgical reconstruction. The operation is a purely elective procedure. We want to answer all of your questions concerning your shoulder problem, the alternatives in its management, and the possible risks and benefits of the surgical treatment. We need you to become an active member of the team.

Surgical Technique

The essential elements of the procedure are reconstruction of the rotator interval capsule–coracohumeral ligament mechanism and reduction of the posteroinferior capsular recess (Fig. 3–39). These goals can only be accomplished through an anterior surgical approach. Thus, we routinely approach a repair for atraumatic instability from the front, even if the predominant direction of instability appears to be posterior. There are additional advantages of the anterior approach: It is cosmetically superior to the posterior approach, and it is accomplished without incising the critical external rotator cuff musculature. Finally, when the capsule is advanced anterosuperiorly on the humeral side, elevation of the arm anteriorly results in additional tightening of the inferior and posterior capsule.

The shoulder is approached through a low anterior axillary incision, entering the deltopectoral groove medial to the cephalic vein. The clavipectoral fascia is divided up to the level of the coracoacromial ligament. The axillary nerve is palpated medially as it courses across the subscapularis and passes inferiorly toward the quadrangular space. The superior edge of the subscapularis is then identified by palpating the rotator interval lateral to the coracoid process and medial to the bicipital groove. The triad of an-

terior humeral circumflex vessels marks the inferior border of the subscapularis. The subscapularis tendon is sharply and carefully dissected from the subjacent capsule.

A substantial defect in the rotator interval is seen consistently in the AMBRII syndrome. This defect is bordered by the capsule adjacent to the supraspinatus overlying the biceps tendon superiorly, the anterior capsule and subscapularis anteroinferiorly, the coracoid process, and the transverse humeral ligament. This defect is accentuated by pushing the humeral head posteriorly. Sutures of No. 2 non-absorbable material are securely placed in the superior edge of the defect and then passed across to the inferior edge of the defect (Fig. 3–40). When these sutures are tied, a strong rotator interval capsule is reconstructed.

The anterior capsule is incised from the humeral neck beginning just below the top of the lesser tuberosity. Traction sutures are placed in the capsule. With the axillary nerve protected and with the arm in adduction and neutral rotation, the anteroinferior and the inferior capsule are incised from the humeral neck. This dissection is continued until superiorly directed traction on the capsular flap causes the capsule to tighten on a finger placed in the posteroinferior capsular recess (Fig. 3–41). Usually this point is reached when the capsule is released just past the inferior (6 o'clock) position on the

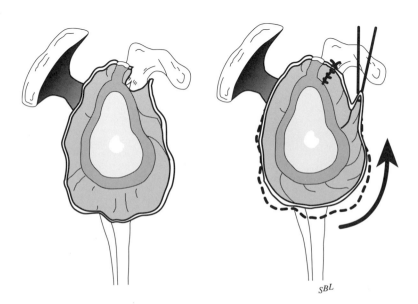

FIGURE 3–39.

The essence of the capsular reconstruction for atraumatic instability is the reduction of the posteroinferior recess by anterosuperior advancement of the capsule combined with closure of the rotator interval capsule. This reconstruction has the advantage of becoming additionally tight as the arm is elevated in anterior planes, where common functions are carried out.

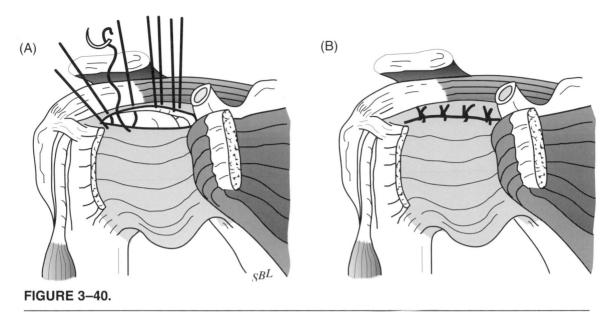

FIGURE 3–40.

Identification of the superior edge of the rotator interval defect and placement of sutures, taking care to protect the long head tendon of the biceps *(A)*. When these sutures are tied, they securely reconstruct the coracohumeral–rotator interval capsular mechanism *(B)*.

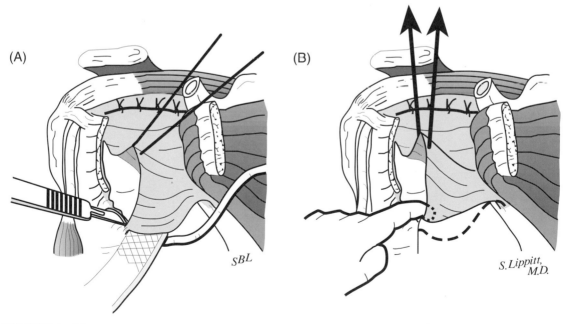

FIGURE 3–41.

Release of the capsule from the humeral neck laterally. This dissection is carried beyond the inferior (6 o'clock) position *(A)* until traction on the anterior capsular flap reduces the posteroinferior recess *(B)*.

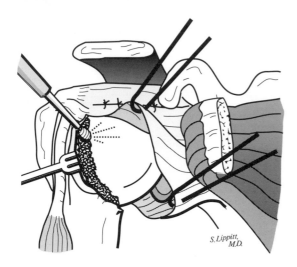

FIGURE 3–42.

Preparation of the humeral neck with a groove at the margin of the articular surface.

FIGURE 3–43.

Sutures are placed through drill holes so that they exit the groove and pass through the advanced capsule and then back out through adjacent drill holes.

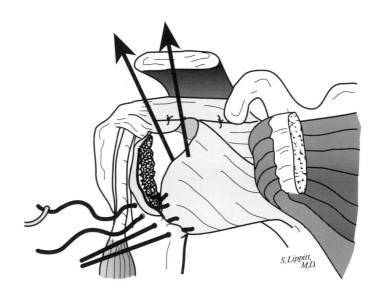

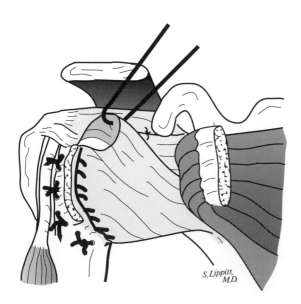

FIGURE 3–44.

Tying the sutures fixes the advanced capsule to the groove.

humeral neck, sectioning the posterior band of the inferior glenohumeral ligament.

After the capsular release, a bony trough is created in the anteroinferior humeral neck adjacent to the articular surface using a power burr (Fig. 3–42). Holes are made in the humeral neck lateral to the groove, and sutures are passed through these holes into the groove for reattachment of the capsule securely to bone. With the arm at the side and in neutral rotation and with strong anterior superior traction on the sutures to obliterate the posterior inferior recess, the sutures from the groove are passed through the lateral edge of the capsule (Fig. 3–43). Tying these sutures securely fixes the capsule in its advanced position (Fig. 3–44). This step needs to be accomplished with excellent direct vision to be sure the bites in the capsule are sufficiently inferior to tighten it to the groove and to ensure the safety of the axillary nerve. The surgeon must ensure that pulling up on these sutures obliterates the posteroinferior recess. If this is not the case, either the inferior capsular release was insufficient or the sutures were not placed sufficiently inferior.

This repair to the groove is continued anteriorly up the humeral neck.

Redundant anterosuperior capsule is folded down over the previous repair to reinforce it (Fig. 3–45). At this point, the shoulder is checked to ensure that internal rotation of the abducted arm is limited to 45 degrees below the horizontal, that the posterior drawer is less than 50 percent of the humeral head diameter, and that external rotation of the arm at the side is 30 degrees. Excessive internal rotation of the abducted arm indicates the inferior capsule was not advanced sufficiently. Excessive translation on the posterior drawer test indicates that the posterior capsule was insufficiently tightened. Excessive limitation of external rotation indicates that the anterior capsule was tightened too much.

The subscapularis is then repaired to its normal anatomic insertion. After a standard wound closure, the arm is placed in a prefitted "handshake" orthosis with the arm in

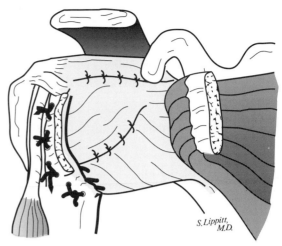

FIGURE 3–45.

Any redundant anterosuperior capsule is folded down to reinforce the previous repair.

neutral rotation and slight abduction (see Fig. 3–38).

Postoperative Rehabilitation

With the arm in the orthosis, the patient is started on grip strengthening, elbow range of motion, isometric external rotation, and isometric abduction shoulder exercises. The brace is usually continued for 1 month, although longer periods may be used for people who are extremely lax, and shorter periods may be used for people older than 25 years of age who may be prone to excessive stiffness.

The patient is then weaned from the orthosis over a period of a week. During this time the patient is taught to elevate the arm in the coronal plane only, to continue the cuff and deltoid strengthening, and to avoid any activities that may challenge the repair. From this point, range of motion is gained only with active exercises; no passive stretching is used. Lifting of more than 10 pounds is delayed for 6 months. Sports are delayed for at least 1 year after surgery and are permitted only if the patient has excellent strength and dynamic control of the shoulder (see Patient Information Form 3–3).

PATIENT INFORMATION 3–3

UNIVERSITY OF WASHINGTON SHOULDER AND ELBOW SERVICE

Rehabilitation After Surgery for Atraumatic Instability

You have had a major reconstruction for instability of your shoulder. You now have the responsibility for taking care of your repair and for the progressive rehabilitation of your shoulder.

Your arm is now in a brace to ensure that it heals properly. If this brace is not comfortable, be sure to let us know immediately.

For 1 month after the operation, your arm must stay in the brace. If someone can hold your arm in the correct position for you during bathing, you may briefly remove the brace for this purpose. Otherwise, you should clean yourself twice a day using an alcohol sponge underneath the straps of the brace. You can put on a shirt if someone can help you by keeping your arm in the correct position while your arm is threaded through the sleeve. Otherwise you should wear loose-fitting clothes over the brace.

Each day you can loosen the forearm straps to put your elbow through a range of motion.

You need to start exercises in your brace right away. First, you need to maintain the strength of your grip by squeezing a ball, sponge, or putty several hundred times a day. Second, you should perform 3 minutes of gentle isometric exercises at least three times a day against some fixed object—pushing your wrist outward, pushing your hand forward, pushing your elbow outward, and pushing the elbow back. These exercises are designed to maintain your muscle tone. The shoulder is not moved during these exercises. They should be comfortable.

You should return to the office 1 month after surgery. If everything is healing properly, you may begin weaning yourself from the brace at that time.

In the weaning process, you will start moving your shoulder out to the side, avoiding the positions that used to be symptomatic for you. You may find it reassuring to sleep in your brace for another week. You will regain your motion on your own, moving your shoulder under its own motor power and specifically avoiding any stretching. You need to continue your previous isometric exercises and can add internal and external rotation strengthening against rubber tubing.

You then progress by using your arm for light activities of daily living, avoiding the positions that used to be unstable. Always avoid "checking" your shoulder to see if it is stable. You must not lift more than 10 pounds for the first 6 months after your surgery.

After 4 months, you can begin gentle, well-controlled, repetitive activities with your shoulder, such as swimming and using a rowing machine, provided that these activities are comfortable for you.

You cannot return to contact sports or heavy work for at least a year after this surgery, and then only if you have excellent strength and coordinated control of your shoulder.

We hope that this provides you with the information you need to successfully rehabilitate your shoulder. If you have any questions at any time, please let us know.

TRAUMATIC INSTABILITY

Traumatic instability is instability that arises from an injury of sufficient magnitude to tear the glenohumeral capsule, ligaments, or rotator cuff or to produce a fracture of the humerus or glenoid. To injure these strong structures, a substantial force must be applied to them. The most common pathologic condition associated with traumatic instability is the avulsion of the anteroinferior capsule and ligaments from the glenoid rim. Substantial force is required to produce this avulsion in a healthy shoulder. Although this load may be applied directly (for example, by having the proximal humerus hit from behind), an indirect loading mechanism is more common. Indirect loading is most easily understood in terms of a simple model of the torques involved. When the upper extremity is abducted and externally rotated by a force applied to the hand, the following equation for torque equilibrium is a useful approximation, *if* we attribute the major stabilizing role to the ligament:

$$I \times R = F \times A$$

or equivalently

$$I = F \times A/R$$

where I is the tension in the inferior glenohumeral ligament, R is the radius of the humeral head, F is the abduction external rotation load applied to the hand, and A is the distance from the center of the humeral head to the hand (Fig. 3–46). If the radius of the humeral head is 2.5 cm and the distance from the head center to the hand is 1 m, this formula suggests that the inferior glenohumeral ligament would experience a load 40 times greater than that applied to the hand. From this example we can see that a much lesser load is required to produce the characteristic lesion of traumatic instability if this load is applied indirectly through the lever arm of the upper extremity.

Avulsion of the anterior glenohumeral ligament mechanism (Fig. 3–47) deprives the joint of stability in positions where this structure is a major stabilizer of the joint, which is typically approaching maximal external rotation and extension of the arm elevated near the coronal plane. These are positions in which stability is dependent on integrity of the capsuloligamentous mechanism. Thus, it is evident that in recurrent traumatic instability, problems are most likely to occur when the arm is placed in a position approximating that in which the original injury occurred. Midrange instability may also result from a traumatic injury if the glenoid concavity is compromised by avulsion of the labrum or fracture of the bony lip of the glenoid. Lessening of the effective glenoid depth compromises the effectiveness of concavity compression, reduces the angles through which the glenoid can balance the net humeral joint reaction

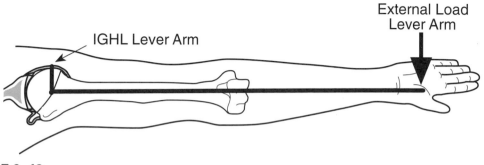

FIGURE 3–46.

In the absence of muscular forces, an external load applied to the hand must be resisted by a force 40 times greater in the anterior band of the inferior glenohumeral ligament (IGHL), as a result of the great difference between the moment arm of the external load (approximately equal to the length of the arm) as compared with the moment arm of the inferior glenohumeral ligament (approximately equal to the radius of the humeral head).

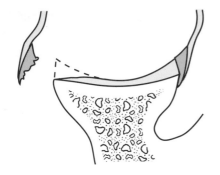

FIGURE 3–47.

Avulsion of the glenoid labrum without or with the anterior lip of the glenoid reduces the size and the depth of the glenoid concavity and also compromises the attachment of the inferior glenohumeral ligament.

force, reduces the surface available for adhesion-cohesion, and compromises the ability of the glenoid suction cup to conform to the head of the humerus.

The corner of the glenoid abuts against the insertion of the cuff to the tuberosity when the humerus is extended, abducted, and externally rotated (Fig. 3–48). Thus, the same forces involved in challenging the strength of the inferior glenohumeral ligament are also applied to the greater tuberosity–cuff insertion area. It is not surprising, therefore, that tuberosity fractures and cuff injuries may be a part of the clinical picture of traumatic instability. The exact location and type of traumatic injury depend on the age of the patient and the magnitude, rate, and

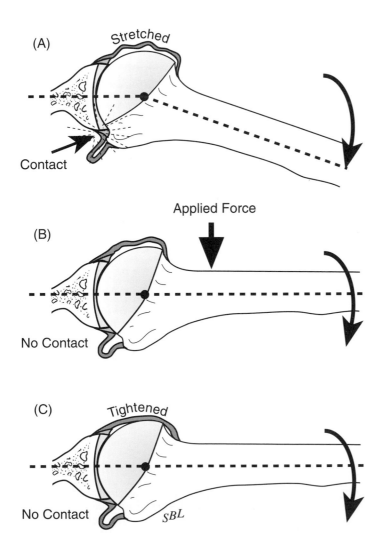

FIGURE 3–48.

Posterior contact between the glenoid lip and the insertion of the cuff to the tuberosity occurs in the "apprehension," or fulcrum, position, especially if the anteroinferior capsule has been stretched, allowing the humerus to extend to an unusually posterior scapular plane. This contact can challenge the integrity of the posterior cuff insertion and the tuberosity *(A)*. Applying a posteriorly directed force on the front of the shoulder may change the humeroscapular position enough to relieve this posterior abutment. This maneuver is similar to that of the "relocation test"; however, this analysis suggests that the mechanism for relief of discomfort is the avoidance of posterior abutment rather than the elimination of subluxation *(B)*. A similar protection from posterior abutment may be achieved by tightening the anterior capsule, preventing the extension of the humerus to a substantially posterior scapular plane *(C)*.

direction of force applied. Avulsions of the glenoid labrum and glenoid rim fractures are more commonly seen in young persons after a major injury. In patients older than 35 years of age, traumatic instability tends to be associated with fractures of the greater tuberosity and rotator cuff tears. This tendency increases with increasing age at the time of the initial traumatic dislocation. Thus, as a rule, younger patients require management of anterior lesions, and older patients require management of posterior lesions.

The posterior lateral humeral head defect is a common feature of traumatic instability. These lesions are often noted after the first traumatic dislocation and tend to increase in size with recurrent episodes. This impaction injury occurs when the anterior corner of the glenoid is driven into the posterior lateral humeral articular surface. It is evident that this injury is close to the cuff insertion. Large head defects compromise stability by diminishing the articular congruity of the humerus.

We refer to the usual type of traumatic instability as the *TUBS syndrome* because it arises from a significant episode of *trauma*, characteristically from abduction and extension of the arm elevated in the coronal plane. The resulting instability is usually *unidirectional* in the anteroinferior direction. The pathologic condition is usually an avulsion of the capsuloligamentous complex from the anteroinferior lip of the glenoid, commonly referred to as a *Bankart* lesion. With functionally significant recurrent trau-

matic instability, a *surgical* repair of this ligament avulsion is frequently required to restore function.

History

The Initial Episode of Instability

Traumatic instability commonly begins with an injury when the patient is between 14 and 34 years of age (Fig. 3–49). In suspected recurrent instability from a traumatic cause, the most important element in the history is the definition of the original injury. As is evident to anyone who has attempted to re-create these lesions in a cadaver, substantial force is required to produce a traumatic dislocation. In characteristic anterior traumatic instability, the structure that is avulsed is the strongest part of the shoulder's capsular mechanism: the anteroinferior glenohumeral ligament. To tear this ligament, substantial force needs to be applied to the shoulder when the arm is in a position to tighten this ligament. Thus, the usual mechanism of injury involves the application of a large extension–external rotation force to the arm elevated near the coronal plane. Such a mechanism may occur in a fall during snow skiing or execution of a high-speed cut in water skiing, in an arm tackle during football, with a block of a volleyball or basketball shot, or in relatively violent industrial accidents with the arm in this position. Awkward lifting and rear-end automobile accidents would not be expected

FIGURE 3–49.

Age distribution of 32 patients with traumatic instability.

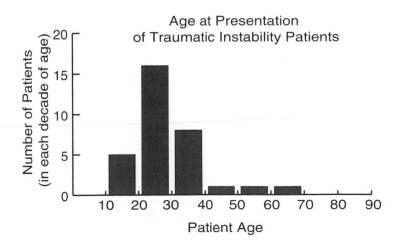

to provide the conditions or mechanism for this injury. We find that direct questioning and persistence are often required to elicit a full description of the initial mechanism of injury, including the position of the shoulder and the direction and magnitude of the applied force at the time of the initial injury, yet this information is critical to establishing the diagnosis.

An initial traumatic dislocation often requires assistance in reduction rather than reducing spontaneously as is usually the case in atraumatic instability. Radiographs from previous emergency department visits may be available to show the shoulder in its dislocated position. Axillary or other neuropathy may have accompanied the glenohumeral dislocation. Any of these findings, individually or in combination, support the diagnosis of traumatic as opposed to atraumatic instability.

Traumatic instability may occur without a complete dislocation. In this situation, the injury produces a traumatic lesion, but this lesion is insufficient to allow the humeral head to completely escape from the glenoid. The shoulder may be unstable because, as a result of the injury, it manifests apprehension or subluxation when the arm is placed near the position of injury. In these instances, there is no history of the need for reduction or radiographs with the shoulder in the dislocated position. Thus, the diagnosis rests to an even greater extent on a careful history that focuses on the position and forces involved in the initial episode.

Subsequent Episodes of Instability

Characteristically, the shoulder with traumatic instability is comfortable when troublesome positions are avoided. However, the shoulder often remains vulnerable to recurrent episodes of instability. These may range from sensations of apprehension or impending dislocation to recurrent complete dislocations requiring manipulative reduction. In this context, recurrent episodes of instability occur most commonly when the shoulder is forced unexpectedly into the abducted, externally rotated position or during sleep when the patient's active guard is less effective. There may be a history of increasing ease of dislocation. We determine whether the patient is reluctant to carry out certain activities or to put the arm in certain positions because of fear of instability. This apprehension may interfere with the patient's ability to use the arm for work, activities of daily living, or sports.

The history must seek to demonstrate the position and forces involved in the initial and subsequent episodes of instability. The examiner must be convinced that these are appropriate and sufficient to tear the normally strong capsuloligamentous structures that stabilize the shoulder at the extremes of motion. This careful history is the foundation on which the diagnosis of traumatic instability rests.

Functional Evaluation

The results from the Simple Shoulder Test evaluations of patients with traumatic anterior glenohumeral instability are shown in Figure 3–50. The most consistent functional impairment was the inability to throw overhand, but many patients also had problems sleeping, putting their hand behind their head, and lifting a filled gallon container to head level.

Physical Examination

The goal of the physical examination is largely to confirm the impression obtained from the history: that a certain combination of arm position and force application produces the actual or threatened glenohumeral instability that is of functional concern to the patient. If the diagnosis has been rigorously established from the history, such as by documented recurrent anterior dislocations, it is not necessary to risk redislocation on the physical examination. If such rigorous documentation is not available, however, we must challenge the ligamentous stability of the shoulder in the suspected position of vulnerability. We seek to have the patient identify the positions and events that are of functional significance.

The most common direction of recurrent traumatic instability is anteroinferior. Stability in this position is challenged by exter-

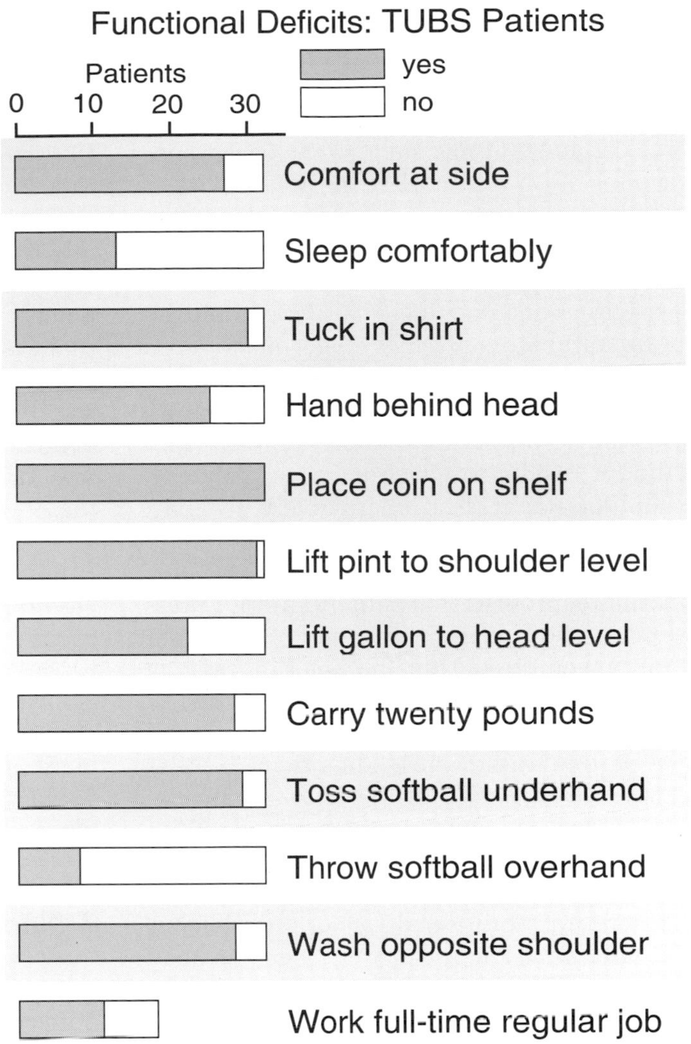

Functional Deficits: TUBS Patients

Patients — yes / no

Comfort at side

Sleep comfortably

Tuck in shirt

Hand behind head

Place coin on shelf

Lift pint to shoulder level

Lift gallon to head level

Carry twenty pounds

Toss softball underhand

Throw softball overhand

Wash opposite shoulder

Work full-time regular job

FIGURE 3–50.

Simple Shoulder Test results from 32 patients presenting with traumatic instability.

nally rotating and extending the arm elevated in the coronal plane. This is conveniently done in the supine position with one of the examiner's hands under the back of the shoulder serving as a fulcrum for the external rotation and extension force. We apply extension and external rotation loads in different positions of elevation to challenge the various parts of the anterior capsular mechanism. The patient often guards against the position of instability by actively limiting the range of humeroscapular motion. For this reason, we may need to hold the arm in the challenging position for 1 or 2 minutes to fatigue the stabilizing muscu-

lature. When the muscle stabilizers tire, the capsuloligamentous mechanism is all that is holding the humeral head in the glenoid. At this moment the patient with traumatic anterior instability becomes apprehensive, recognizing that the shoulder is about to come out of joint. This recognition is strongly supportive of the diagnosis of traumatic anterior instability.

Standard tests of glenohumeral laxity are of limited value in the diagnosis of traumatic instability. As described earlier, the *magnitude* of translation on the standard tests of glenohumeral laxity does not distinguish stable from unstable shoulders. The magnitude of translation on some clinically stable shoulders may be as great or greater than that on shoulders with traumatic instability. However, the experienced examiner may detect certain findings such as increased *ease* of translation on the anterior drawer test or grinding as the humeral head slides over a bony edge of the glenoid from which the labrum has been avulsed. There may also be a catching or a locking of a torn glenoid labrum, producing findings analogous to those of a torn meniscus in the knee.

We do not consider pain on abduction, external rotation, and extension to be specific for instability. Such pain may relate to shoulder stiffness or, alternatively, to abutment of the glenoid against the cuff insertion to the head posteriorly (see Fig. 3–48). Furthermore, relief of this pain by anterior pressure on the humeral head may result from diminished stretch on the anterior capsule or from relief of the abutment posteriorly.

In all patients with traumatic instability, but particularly in those older than 35 years of age, the strength of the internal and external rotation must be examined. With increasing age, there is an increasingly common association between traumatic glenohumeral instability and rotator cuff defects. Patients with significant cuff lesions may demonstrate atrophy of the spinatus muscles as well as pain and/or weakness on resisted abduction or external rotation. Any rotator cuff pathologic changes must be recognized and incorporated in the treatment plan.

Finally, the brachial plexus is carefully examined to ensure that the episodes of traumatic instability have not compromised its function.

Radiographs

Radiographs frequently help to provide confirmation of traumatic glenohumeral instability. The findings may include an indentation or impaction in the posterior aspect of the humeral head from contact with the anteroinferior corner of the glenoid when the joint is dislocated. Radiographs may also reveal a periosteal reaction to the ligamentous avulsion at the glenoid lip or, occasionally, a fracture of the glenoid rim.

These lesions are usually revealed by an anteroposterior view in the plane of the scapula and a proper axillary view. We have not found additional radiographic views, CT, arthrography, or MRI to be cost effective in the evaluation of shoulders with characteristic traumatic instability. We occasionally use CT to define the magnitude of bone loss when sizable humeral head or glenoid defects have been identified on a series of plain radiographs.

In a patient whose onset of traumatic instability occurred after age 35, there may be evidence on history and physical examination of rotator cuff pathologic changes. In these situations, preoperative imaging of cuff integrity may play an important role in surgical planning: The approach for rotator cuff repair is quite different from the approach for the repair of an anteroinferior capsular lesion.

Electromyography may be helpful in the evaluation of the patient with recurrent traumatic instability if the history and physical examination suggest residual brachial plexus lesions.

Treatment

A patient with traumatic anterior glenohumeral instability has symptoms of instability (apprehension, subluxation, or dislocation) when the arm is elevated near the coronal plane, extended, and externally rotated. Characteristically, the shoulder is relatively asymptomatic in other extreme positions or in midrange positions. Thus, for some patients appropriate management may consist solely of education about the nature of the lesion and identification of the positions and activities that need to be avoided. Strengthening the shoulder musculature may help prevent the shoulder from being forced into positions of instability. The exercise program suggested for atraumatic instability may be considered as an option for traumatic instability as well. "Training tape" may be applied to the anterior aspect of the shoulder as a reminder to avoid abduction, external rotation, and extension of the shoulder.

We consider surgical treatment for informed patients who are unwilling to accept the functional limitations imposed by recurrent traumatic instability.

Surgical Management of Traumatic Anterior Glenohumeral Instability

This section on surgical treatment concerns the management only of patients who have traumatic anteroinferior glenohumeral instability that has been established preoperatively by careful history and physical examination. The indications for surgical treatment of this lesion are persistent significant functional deficits (apprehension, subluxation, dislocation) in abduction, external rotation, and extension resulting from an initial episode that was sufficiently traumatic to tear part of the major capsuloligamentous supporting structures of the glenohumeral joint. For patients not meeting these strict criteria, we use the methods for treatment of atraumatic instability presented previously.

The goals of treating traumatic anteroinferior glenohumeral instability are to repair the traumatic lesion safely, restoring the attachment of the glenohumeral ligaments, capsule, and labrum to the rim of the glenoid. By ensuring that reattachment occurs to the rim, the effective depth of the glenoid is restored. By definition, these patients do not have a functional problem with capsular laxity; thus, capsular reefing is not a part of this procedure.

Preoperative patient education includes the information provided in Patient Information 3–4.

Surgical Technique

The goal of the surgical treatment of traumatic anterior glenohumeral instability is the safe and secure reattachment of the detached glenohumeral ligaments to the lip of the glenoid from which they were avulsed (see Figs. 3–18 and 3–51). No attempt is made to modify the normal laxity of the anterior capsule. This anatomic reattachment should reestablish not only the capsuloliga-

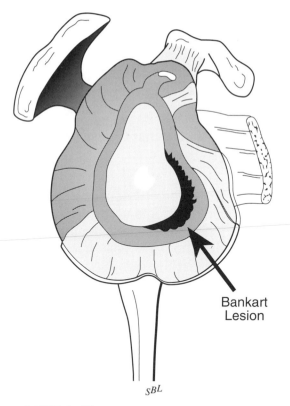

Bankart Lesion

FIGURE 3–51.

The capsulolabral detachment typical of traumatic instability.

mentous checkrein but also the fossa-deepening effect of the glenoid labrum. A repair that is secure from the time of surgery is highly desirable in that it allows patients to resume many of their activities of daily living while the repair is healing. A repair that is secure from the time of surgery also allows controlled mobilization, thereby minimizing the possibility of unwanted stiffness.

We approach the shoulder through the dominant anterior axillary crease to facilitate a cosmetically acceptable scar. The deltopectoral groove is entered, retracting the cephalic vein laterally with the deltoid. The clavipectoral fascia is incised just lateral to the short head of the biceps, up to but not through the coracoacromial ligament. We routinely palpate the axillary nerve as it crosses the anteroinferior border of the subscapularis. The anterior humeral circumflex vessels can usually be protected by bluntly dissecting them off the subscapularis muscle

UNIVERSITY OF WASHINGTON SHOULDER AND ELBOW SERVICE

Traumatic Anteroinferior Glenohumeral Instability

When a major force is applied to the arm, the supporting ligaments of the shoulder joint may be torn. Sometimes these ligaments heal spontaneously in the proper location so that the stability of the shoulder is regained. On other occasions, strong healing to the appropriate location does not occur, leaving the shoulder unstable when it is put in certain specific positions. We refer to this as *traumatic instability of the shoulder.* These injuries most commonly arise from situations in which the elevated arm is forced violently backward, such as in a fall while skiing. If this is your situation, you may elect to avoid the positions in which the shoulder feels unstable, recognizing that this may require giving up certain activities. Alternatively, you may seek a surgical repair of the torn structures with a goal to regain some of the functional abilities you lost.

The ligaments are almost always torn from the front bottom part of the socket of the shoulder. We can often repair this injury by sewing the ligaments back to the bone from which they were torn. We make an incision in the lower front skin crease of the shoulder and gain access to the joint between two of its major muscles: the deltoid and the pectoralis major. The ligaments are reattached by roughening up the edge of the bony socket and placing small drill holes in the lip of this socket. Sutures are passed through these drill holes and through the ligaments so that when the sutures are tied the ligaments are held in the appropriate place for healing.

For 3 to 4 weeks after the surgery, you must protect your shoulder from elevation above the horizontal and from rotation away from the body. You will need to carry out isometric strengthening exercises, which are done with your arm in a sling. After this first period of protection, you will be given gentle range of motion and additional strengthening exercises.

During the second 6 weeks, we will emphasize shoulder range of motion, strength, endurance, and coordination. Usually, patients can resume rigorous physical activities 3 months after the operation, provided they have regained excellent strength, coordination, endurance, and a near-normal range of motion of the shoulder.

The risks of this surgery include but are not confined to infection, injury to nerves and blood vessels around the shoulder, unwanted shoulder stiffness, persistent instability of the shoulder, pain, complications of anesthesia, and the need for revision surgery.

If you have questions about your shoulder problem or the alternatives in its treatment, you are invited to ask us at any time.

at its inferior border. The subscapularis tendon and the subjacent capsule are incised 5 mm medial to their insertion at the lesser tuberosity. This incision starts superiorly at the upper rolled edge of the subscapularis and extends inferiorly to the bottom of the lesser tuberosity. It is important that the incision through the subscapularis tendon leaves strong tendinous material on both sides of the incision to facilitate a secure repair at the conclusion of the procedure. We examine the joint for loose bodies, for displaced fragments of glenoid labrum, and, particularly in older patients, for evidence of rotator cuff tears. We can usually palpate a posterior lateral humeral head defect. The capsule and subscapularis are then retracted medially as a unit, and a humeral head retractor is placed in the joint. An angled retractor is used to expose the glenoid lip and to identify the capsuloligamentous avulsion. Occasionally, flimsy attempts to heal the lesion temporarily obliterate the defect. However, in these instances, a blunt elevator easily reveals the typical lesion in the anteroinferior quadrant of the glenoid. A spiked retractor is then placed through the ligamentous avulsion to expose the glenoid lip.

We roughen the anterior, non-articular aspect of the glenoid lip with a curette or a motorized burr, taking care not to compromise the bony strength of the glenoid lip

(Fig. 3–52). We then place holes on the articular aspect of the glenoid 3 to 4 mm back from the edge of the lip to ensure a sufficiently strong bony bridge. We place these holes 5 to 6 mm apart; thus, the size of the defect dictates the number of holes used for reattachment of the avulsed capsule. Corresponding slots are placed on the anterior non-articular aspect of the glenoid. Using a 000 angled curette, we establish continuity between the corresponding slots and holes (Fig. 3–53).

We then pass a strong No. 2 nonabsorbable braided suture through the holes in the glenoid lip using a trocar needle and an angled needle holder. After each suture is placed through the glenoid lip, the integrity of the bony bridge is checked by a firm pull on the suture.

The spiked retractor is then removed from the lesion, and an angled retractor is used to expose the trailing medial edge of the avulsed capsule. Next, using the trocar needle, we pass the end of the suture, exiting the anterior non-articular aspect of the glenoid lip through the trailing medial edge of the capsule, taking care to include the glenoid labrum, if present, and the strong medial edge of the capsule (Fig. 3–54). We avoid including any more capsule than necessary to obtain a firm purchase; this prevents unwanted tightening of the anteroinferior capsule. In larger glenohumeral

FIGURE 3–52.

Roughening of the anterior, non-articular surface of the glenoid using a pine cone burr. The capsule and subscapularis are retracted medially with a sharp-tipped retractor. The humeral head is retracted laterally with a humeral head retractor.

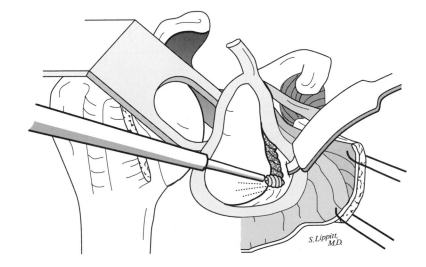

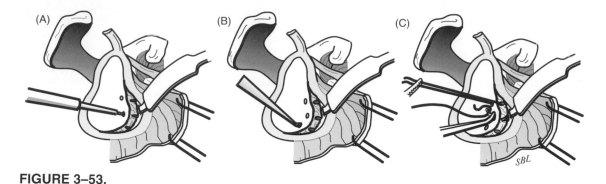

FIGURE 3–53.

Drill holes are made in the lip of the articular surface of the glenoid 4 mm from the edge and 6 mm apart *(A)*. These drill holes are completed to the anterior aspect of the glenoid using a 000 angled curette *(B)*; a non-absorbable suture is then passed through the drill holes *(C)*.

ligament avulsions, the detached medial edge of the capsule tends to sag inferiorly; thus, in these larger lesions, an effort needs to be made to pass the needle through the capsule slightly inferior to the bony holes in the glenoid. At the time of closure, the inferiorly sagging medial capsule will be repositioned anatomically.

Once the sutures have been passed through the capsule, they are tied so that the labrum and medial edge of the capsule are positioned on the glenoid lip. The knots are tied so that they come to rest over the capsule rather than on the articular surface of the glenoid (Fig. 3–55).

Once these sutures are tied, the smooth continuity between the articular surface of the glenoid fossa and the capsule should be reestablished. No stepoff, or discontinuity, in the capsule should be present. If such a

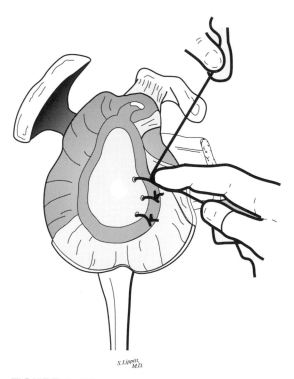

FIGURE 3–55.

Tying the suture over the capsule securely reapproximates the detached tissues to the roughened glenoid edge, restoring the fossa-deepening effect of the capsule and labrum.

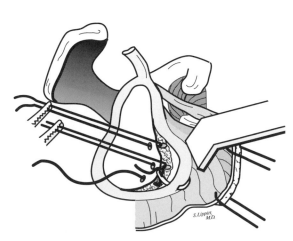

FIGURE 3–54.

The sutures (shown in Fig. 3–53) are then passed through the trailing medial edge of the capsule and the labrum.

discontinuity is noted, the sutures are replaced so that they obliterate the defect.

At the conclusion of the surgical repair the capsule and subscapularis tendon are repaired anatomically to their mates at the lesser tuberosity. The shoulder should have at least 30 degrees of external rotation at the side after the subscapularis-capsular repair. A standard wound closure is carried out, using a subcuticular suture, which is removed 3 days later.

Within the first few days after surgery, reliable patients are encouraged to use the arm up to 90 degrees of elevation in the anterior plane and out to zero degrees of external rotation. This allows sufficient range of motion to perform most activities of daily living, such as eating and personal hygiene, as well as certain vocational activities, such as writing and typing. Gripping, isometric external rotation, and isometric abduction exercises are started immediately after surgery to minimize the effects of disuse. If a patient does not appear able to comply with this restricted-use program, we require that the arm be kept in a sling for 3 weeks.

At 3 weeks the patient should return for an examination and should have at least 90 degrees of elevation and external rotation to zero degrees. From 3 to 6 weeks postoperatively, the patient is instructed to increase the range of motion to 140 degrees of elevation and 40 degrees of external rotation. At 6 weeks after surgery, if there is good evidence of active control of the shoulder, gentle repetitive activities such as swimming and using a rowing machine may be instituted to help with coordination, strength, and endurance of the shoulder. More vigorous activities, such as basketball, volleyball, throwing, and serving in tennis, should not be started until 3 months and then only if there is excellent strength, endurance, range of motion, and coordination of the shoulder.

Patients are usually able to conduct their own postoperative rehabilitation program with instructions from a physical therapist or a physician. These instructions are included in the Patient Information 3–5.

Vigilance must be exercised for patients older than 35 years of age to be sure that they do not develop unwanted postoperative stiffness. Thus, particularly for these pa-

tients, the 3-week and 6-week checks are important to make sure that the ranges of elevation and external rotation are, respectively, 90 and zero degrees at 3 weeks and 140 and 40 degrees at 6 weeks.

This section has described the pathologic changes, diagnosis, and management of shoulders with traumatic instability. This diagnosis is made predominately on the basis of the history of the initial and subsequent episodes of instability and is corroborated by the physical examination and often by bony changes on plain radiographs. The goal of the surgical repair is to restore anatomically the continuity of the capsuloligamentous and labral complex with the cartilage of the glenoid fossa and to avoid limitation in range of motion from unnecessary capsular tightening. It is also important that the surgical repair be sufficiently strong that early protected use of the shoulder can be instituted while the tissues are held in secure anatomic position to the bone of the glenoid. With this approach, more complicated and complication-prone procedures such as capsular tightening, coracoid osteotomy, coracoid transfer, metal fixation, bone blocks, and osteotomies can be avoided. It is to be reemphasized that satisfactory treatment of this entity depends on a precise diagnosis, which is established by the history and physical examination prior to the patient's arrival in the operating room.

Intermediate Types of Recurrent Instability

The AMBRII and TUBS syndromes represent clearly defined clinical pathologic entities, each of which has specific diagnostic features and treatment strategies. Together, they constitute the great majority of patients who present with glenohumeral instability. Patients who do not fit into one of these two categories have highly individualized problems and cannot be grouped effectively together. In evaluating these patients, a meticulous history and physical examination assume even greater importance. When there has been an initiating injury, it is essential to determine the position of the arm and the direction and magnitude of the force

UNIVERSITY OF WASHINGTON SHOULDER AND ELBOW SERVICE

Rehabilitation After Surgery for Traumatic Instability

You have had a repair for instability of your shoulder. You now have the responsibility for taking care of your repair and for the progressive rehabilitation of your shoulder.

Your arm is now in a sling to ensure that it heals properly. If this sling is not comfortable, be sure to let us know immediately.

You may remove your arm from the sling to perform your exercises. These include lying down on your back and lifting your arm so that the elbow points straight up. In the second exercise, also performed lying on your back, you rotate your forearm away from your stomach until it points straight ahead.

You need to start exercises in your sling right away. First, you need to maintain the strength of your grip by squeezing a ball, sponge, or putty several hundred times a day. Second, you should perform 3 minutes of gentle isometric exercises at least three times a day against some fixed object—pushing your wrist outward, pushing your hand forward, pushing your elbow outward, and pushing the elbow back. These exercises are designed to maintain your muscle tone. The shoulder is not moved during these exercises. They should be comfortable.

You will return to the office 3 weeks after surgery. If everything is healing properly, you will begin weaning yourself from the sling at that time.

At 3 weeks after surgery, you can increase your overhead reach until your arm is close to your ear and until your forearm can be externally rotated 40 degrees from the straight-ahead position. You need to continue your previous isometric exercises and can add internal and external rotation strengthening using rubber tubing.

You then progress by using your arm for light activities of daily living, avoiding the positions that used to be unstable. Always avoid "checking" your shoulder to see if it is stable. You must not lift over 10 pounds for the first 3 months after your surgery.

After 6 weeks, you can begin gentle, well-controlled, repetitive activities with your shoulder, such as swimming and using a rowing machine, provided that these activities are comfortable for you.

You cannot return to contact sports or heavy work for at least 3 months after this surgery, and then only if you have excellent strength and coordinated control of your shoulder.

We hope that this provides you with the information you need to successfully rehabilitate your shoulder. If you have any questions at any time, please let us know.

producing the injury so that the likelihood of a capsular tear can be determined. Unless this is clearly the case, the default assumption is that the shoulder has become dysfunctional without a substantial anatomic lesion and therefore needs to be managed with a rehabilitative approach emphasizing strength, balance, endurance, and good technique. Unless a functionally significant instability can be determined on history and physical examination, the emphasis on rehabilitation must continue. When the history and physical examination do not indicate the nature of the functional instability, "studies" such as contrast CT, MRI, examination under anesthesia, and arthroscopy are unlikely to be helpful in determining the treatment. "Findings" on these tests, such as "increased translation," "a large axillary pouch," or "labral fraying," may be identified even in functionally normal shoulders and, as such, may have no relation to the patient's functional problem. The risk, therefore, is that findings on these tests may distract the clinician from findings on history and physical examination. Unless the functional instability can be rigorously characterized by the history and physical examination, it is unlikely that surgical treatment will be curative.

The history and physical examination constitute the most efficient and cost-effective mechanisms for identifying treatable problems of glenohumeral instability. When these clinical tools do not clearly define the nature of the patient's functional problem, management by techniques other than physical rehabilitation and activity modification is unlikely to be effective. When this approach is used, the need for expensive diagnostic procedures in cases of suspected instability is reduced to a minimum and surgery is reserved for those patients who can most benefit from it. This highly selective approach improves the overall results of surgical treatment of instability by helping avoid the situation in which a well-done operation fails to restore the patient's function.

CHAPTER

4

Strength

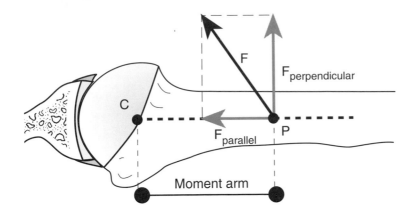

FIGURE 4–1.

The moment arm is the distance between the point of application of a force (P) and the center of movement (C). *Torque* is the product of the moment arm and the component of the muscle force perpendicular to it ($F_{perpendicular}$). The component of the muscle force that is parallel to the moment arm ($F_{parallel}$) can contribute to joint stability through concavity compression.

Strength is essential to carry out the functions of the shoulder. A stable joint with normal passive motion is not functional unless its musculature can position and move it effectively.

Many different muscles are required to power the shoulder because of the need to control both humeroscapular and scapulothoracic positions and to allow the vast range of motions of these articulations. For normal individual function each muscle must be intrinsically healthy, conditioned, attached securely to bone at both ends, and connected to the central nervous system by a healthy nerve supply. To contribute properly to the function of the shoulder, all the muscles around the shoulder must be activated by coordinated input from the central nervous system.

The strength of a given shoulder action is determined by the net torque created by the muscles responsible for this action. The torque resulting from a muscle's action is determined by the magnitude and direction of the muscle force and by the distance between the point of application of this force and the center of movement (the moment arm) (Fig. 4–1).

The magnitude of force deliverable by a muscle is determined by its size, health, and condition. It is also affected by the length of the muscle in the specified position of the shoulder—muscles are usually stronger near the middle of their excursion (Fig. 4–2).

The points of application of a muscle force are not necessarily the same as that muscle's anatomic origin and insertion. For example, the *effective* humeral point of application for cuff tendons wrapping around the head is on the articular surface of the humeral head (Fig. 4–3).

Finally, the direction of a given muscle force is also determined by the position of the joint. The anterior deltoid is a more effective internal rotator when the arm is in external rotation (Fig. 4–4).

Changes in the direction and the point of application of a muscle force in different joint positions have a profound effect on the moment arm and, therefore, the torque that results from a given magnitude of muscle force.

Thus, we see that each of the major determinants of a given muscle's contribution to torque is affected by joint position. It is apparent that maximizing shoulder strength must include positioning to optimize the contributions of the component muscles.

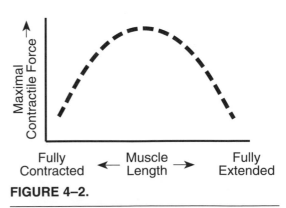

FIGURE 4–2.

A typical relationship between a muscle's length and the maximal force it can produce.

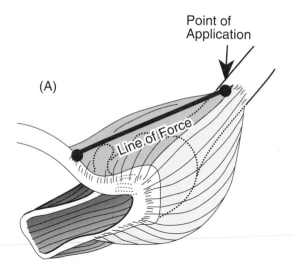

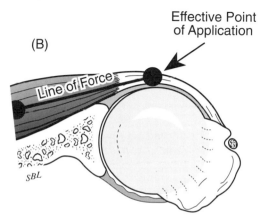

FIGURE 4–3.

Point of application of muscle force. *A,* The line of anterior deltoid force is collinear with its origin and insertion. *B,* The rotator cuff tendons wrap around the head of the humerus so that their effective point of attachment may lie on the humeral articular surface.

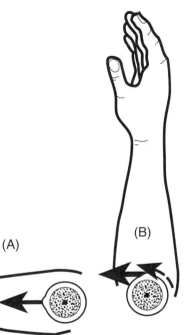

FIGURE 4–4.

Arm position affects the direction of the muscle force. For example, the anterior deltoid is a less effective internal rotator when the arm is in internal rotation *(A)* than when it is in external rotation *(B).*

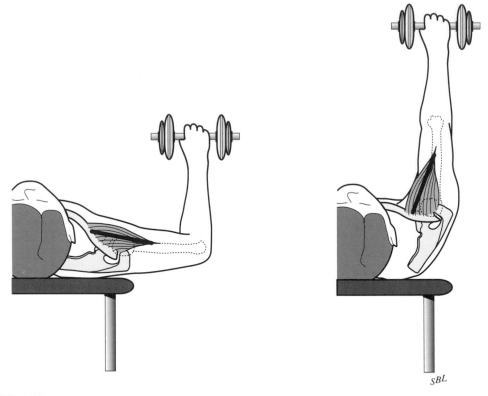

FIGURE 4–5.

Scapular protraction during bench press keeps the deltoid within its optimal length range. If this degree of scapular mobility were absent, the arc through which power could be achieved would be much less.

This positioning is facilitated by the mobility of the scapula, which, for example, enables the anterior deltoid to remain within an optimal length range as the arm is moved forward in an activity such as the bench press (Fig. 4–5).

One of the relatively unexplored facets of active shoulder motion is the requirement for strict muscular balance. In the knee, the muscles generate torques primarily about a single axis: that of flexion-extension. If the quadriceps pull is slightly off-center, the knee still extends. In the shoulder, no such fixed axis exists. In a specified position, each muscle creates a unique set of rotational moments. The anterior deltoid exerts moments in forward elevation, internal rotation, and cross-body movement (Fig. 4–6). If elevation without rotation in the plus 90 degree (sagittal) plane is desired, the cross-body and internal rotation moments of this

muscle must be resisted by other muscles (such as the posterior deltoid and infraspinatus) at an additional energy cost (Fig. 4–7). As another example, the latissimus dorsi cannot internally rotate the elevated arm unless other muscles resist its adduction moment. Conversely, it cannot act as a pure adductor unless other muscles resist its internal rotation moment.

The timing and magnitude of these balancing muscle effects must be precisely coordinated to avoid unwanted directions of humeral motion. For a ballerina to hold her arm motionless above her head, all the forces and torques exerted by each of her shoulder muscles must add up to zero. Thus, the simplified view of muscles as isolated motors must give way to an understanding that the shoulder muscles function together in a precisely coordinated way to yield the desired effect. Opposing muscles work to

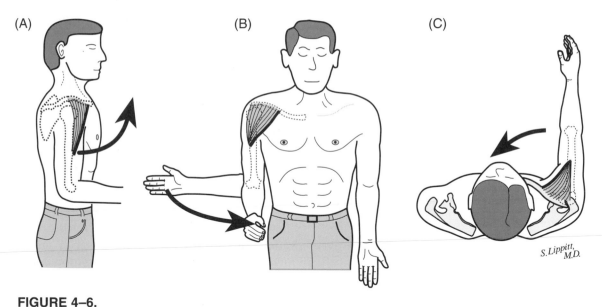

FIGURE 4–6.

The anterior deltoid generates moments in forward elevation *(A)*, internal rotation *(B)*, and cross-body movement *(C)*.

cancel out undesired effects. Even the concept of force couples may be an oversimplification. Perhaps the best way to present the concept of muscle balance is to state that the

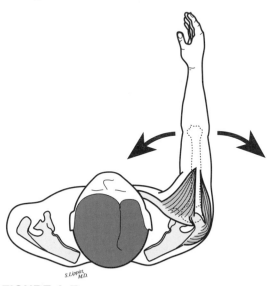

FIGURE 4–7.

Pure elevation requires that the internal rotation and cross-body moments of the anterior deltoid be opposed by other muscle action. For example, even though it is an "antagonist" to the anterior deltoid, the posterior deltoid must contract during elevation in a plus 90 degree thoracic plane to resist the cross-body moment of the anterior deltoid.

summation of all the muscle actions around the joint must provide (1) joint stability and (2) the torque necessary to carry out only the action desired. This degree of coordination requires a preprogrammed strategy or pattern that must be established before the motion is carried out.

ACTIVITY

Take a yo-yo. Wind some of the string about the axle. Apply a force to the string to lift it: the yo-yo unwinds and falls instead. Tape a small weight on the edge where the string enters the yo-yo so that it balances the tendency to unwind. Now, lifting the string lifts the yo-yo. What is the ideal mass of the balancing weight? (Answer: the mass of the yo-yo times the radius of the axle divided by the difference in the radius of the yo-yo and the radius of the axle.)

Rotator Cuff

The four muscles of the rotator cuff are uniquely adapted to contribute to muscle

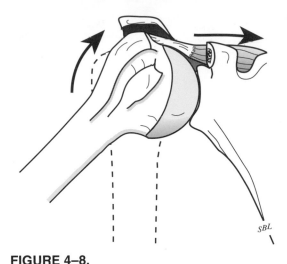

FIGURE 4–8.

Concentric action of the cuff muscles: the muscle shortens under active tension.

balance. These muscles are relatively small in size and have small moment arms in comparison with the deltoid and the pectoralis major. Through their role in muscle balance, these muscles make a major contribution to shoulder strength. Their insertion into a continuous cuff around the humeral head permits these muscles to provide an infinite variety of moments to oppose unwanted components of the stronger motors. To hold a glass of water straight out in front of the body, for example, one needs to use the infraspinatus to balance the internal rotation

moment of the anterior deltoid. When the function of the cuff muscles is compromised, the shoulder loses both the cuff's direct contribution to strength and the effectiveness of the muscles that the cuff balances.

The fibers of the cuff are subjected to many different challenges. They sustain concentric loads when moving the humerus actively (Fig. 4–8), and they sustain eccentric loads when resisting humeral motion or displacement (Fig. 4–9). The tendon fibers are subjected to bending loads when the humeral head rotates with respect to the scapula (Fig. 4–10). The glenoid rim abuts against the deep surface of the tendon insertion when the humeral head is rotated beyond the limits of the glenohumeral articular surfaces (Fig. 4–11) (see Chapter 2). In certain circumstances, the superficial fibers of the cuff may be abraded by the coracoacromial arch (Fig. 4–12). Like the rest of

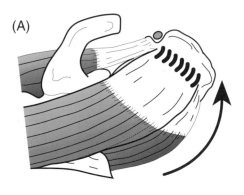

(A)

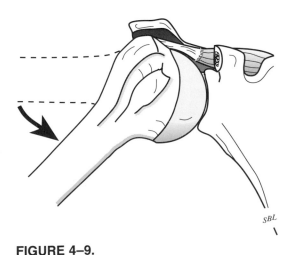

FIGURE 4–9.

Eccentric action of the cuff muscles: the muscle lengthens under active tension.

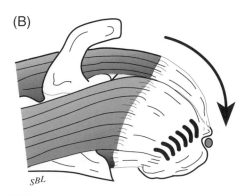

(B)

FIGURE 4–10.

The cuff fibers bend at their insertion as the humerus rotates from internal rotation (A) to external rotation (B).

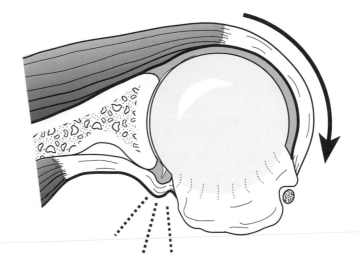

FIGURE 4–11.

Abutment of the deep surface of cuff insertion against the glenoid rim at the extremes of motion.

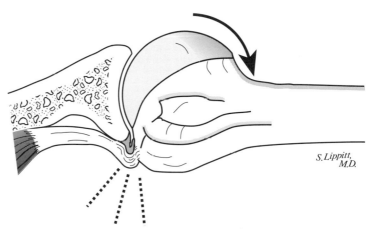

S.Lippitt, M.D.

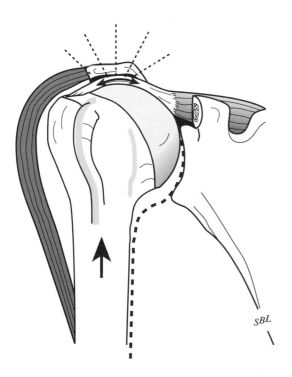

SBL

FIGURE 4–12.

Abrasion of the superficial surface of the cuff by the coracoacromial arch resulting from slight superior displacement of the head relative to the glenoid.

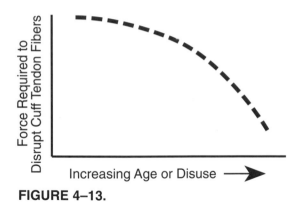

FIGURE 4–13.

The force necessary to disrupt the rotator cuff tendon fibers diminishes with age, disuse, or both.

the body's connective tissues, rotator cuff tendon fibers become weaker with disuse and age. As they become weaker, less force is required to disrupt them (Fig. 4–13).

Rotator Cuff Fiber Failure

The young healthy cuff is highly resistant to disruption or degeneration. For this reason, full thickness cuff lesions are most unusual in people younger than 40 years of age (Fig. 4–14). When cuff lesions occur in the younger age group, they may be only partial thickness, or they may include the avulsion of bone from the tuberosity (Fig. 4–15). Disuse and scarring of the partial thickness lesion may lead to stiffness limiting the range of elevation, cross-body adduction, and internal rotation.

With increasing age and disuse, less force is required to tear the cuff. Often, the acute symptoms from progression of the cuff defect are dismissed as "tendinitis" or "bursitis." Once these transient symptoms resolve, the shoulder becomes asymptomatic, except for a relatively imperceptible increment in weakness. Thus, we often encounter patients with large cuff defects and minimal symptoms. If these shoulders remain stable with the humeral head centered in the glenoid, they can demonstrate an astounding degree of function. Bilateral degenerative cuff defects are common. In one of our studies, we found that 55 percent of patients presenting with a symptomatic cuff tear on one side also had a tear on the opposite side.

Cuff failure may progress as major episodes of tendon tearing (Fig. 4–16) or as creeping tears involving relatively few fibers at a time (Fig. 4–17) with thinning of the cuff tendon. Degenerative lesions of the cuff typically start at the deep surface of the anterior insertion of the supraspinatus near the long head of the biceps (Fig. 4–18). Once these lesions begin, it is difficult for them to heal because of the hostile environment, the compromised vascularity, the large loads, and the large deformations that the healing tissue must endure. Failure of one fiber or of groups of fibers places greater loads on the adjacent fibers, favoring their failure (the "zipper" phenomenon). When a tendon fiber fails, the muscle fiber to which it attaches produces retraction away from the site of disruption, increasing the gap need-

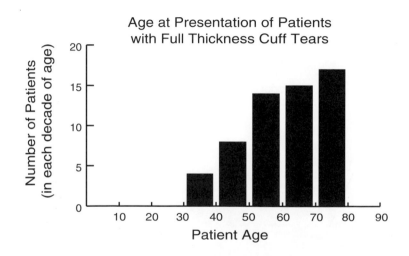

FIGURE 4–14.

The age at the time of presentation for 58 patients with full thickness cuff tears.

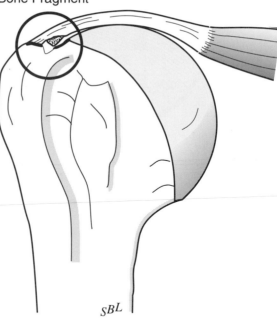

Avulsion with
Bone Fragment

FIGURE 4–15.

Partial thickness cuff tear with avulsion of bony fragment from the tuberosity.

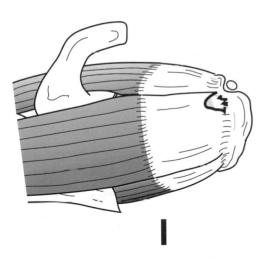

Acute Extension of Tear

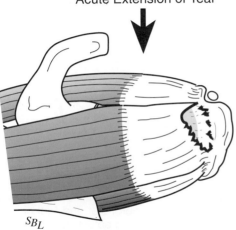

FIGURE 4–16.

Acute extension of a defect in the rotator cuff.

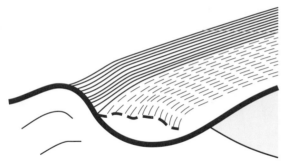

FIGURE 4–17.

In degenerative cuff disease, the tendon fibers fail a few at a time.

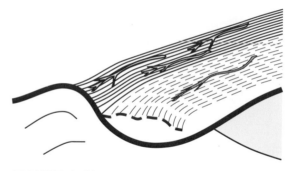

FIGURE 4–19.

Excessive tension at the margin of the tear can compromise the local tendon circulation.

ing to be closed. This retraction also places tension on the local vasculature, leading to limitation of tendon blood flow in the area where healing is needed (Fig. 4–19). Rotator cuff tendon defects are subject to the effects of synovial fluid on both their articular and bursal sides; the fluid and its enzymes may remove the fibrin clot necessary for healing of the cuff lesion (Fig. 4–20). In the absence of repair, the degenerative process tends to continue through the substance of the supraspinatus tendon to produce a full thickness defect in the anterior supraspinatus tendon (Fig. 4–21). This full thickness defect tends to concentrate loads at its margin, facilitating additional fiber failure with smaller

loads than those that produced the initial defect (Fig. 4–22).

ACTIVITY

The "notch effect": Take an intact piece of paper. Pull on its corners, noting the force necessary to initiate a rip. Then, repeat the experiment after creating a small notch in the edge of the paper.

Once a supraspinatus defect is established, it typically propagates posteriorly

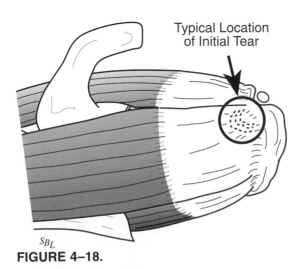

Typical Location of Initial Tear

S_{BL}

FIGURE 4–18.

Rotator cuff defects usually begin at the deep surface of the supraspinatus, near the long head of the biceps.

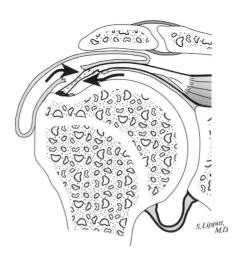

S. Lippitt, M.D.

FIGURE 4–20.

The tendon defect is bathed in joint fluid, preventing the formation of a fibrin clot and further compromising the tear's healing potential.

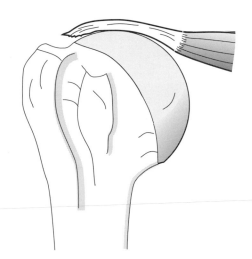

FIGURE 4–21.

Full thickness defect in the supraspinatus tendon.

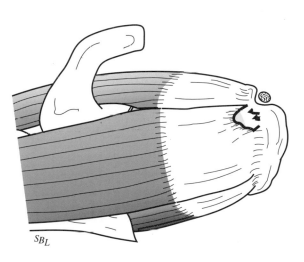

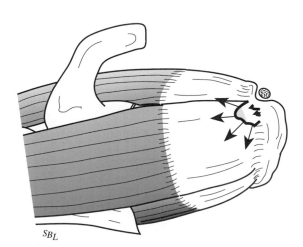

FIGURE 4–22.

The notch phenomenon: the stress on the tendon is channeled toward the edges of the defect, leading to further fiber failure.

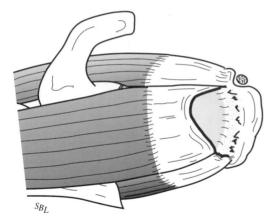

FIGURE 4–23.

The defect propagates through the remainder of the supraspinatus and into the infraspinatus tendon.

through the remainder of the supraspinatus, then into the infraspinatus and teres minor (Fig. 4–23). Further propagation of the cuff defect crosses the bicipital groove to involve the subscapularis, starting at the top of the lesser tuberosity and extending inferiorly. As the defect extends across the bicipital groove, it may be associated with rupture of the transverse humeral ligament and destabilization of the long head tendon of the biceps (Fig. 4–24).

The concavity compression mechanism is compromised by cuff disease. Beginning with the early stages of cuff fiber failure, the compression of the humeral head becomes less effective in resisting the upward pull of the deltoid. Partial thickness cuff tears cause pain on muscle contraction similar to that seen with other partial tendon injuries (such as those of the Achilles tendon and extensor carpi radialis brevis). This pain produces reflex inhibition of the muscle action. In turn, this reflex inhibition, along with the absolute loss of strength from fiber detachment, makes the muscle less effective in balance and stability. The weakened cuff function allows the humeral head to rise under the pull of the deltoid, squeezing the cuff between the head and the coracoacromial arch. Under these circumstances, abrasion occurs with humeroscapular motion, further contributing to cuff degeneration. Degenerative traction spurs develop in the coracoacromial ligament, which is loaded by pressure from the humeral head (analogous to the calcaneal traction spur that occurs with chronic strains of the plantar fascia). Upward displacement of the head also wears on the upper glenoid lip and labrum, reducing their contributions to the effective depth of the upper glenoid and to glenohumeral stability from concavity compression. Further deterioration of the cuff allows the tendons to slide down below the center of the humeral head, producing a "boutonniere" deformity (Fig. 4–25). The cuff tendons become head

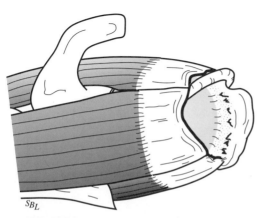

FIGURE 4–24.

The defect further propagates across the bicipital groove to the subscapularis, destabilizing the tendon of the long head of the biceps.

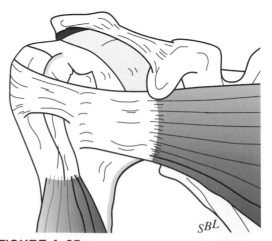

FIGURE 4–25.

The boutonniere deformity, in which the subscapularis and infraspinatus tendons slide below the center of the humeral head.

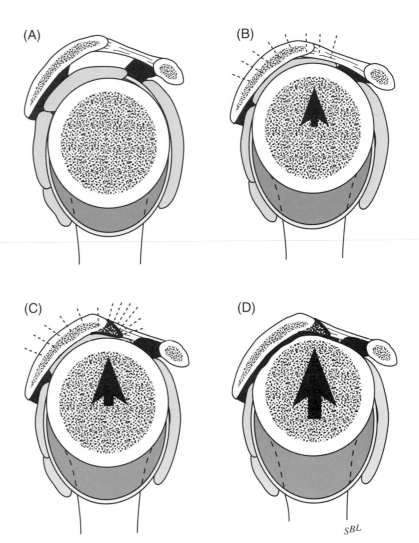

FIGURE 4–26.

With progressive cuff fiber failure, the head moves upward against the coracoacromial arch. *A,* Normal relationships of the cuff and the coracoacromial arch. *B,* Upward displacement of the head, squeezing the cuff against the acromion and the coracoacromial ligament. *C,* Greater contact and abrasion, giving rise to a traction spur in the coracoacromial ligament. *D,* Still greater upward displacement, resulting in abrasion of the humeral articular cartilage and cuff tear arthropathy.

elevators rather than head compressors. Once the full thickness of the cuff has failed, abrasion of the humeral articular cartilage against the coracoacromial arch may lead to a secondary degenerative joint disease known as *cuff tear arthropathy* (Fig. 4–26).

The progression from partial thickness tear toward cuff tear arthropathy can take place as a subtle and even subclinical degenerative process, with a few fibers giving way at a time (see Fig. 4–17). It can also progress as a series of episodes interpreted as "tendinitis," "bursitis," or "impingement syndrome." A more significant injury can produce an acute extension of the defect (see Fig. 4–16). It is important to note that cuff defects arising with minimal or no injury

suggest that the cuff tissue is of poor quality and thus is more likely to fail again after surgical repair. By contrast, acute tears resulting from major injuries are more likely to involve robust tissue that is more amenable to a durable repair.

The resulting disuse leads to scarring and atrophy of tendon and muscle. Loss of cuff material from the degenerative process limits what is available for repair. Local injections of steroids may further compromise the healing potential of failed cuff fibers. Once the humeral head has started to subluxate superiorly, increased stretching loads are placed on the residual tendons, tending to exacerbate the cuff defect. Long-standing superior subluxation leads to erosion of the upper glenoid lip, favoring continued superior subluxation even after cuff repair. Once the process of superior subluxation is established, stabilization of the humeral head in its normal position is difficult even if a cuff repair is achieved (see Chapter 3).

Shoulder Weakness

Weakness of the shoulder can come from deficits in any of the elements contributing to shoulder strength. These deficits include myopathy, disuse, tendon lesions, peripheral nerve lesions, and poor neuromuscular control. We will confine our discussion to the evaluation and management of the most common mechanical cause of shoulder weakness: rotator cuff fiber failure. The necessary and sufficient criteria for complete and incomplete cuff failure are listed in Table 4–1.

History

Figure 4–14 shows the age distribution of patients presenting for evaluation of full thickness rotator cuff tears.

A typical history for degenerative cuff fiber failure in an older person reveals an insidious onset of weakness of flexion and external rotation, perhaps punctuated by episodes of "bursitis" or "tendonitis." Failure of weakened tendon tissue may not produce much in the way of pain, bleeding, or swelling. The shoulder may have been treated with steroid injections with some relief of discomfort but without improvement in strength. More acute incremental losses of strength from tear propagation may follow lifting or falls.

A greater injury is required to tear the cuff of persons at the younger end of the age distribution. A history of sudden eccentric loading, such as trying to support a falling load or trying to cushion a fall with the arm, is commonly given by younger patients with cuff tears. Traumatic glenohumeral dislocations in persons older than 40 years of age have a strong association with rotator cuff tears. These traumatic cuff tears may also

TABLE 4–1. Necessary and Sufficient Diagnostic Criteria for Full Thickness and Partial Thickness Rotator Cuff Lesions

I. Full Thickness Rotator Cuff Tear
  A. History
    1. Functionally significant weakness of glenohumeral elevation and/or rotation
    2. Age over 30 years, usually over 40 years
    3. Diagnosis is supported by a history of sudden, unexpected loading of the arm followed by shoulder weakness
  B. Physical Examination
    1. Weakness on elevation and/or rotation
    2. Diagnosis is supported by supraspinatus and/or infraspinatus atrophy, subacromial crepitance, and/or palpable defect in rotator cuff
  C. Radiographs
    1. Diagnosis is supported by upward displacement of the humeral head in relation to the acromion and by acromial spurring
  D. Definite identification of a full thickness cuff defect by an expert observer using one of the following: ultrasonography, arthrography, MRI, arthroscopy, or open surgery
II. Incomplete Thickness Cuff Lesion
  A. History
    1. Compromise of shoulder function in activities requiring rotator cuff function
    2. Mechanism for damaging the rotator cuff, such as an unanticipated eccentric load applied to the elevated arm
  B. Physical Examination
    1. Pain and weakness on tests of rotator cuff function, such as resisted elevation and resisted external rotation
    2. Diagnosis is supported by subacromial crepitance
  C. Radiographs
    1. Diagnosis is supported by upward displacement of the humeral head in relation to the acromion and by acromial spurring
  D. Definite identification of an incomplete thickness cuff lesion by an expert observer using one of the following: arthrography, arthroscopy, or open surgery

involve the subscapularis, producing weakness in internal rotation.

Characteristic elements in the history of other common causes of shoulder weakness include the following:

1. Long thoracic nerve palsy—posterior protrusion of the scapula on attempts to elevate the arm.
2. Cervical radiculopathy—pain on top of the shoulder with radiation down the arm below the deltoid tubercle, weakness of the biceps, diminished biceps reflex, and sensory changes on the lateral forearm.

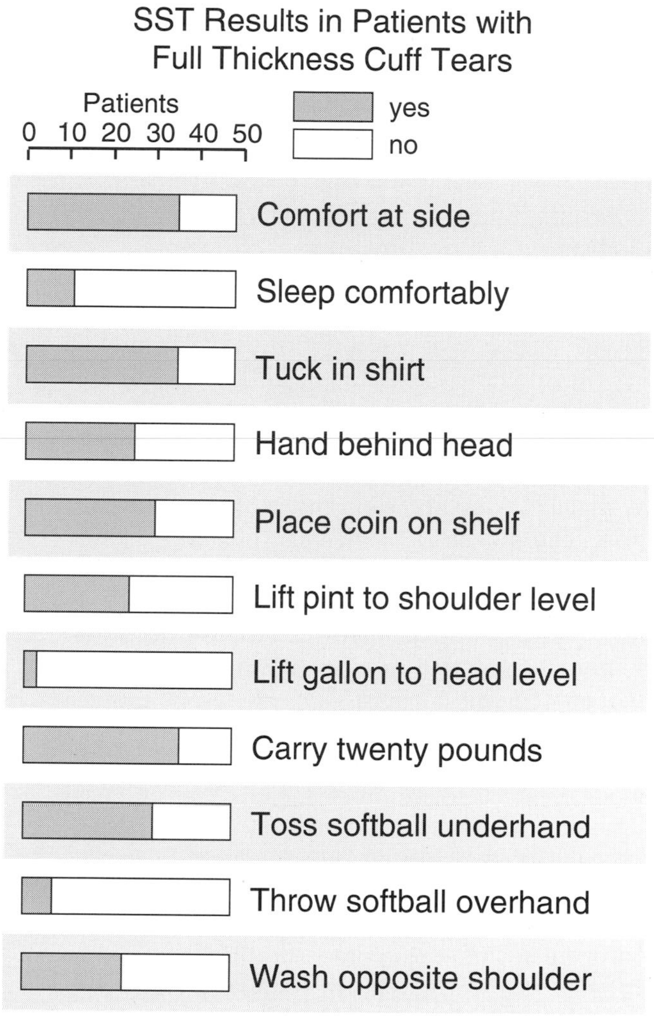

SST Results in Patients with Full Thickness Cuff Tears

Patients: 0 10 20 30 40 50

yes / no

- Comfort at side
- Sleep comfortably
- Tuck in shirt
- Hand behind head
- Place coin on shelf
- Lift pint to shoulder level
- Lift gallon to head level
- Carry twenty pounds
- Toss softball underhand
- Throw softball overhand
- Wash opposite shoulder

FIGURE 4–27.

The Simple Shoulder Test results demonstrate the functional deficits of 48 patients presenting with full thickness cuff defects.

3. Suprascapular neuropathy from brachial neuritis—acute onset of pain lasting several weeks followed by profound weakness of external rotation.
4. Suprascapular neuropathy from traction—external rotation weakness following an injury in which the shoulder was forced down and the neck forced to the opposite side (may be part of a full Erb's palsy).
5. Suprascapular neuropathy from compression-entrapment—insidious onset of external rotator weakness.

Facioscapulohumeral muscular dystrophy is suggested by the atraumatic onset of bilateral symmetrical weakness of the scapular musculature.

The Simple Shoulder Test provides a set of data for characterizing some functional impairment from rotator cuff tears (Fig. 4–27). It is evident that sleeping on the affected side, placing the hand behind the head, lifting 8 pounds, and throwing overhand are particularly compromised by cuff tears.

Substantial information bearing on the reparability of a rotator cuff defect can also be determined from the history. Acute tears in younger, healthy persons without prior shoulder disease are likely to be reparable. Long-standing tears associated with major weakness in older patients carry a poor prognosis. The prognosis for a durable repair is even worse if the history reveals local or systemic steroids, smoking, or difficulties in healing previous injuries or surgical procedures. The surgeon can also determine preoperatively the patient's goals and functional expectations for surgical treatment to see whether these are reasonable in view of the likely prognosis.

Physical Examination

Chronic rotator cuff tears are accompanied by atrophy of the spinatus muscles. Subtle atrophy can be seen most easily by casting a shadow from a light over the head of the patient. Rupture of the long head of the biceps is frequently evident on inspection of shoulders with rotator cuff tears. Defects in the cuff can often be palpated by rotating the proximal humerus under the examiner's finger placed at the anterior corner of the acromion. The defect is usually just posterior to the bicipital groove and medial to the greater tuberosity. Crepitance on rotation of the arm elevated to shoulder height may result from the abrasion of torn tendon margins against the coracoacromial arch (a positive "abrasion sign") (Fig. 4–28). A boutonniere deformity is evident when no cuff can be palpated over the humeral head. Chronic massive cuff defects may present with anterosuperior instability of the humeral head on attempted elevation of the arm. This may be particularly severe after previous surgical compromise of the coracoacromial arch. Cuff tear arthropathy is indicated by bone-on-bone crepitance when the humeral head is rotated beneath the coracoacromial arch.

Three isometric tests are used to evaluate the strength of the different components of the cuff. Weakness or effort-limiting pain on isometric testing is considered a positive "tendon sign" (Fig. 4–29). The supraspinatus is challenged by isometric flexion of the internally rotated arm that is elevated 90 degrees in the plane of the scapula. The infraspinatus is challenged by isometric external rotation with the arm in neutral rotation at the side. The subscapularis is challenged by isometric internal rotation, pushing the hand away from the waist in the posterior midline. The size of the cuff tear can be estimated by physical examination. Partial tears tend to demonstrate relatively more pain with minimal loss of strength. Small tears usually compromise only the function of the supraspinatus. Large tears involve the infraspinatus and compromise ex-

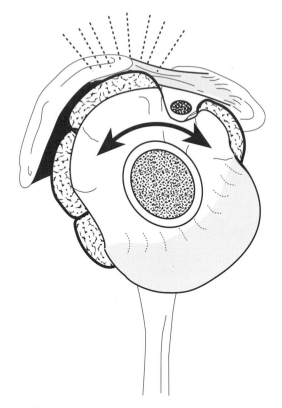

FIGURE 4–28.

Abrasion sign: symptomatic subacromial crepitance on rotation of the arm elevated to 90 degrees with respect to the thorax, a position in which the capsule and ligaments are normally not under tension.

ternal rotation. Massive tears compromise the subscapularis and weaken internal rotation.

Shoulders with incomplete thickness cuff lesions often manifest limitation of motion, particularly in flexion, internal rotation, and cross-body movement owing to selective contracture of the posterior capsule.

The examination of a patient with a weak shoulder must include the neck and the brachial plexus. Placing the head in extension and rotating the chin to the affected side usually exacerbates symptoms of cervical radiculopathy. The neurologic examination tests the cutaneous distribution of the nerve roots from C5 to T1. The biceps and the triceps reflexes help screen C5–6 and C7–8, respectively. The next component of the neurologic examination requires recognition

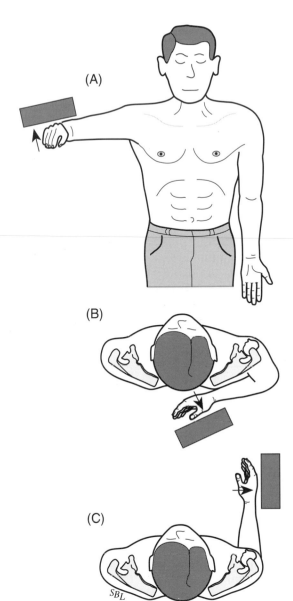

FIGURE 4–29.

Tendon signs: *A,* Supraspinatus tendon sign: pain and weakness on isometric elevation of the arm that is internally rotated and elevated to the horizontal position in the plane of the scapula. *B,* Subscapularis tendon sign: pain and weakness on isometric internal rotation of the arm with the hand held away from the body at the posterior waist. *C,* Infraspinatus tendon sign: pain and weakness on isometric external rotation with the arm at the side and the forearm pointing ahead.

of the segmental innervation of joint motion, as follows:

Shoulder abduction—C5
Shoulder adduction—C6, C7, and C8
Shoulder external rotation—C5
Shoulder internal rotation—C6, C7, and C8
Elbow flexion—C5 and C6
Elbow extension—C7 and C8
Wrist extension and flexion—C6 and C7
Finger flexion and extension—C7 and C8
Finger adduction and abduction—T1

ACTIVITY

Perform the motions in the previous list as a "dance," calling out the segmental innervation of each movement as you do it.

A set of screening tests checks the motor and sensory components of the major peripheral nerves: (1) the axillary nerve (the anterior, middle, and posterior parts of the deltoid and the skin just above the deltoid insertion); (2) the radial nerve (the extensor pollicis longus and the skin over the first dorsal web space); (3) the median nerve (the opponens pollicis and the skin over the pulp of the index finger); (4) the ulnar nerve (the first dorsal interosseous and the skin over the pulp of the little finger); and (5) the musculocutaneous nerve (the biceps muscle and the skin over the lateral forearm). The long thoracic nerve is checked by having the patient elevate the arm 60 degrees in the anterior sagittal plane while the examiner pushes down on the arm, seeking winging of the scapula posteriorly. The nerve of the trapezius is checked by observing the strength of the shoulder shrug. Lesions of the suprascapular nerve produce weakness of elevation and external rotation without sensory loss.

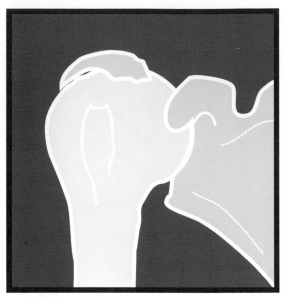

FIGURE 4–30.

Radiographic appearance of cuff tear arthropathy with "acetabularization" of the upper glenoid and the coracoacromial arch and "femoralization" of the proximal humerus.

Radiographs

Standard radiographs are of limited assistance in evaluating shoulder weakness. Small avulsed fragments of the tuberosity may be seen in younger patients with cuff lesions. Chronic cuff disease may be accompanied by sclerosis of the undersurface of the acromion or traction spurs in the coracoacromial ligament from forced contact with the cuff and the humeral head. In large cuff tears, the head of the humerus may be subluxated upward toward or against the undersurface of the acromion. In cuff tear arthropathy, the humeral head may have lost the prominence of the tuberosities (become "femoralized"), and the coracoid, acromion, and glenoid may have formed a deep socket (become "acetabularized") (Fig. 4–30).

Cuff Imaging

A number of different studies are available for imaging the rotator cuff. The single contrast arthrogram can expose full thickness cuff defects by revealing leakage of injected contrast material from the joint into the subacromial subdeltoid bursa. MRI can reveal some information about the tendon and muscle. Ultrasonography can reveal the thickness of the various components of the cuff and the extent of cuff defects. Each of these tests adds expense to the evaluation of the patient. Resources can be conserved by not ordering imaging tests unless doing so will change the management of the patient. Patients younger than 40 years of age without a major injury are unlikely to have significant cuff defects; thus, cuff imaging will not be helpful in their evaluation. At the other extreme, patients with weak external rotation and atrophy of the spinatus muscles whose plain radiographs show the head of the humerus in contact with the acromion do not need cuff imaging to establish the obvious diagnosis of a rotator cuff defect. Finally, the management of patients with nonspecific shoulder symptoms and an unremarkable physical examination is unlikely to be changed by the results of a cuff imaging test. In summary, cuff imaging is usually not needed when a cuff tear is very unlikely (such as in a 35-year-old person with the minimally traumatic onset of shoulder pain) or when it is very likely (such as in a 70-year-old person with gradual onset of shoulder weakness, spinatus atrophy, and radiographic evidence of contact between the head of the humerus and the acromion). The primary indication for cuff imaging is to establish the diagnosis in situations when it would affect treatment, such as a 47-year-old person with weakness of flexion and external rotation after a major fall on the outstretched arm.

Electromyography

Electromyography can be an important diagnostic test for the patient with shoulder weakness in the absence of cuff lesions. It is particularly helpful in patients with a history suggestive of cervical radiculopathy or suprascapular nerve lesions and a physical examination showing neurologic signs.

Treatment

At the outset, we emphasize that although cuff repair may increase the strength of the shoulder, our preference is to avoid having the patient return to heavy lifting, pushing, pulling, or overhead work after a major cuff repair. Thus, we attempt to initiate vocational rehabilitation as soon as the diagnosis of cuff tear is made, indicating that in spite of optimal treatment, there is a substantial risk of retearing if the repaired cuff is subjected to major loads. It is important to remind both the patient and the employer that a cuff tear usually occurs through an abnormal cuff tendon. Repairing the tear does not restore the quality of the tendon tissue; thus, the repaired cuff remains vulnerable to sudden or large loads.

Patients with rotator cuff tears may present with problems of shoulder stiffness or shoulder roughness. These aspects are discussed in Chapters 2 and 5, respectively. In this chapter we are concerned with the potential for improving strength through rotator cuff repair. Critical determinants of the success of operative treatment are the quality of the tendon and muscle and the amount of cuff tendon tissue that has been lost. As we have seen previously, the expected strength of the cuff diminishes with age and

disuse. Thus, the chances of a durable cuff repair likewise decrease in older and less active shoulders. This is particularly the case if the cuff defect has been long-standing.

Table 4–2 describes the factors that contribute to a durable repair, together with those that make a successful outcome unlikely. None of the factors in this table requires special imaging of the rotator cuff; all are discernible from the history, physical examination, and plain radiographs. MRI is not necessary to determine muscle atrophy. Although none of these factors is a contraindication to surgery, each works to some degree against the chances of a durable repair.

Treatment of shoulder weakness caused by cuff failure is determined by the functional needs of the patient and the likeliness of a durable surgical repair. Patients with low functional requirements and a substan-

TABLE 4–2. Prognostic Factors Related to the Durability of Cuff Repair

Encouraging	Discouraging
History	
Age under 55 years	Age over 65 years
Acute traumatic onset	Insidious atraumatic onset
Short duration of weakness	Weakness longer than 6 months
No history of smoking	Many smoking pack-years
No steroid injections	Repeated steroid injections
No major medications	Systemic steroids or antimetabolites
No concurrent disease	Inflammatory joint disease, other chronic illnesses
No infections	History of previous shoulder infection
No previous shoulder surgery	Previous cuff repair attempts
Benign surgical history	History of failed soft tissue repairs (e.g., dehiscence, infections)
Physical Examination	
Good nutrition	Poor nutrition
Mild to moderate weakness	Severe weakness
No spinatus atrophy	Severe spinatus atrophy
Stable shoulder	Anterior superior instability
Intact acromion	Previous acromial resection
No stiffness	Stiffness
X-rays	
Normal radiographs	Upward displacement of the humeral head against the coracoacromial arch
	Cuff tear arthropathy

tial number of the "discouraging" factors shown in Table 4–2 are given a nonoperative program to help optimize the strength and coordination of the muscles about the shoulder that remain intact. At the opposite extreme, patients with major functional demands and mostly "encouraging" factors are presented with the option of an attempted surgical repair and are informed that the success of this repair will be determined primarily by the quality of the tendon and muscle and the amount of tissue lost.

Cuff repair is a shoulder-tightening operation. It is not a treatment for the shoulder with functional limitation caused by tightness, even if a cuff defect is present. If the shoulder demonstrates stiffness, especially of the posterior capsule, a shoulder mobilization program is instituted before consideration of surgery (see Chapter 2, Patient Information 2–1: Home Exercise Program for the Stiff Shoulder).

In chronic cuff deficiency, surgical repair is not an emergency; there is time to explore nonoperative management, including a general shoulder strengthening program along with the stretching program. This non-operative program may be the treatment of choice in patients with chronic weakness who are not candidates for surgery or for those in whom achieving a durable repair seems unlikely. This program emphasizes strengthening the muscle groups that provide elevation of the shoulder (Patient Information 4–1).

Surgical Treatment

Surgical exploration and attempted cuff repair is an option for the patient who understands the limitations of this procedure. Prompt surgical exploration of the rotator cuff is considered for physiologically young patients with acute tears. Repair should be carried out before tissue loss, retraction, and atrophy occur. For tears older than 12 months, a period of stretching and gentle strengthening exercises can indicate the potential for non-operative management. Exploration is considered for patients with functionally significant weakness from tears older than 12 months refractory to non-op-

erative management, provided that their expectations are realistic. We use Patient Information 4–2 to help communicate the important considerations surrounding surgical repair.

Rotator Cuff Repair

The goal of cuff repair surgery is to improve the strength and muscular balance of the shoulder. This operative procedure is considered when the shoulder demonstrates weakness from a cuff defect and when there appears to be a substantial chance of achieving a durable functional repair. These conditions are most likely met in a traumatic tear where a physiologically sound cuff has been torn acutely by a substantial injury. In this situation, the quality and quantity of tendon for repair should be excellent. In contrast, with chronic massive degenerative tears, the quantity and quality of the cuff are less likely to be optimal for surgical repair. In this situation, the surgeon and the patient must understand preoperatively the potential limitations imposed by the tissue in the shoulder.

There are several ways in which surgery may worsen the function of a cuff-deficient shoulder, and these need to be reviewed before each cuff operation. The most serious is compromise of the deltoid muscle. The deltoid may be compromised by nerve injury. This injury may involve the intramuscular motor branches to the anterior third of the muscle resulting from a too distal split of the muscle in the surgical approach. Deltoid denervation may also arise from axillary nerve injury during a search for cuff tendons laterally and posteriorly around the quadrangular space. Normally, the deltoid has a strong tendon of origin between its anterior and middle thirds. This tendon attaches to the anterior lateral corner of the acromion. Postoperative function of the deltoid may be compromised by failure to achieve a strong reattachment of this tendon and the anterior muscle fibers after acromioplasty. This is particularly problematic when a large anterior acromial resection is performed requiring stretch of the deltoid for reattachment. Failure of the anterior deltoid origin devas-

Text continued on page 135

UNIVERSITY OF WASHINGTON SHOULDER AND ELBOW SERVICE

Home Exercise Program for the Weak Shoulder

The strength of your shoulder depends on the coordinated working of several groups of muscles, including the muscles of the rotator cuff, the deltoid and pectoralis major, and the muscles that power the shoulder blade. The simple exercises described here are designed to help you optimize the strength and coordination of these muscle groups.

The primary exercise is called the *progressive supine press* (Fig. 4–31). It is most effective for helping you regain the ability to use your arm in an elevated position. The nice things about this exercise

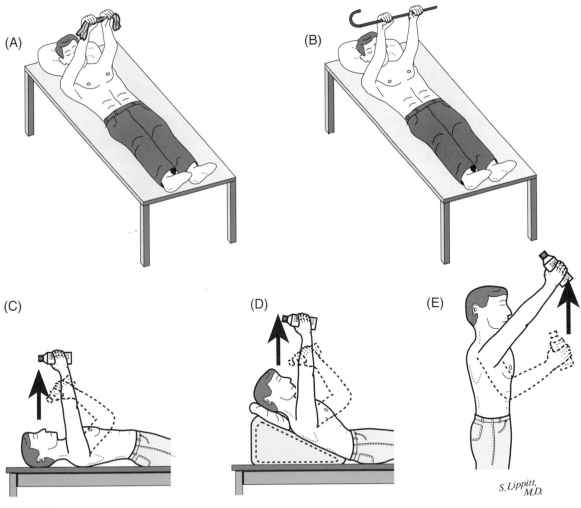

FIGURE 4–31.

Progressive supine press exercises to strengthen flexion. The motion is always pushing up toward the ceiling, ending with a lift of the shoulder blade off the bed. *A,* Start with two hands together holding a wash cloth; *B,* then two hands apart; *C,* then one hand with a 1-pint (i.e., 1-lb) weight; *D,* then one hand with a 1-pint weight with greater degrees of sitting up; and finally, *E,* one hand with a 1-pint weight while standing.

are that you can do it by yourself, and you can adjust your rate of progress according to what is most comfortable for you. The exercise proceeds in small steps.

Start by lying on your back, grasping a washcloth with both hands together. Push the cloth straight up toward the ceiling. At the end of each push, lift your entire shoulder off the bed or floor. When you can do this 20 times easily, separate your hands an inch or so when you push the cloth toward the ceiling. This places slightly more of the load on the muscles of your weaker shoulder. As the exercise gets easier, separate your hands more on the washcloth until you can push your hand toward the ceiling without any assistance from the opposite arm. Practice this exercise with nothing in your hand until you are able to repeat it 20 times. Then, take an empty pint container and perform the same movement, pushing it toward the ceiling. Add water to increase the resistance slowly. When the container is full of water, the weight is about 1 pound. Make sure that with each press-up you end by lifting your shoulder blade up off the bed or floor. We call this the *"press plus."* Be sure that you can perform the movement comfortably 20 times at each

stage before advancing to the next stage. When you can press 1 pound toward the ceiling 20 times, the next step is to perform the exercise with your back propped up slightly on pillows or by using a recliner or lawn chair. When 20 comfortable repetitions are possible, increase the degree to which your back is propped up. At each level, push the shoulder all the way up: "press plus." Continue this process until you are able to push the 1-pound weight 20 times toward the ceiling in a sitting position. Work for smooth, slow, controlled motions. This program optimizes the mechanics of your shoulder and gives you the best chance of regaining good function.

You should add other strengthening exercises as your shoulder permits. The trapezius is strengthened by shoulder shrugs made with the arms holding some weight at the side. The internal and external rotator cuff muscles are strengthened using rubber tubing. General shoulder strengthening exercises, such as swimming, light-resistance rowing machine, cross-country skiing simulators, and brisk walking, are excellent for this purpose as well as for restoring coordination, endurance, and general well-being.

UNIVERSITY OF WASHINGTON SHOULDER AND ELBOW SERVICE

Rotator Cuff Surgery

The rotator cuff is composed of four tendons that blend together to help stabilize and move the shoulder. Loss of the integrity of the rotator cuff is a common cause of shoulder weakness. Shoulders with large rotator cuff defects have difficulty raising the arm or rotating it out to the side.

Strong rotator cuff tissue requires a major force to tear it. Weakened degenerative cuff tissue can be torn easily, even while carrying out activities of daily living.

When rotator cuff tears are relatively recent and when a significant force was required to tear the tendon, the chances of regaining shoulder strength by rotator cuff repair surgery are good. Conversely, when the defect is long-standing and occurred without a major injury, the quality and quantity of tissue available for repair may not be sufficient for the restoration of good shoulder function. Thus, with long-standing shoulder weakness from rotator cuff defects, a good try at strengthening the remaining muscles may be worthwhile before considering surgical repair.

The goal of the surgical repair of a rotator cuff defect is to reestablish the connection between the torn tendon and the bone. If the tendon heals securely and durably to the bone, the force of the muscle can be effectively transmitted to the arm.

The rotator cuff is surgically exposed by an incision near the top of the shoulder. Access is gained by splitting part of the deltoid muscle and by shaving the undersurface of the bone at the top of the shoulder known as the *acromion.* The torn edges of the tendon are identified and the quality of the tendon tissue evaluated. If the tendon will not reach to its normal bony attachment site, a special tissue releasing technique may help bridge the defect. If sufficient quality and quantity of tendon can be mobilized, the tendon is implanted into the groove in the arm bone at its normal attachment site and held in position with sutures. A strong repair helps facilitate immediate postoperative motion, which in turn helps inhibit scarring and adhesions after surgery. However, even the best surgical repair is too weak to allow the muscle to raise the arm from the side. This must await full healing of the tendon.

Healing of the repaired tendon is slow, and the loads applied to the tendon are large. Thus protection of your repair is required for many months (sometimes as long as 6 to 12) after the repair. This means that while the shoulder may be moved using the other arm for support, the muscles in the repaired shoulder must not be used to lift the arm or to rotate it against resistance for fear of disrupting the repair. Thus, the postoperative program ideally includes early *passive* motion of the arm to prevent scar tissue and adhesions, but delayed *active* motion. The rehabilitating exercises are learned while you are still in the hospital, and discharge is delayed until comfortable passive motion, including elevation to 140 degrees and external rotation to 40 degrees, is achieved.

Strengthening exercises are delayed until 3, 6, or 12 months after the repair, depending on the size of the defect repaired and the quality of the tissue.

Sometimes, the quality of the tissue is insufficient to hold the suture, or there may not be enough tissue to close the defect. This situation is much like trying to repair a sail when the basic cloth of the sail has deteriorated. Under these circumstances, it may be preferable to clean up the frayed edges of the tendon and leave all or part of the defect unrepaired. In this circumstance, the shoulder is moved immediately after surgery to prevent unwanted scarring, but the need for postoperative protection is less, usually only 6 to 8 weeks.

The potential complications of rotator cuff surgery include infection, nerve injury, blood vessel injury, stiffness of the shoulder, inability to obtain a durable repaired tendon, pain, and the need for revision surgery.

If questions arise concerning your shoulder or the alternatives in its treatment, please ask us at any time.

tates the most important motor for shoulder elevation.

Scarring in the humeroscapular motion interface (see Chapter 2) between the acromion and deltoid and the cuff and humerus can restrict humeroscapular motion, negating any benefit achieved from restoring cuff integrity. This complication results from immobilization of the cuff against the acromion and deltoid after surgery.

Loss of superior stability can result when the coracoacromial arch is sacrificed without reestablishing stability with a durable cuff repair. In this situation, deltoid contraction pulls the head of the humerus anterior superiorly rather than elevating it. The deltoid becomes stretched so that the humeral head seems to be just below the skin. Patients who lose stability and deltoid func-

tion are some of the most unhappy we encounter after previous repair attempts. *Primum non nocere* ("First of all, do no harm").

Surgical Technique

The cuff is approached though an acromioplasty incision in the skin lines perpendicular to the deltoid fibers (Fig. 4–32). This incision offers an excellent exposure and the opportunity for a cosmetic closure, particularly in comparison with the skin incisions parallel to the deltoid fibers. Great care is taken to preserve the tendon fibers of the deltoid origin to permit a strong repair. The deltoid has an important tendon of origin between its anterior and middle thirds. Aris-

FIGURE 4–32.

Deltoid on approach. *A*, Skin incision in Langer's lines across the front of the acromion. The deltoid is split along the tendon at the junction of the anterior and middle thirds. *B*, The deltoid origin is sharply dissected from the acromion, preserving Sharpey's fibers of origin on the muscle and continuity with trapezius insertion.

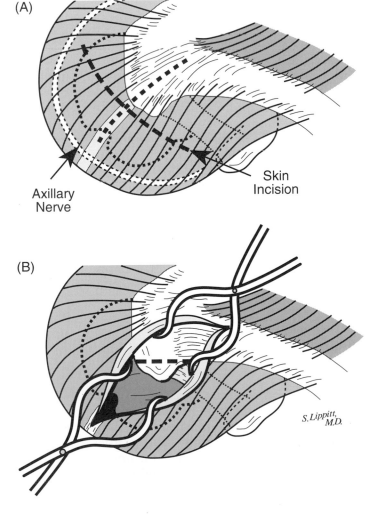

ing from the anterior lateral corner of the acromion, this tendon is not only the guide to exposure of the cuff but is also the key to reattachment of the deltoid origin at the conclusion of the surgery. This tendon is surgically split longitudinally for 2 cm distal to the acromion in line with its fibers, taking care to leave some of the tendon on each side of the split. The split is continued up over the acromion and into the trapezius insertion. For 1 cm on either side of this split, the deltoid origin is sharply dissected off the acromion, so the strong bony attachment fibers remain with the muscle. These fibers provide a strong "handle" on the muscle, so a solid repair can be achieved. Splitting the parietal layer of the bursa on the deep aspect of the deltoid provides a view of the rotator cuff. *Before* a "reflex" acromioplasty is performed, the quality and quantity of the cuff tissue are observed to determine the likelihood of cuff reparability. Hypertrophic bursa and scar tissue are resected to allow a good view of the cuff tissue. We characterize cuff tears using a simple system based on the number of tendons torn. In Type 1, only one tendon (almost always the supraspinatus) is torn. In Type 2, two tendons (usually the supraspinatus and infraspinatus) are torn. In Type 3, the supraspinatus, infraspinatus, and subscapularis are torn. Type 1 is broken down into Type 1A—a partial thickness tear—and Type 1B—a full thickness tear confined to a single tendon. We judge the quality of the cuff tissue in terms of its ability to hold a strong pull applied to a suture passed through its edge. Finally, it is critical to note the amount of tissue that has been lost. The extent of tissue loss and the ability of the remaining tissue to hold suture are the major determinants of cuff reparability.

When Cuff Repair Cannot Be Achieved

If there is major tissue loss and residual tendon of poor quality, it becomes evident that a robust repair cannot be performed. In this situation, when primary stability from an intact cuff cannot be restored, it is important *not* to perform a routine acromioplasty, which would jeopardize the secondary sta-

bilization offered by the coracoacromial arch. Under these circumstances, sacrifice of coracoacromial arch support deprives the shoulder of its last vestige of superior stability, allowing anterosuperior "escape" of the humeral head when elevation is attempted. For this reason, when a strong rotator cuff repair is impossible as a result of the limited quantity and quality of the residual cuff tissue, we do not perform a routine acromioplasty. Instead, we perform only a smoothing of the undersurface of the coracoacromial arch to allow unimpeded passage of the humeral head and residual cuff beneath. Any debris, scar, or thickened bursa in the subacromial area is excised. It is often helpful to smooth the upper surface of the uncovered proximal humerus, particularly if the uncovered tuberosities are prominent or irregular.

A strong repair of the deltoid to the acromion is then carried out. Depending on the quality of the tissues, this may be accomplished by a side-to-side repair of the surgical split in the deltoid tendon and trapezius fascia. Drill holes in the acromion are used as necessary for secure reattachment. The full thickness of the deltoid, including the deltoid side of the bursa, is incorporated in the sutures to be certain that it does not impede smooth motion in the humeroscapular motion interface (Fig. 4–33).

A subcuticular skin closure reinforced with paper tapes provides optimal cosmesis. The patient is returned to the post anesthesia care unit with the arm in continuous pas-

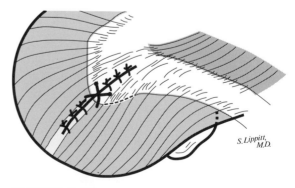

FIGURE 4–33.

Deltoid repair. A secure repair is accomplished by a side-to-side closure with a criss-cross repair to bone: anterior deltoid to more posterior acromion and middle deltoid to more anterior acromion.

sive motion from zero to 90 degrees of flexion to minimize the tendency to form adhesions in the humeroscapular motion interface.

The patient is taught passive mobilization of the shoulder to 140 degrees of elevation and 40 degrees of external rotation and is discharged when these goals are achieved comfortably. Light use of the shoulder with the arm at the side is allowed as comfort permits. Sling immobilization is unnecessary. Strengthening of the deltoid and residual cuff muscles is started 6 weeks after surgery. The best exercise we have found for optimizing active elevation is the progressive supine press that is described in Patient Information 4–1. In this exercise, small increments are used to train the remaining muscles to optimal advantage. Note that the scapular muscles are also put to work in these exercises. This program is easy for the patient to learn and to carry out alone.

When Cuff Repair Is Possible

If inspection of the cuff at surgery reveals good-quality tissue in sufficient quantity for a robust repair, primary glenohumeral stability from concavity compression can usually be restored. Thus, a standard anteroinferior acromioplasty is performed to improve exposure and to protect the repair from abrasion. A flexible osteotome is directed so that the anterior undersurface of the acromion is resected in the same plane as the posterior acromion. Rough spots are smoothed with a motorized burr (Fig. 4–34).

The goal of repair is a strong fixation of the tendon to the humerus under normal tension with the arm at the side. The desired attachment site is at the sulcus near the base of the tuberosity. This goal is facilitated by using three stages of sequential release. These releases are required because the cuff is usually retracted and because tissue is lost in chronic cuff disease. Unless these releases are carried out, increased tension in the repaired tendon will predispose to tightness of the glenohumeral joint and will additionally challenge the repair site. The humeral head is rotated to present the different margins of the cuff defect through the incision rather than enlarging the exposure to show the entire lesion. The deep surface of the cuff is searched for retracted laminations. All layers of the cuff are assembled and tagged with sutures. By applying traction to these sutures, the cuff is mobilized sequentially as necessary to allow the torn tendon edge to reach the desired insertion at the base of the

FIGURE 4–34.

Acromioplasty. The anteroinferior acromion is resected in line with the posterior acromion using an osteotome (A). The undersurface is smoothed with a power burr (B).

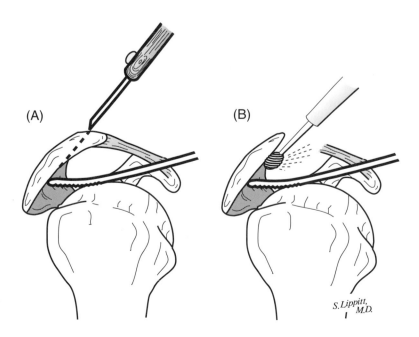

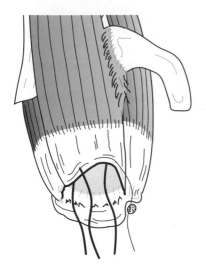
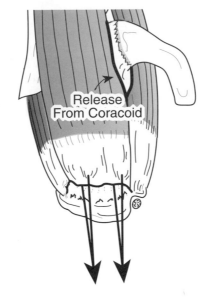

FIGURE 4–35.

Release of the cuff tendons from the coracoid allows their lateral advancement.

tuberosity. First, the humeroscapular motion interface is freed between the cuff and the deltoid, the acromion, the coracoacromial ligaments, the coracoid, and the coracoid muscles. Next, the coracohumeral ligament–rotator interval capsule is sectioned around the coracoid process to eliminate any restriction to the excursion of the cuff tendons and to minimize tension on the repair during passive movement (Fig. 4–35). This release of the coracohumeral ligament and rotator interval capsule also contributes to the comfort and ease of motion after the surgical repair by minimizing the capsular tightening effect of cuff repair. At this point the ease with which the cuff margins can be approximated to their anatomic insertion at the base of the tuberosity is evaluated. If good tissue cannot reach the sulcus, the third release is carried out. This release divides the capsule from the glenoid just outside the glenoid labrum (Fig. 4–36), allowing the capsule and tendon of the cuff to be drawn further laterally toward the desired tuberosity insertion without restricting range of motion.

After the necessary releases have been completed, a judgment is made concerning the site at which the cuff can be implanted into the bone without undue tension while the arm is at the side. Ideally, the site of implantation will be in the sulcus at the base of the tuberosity. In large cuff defects, a somewhat more medial insertion site may be necessary. Often, when a medial insertion site is required for a large cuff defect, the new insertion lies in an area where the articular cartilage has been damaged by abrasion against the undersurface of the acromion.

The repair is accomplished as a tongue-in-groove, with the cuff tendon drawn into a trough near the tuberosity, providing a smooth upper surface to glide beneath the acromion (Fig. 4–37). This groove provides the additional advantage that if some slippage occurs in the suture fixation of the cuff

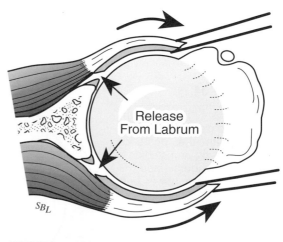

FIGURE 4–36.

Release of the capsule from the labrum allows further lateral advancement.

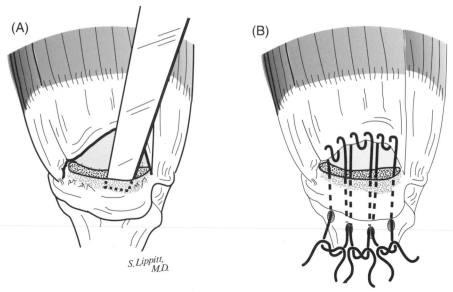

FIGURE 4–37.

A, A groove is created in the sulcus just lateral to the articular surface. *B,* Sutures draw the tendon edge into this groove.

to bone, contact between tendons and bone is not lost. Nonabsorbable sutures passed through the tendon margin are passed through drill holes in the distal tuberosity so that the knots will not catch beneath the acromion (Fig. 4–38). The knots are tied over the tuberosities so that they will lie out

of the subacromial space. If there is a longitudinal component to the tear, it is repaired side to side, with the knots buried out of the humeroscapular motion interface. The repair is checked throughout a range of motion to 140 degrees of elevation and 40 degrees of external rotation to ensure that it is strong

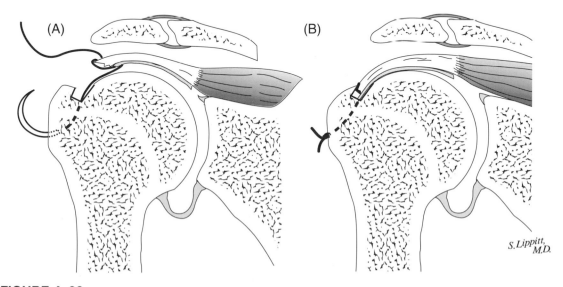

FIGURE 4–38.

The sutures are placed low on the tuberosity *(A)* and tied laterally *(B)* to leave a smooth upper surface for the cuff insertion. The bony eminence above the groove is smoothed as necessary.

and not under excessive tension and that it will permit smooth subacromial motion. If additional resection of the undersurface of the acromion is required to allow smooth passage of the repaired tendon, it is performed at this time.

After a careful and robust deltoid repair using nonabsorbable sutures and cosmetic skin closure, the patient is returned to the post anesthesia care unit with the affected arm in zero to 90 degrees of continuous passive motion. Immediate postoperative motion is valuable because there is a tendency for scarring between the raw undersurface of the acromion and the upper aspect of the rotator cuff or proximal humerus. Immediate postoperative continuous passive motion is facilitated if the surgery is performed under a brachial plexus block, which provides analgesia for up to 18 hours after surgery. Continuous passive motion is continued for as long as 48 hours after surgery but does not appear to be necessary after that. The patient is expected to perform passive exercises in flexion and external rotation. Before discharge, the patient should be able to attain comfortably 140 degrees of passive flexion and 40 degrees of passive external rotation. A progress chart mounted on the patient's wall helps to document progress toward these discharge goals (see Chapter 2).

Post-discharge management must consider the magnitude of the tear and the strength of the repair. It is unlikely that the repair will have substantial strength until at least 3 months after surgery. As is the case with repairs of the anterior cruciate ligament, major cuff repairs require 6 to 12 months to regain useful strength. Thus, in the first several postoperative months, the emphasis is placed on maintaining passive motion and avoiding loading of the repair (see Patient Information 4–3).

Partial Thickness Cuff Tears

Partial thickness defects of the cuff may manifest clinically as the inability to use the cuff forcefully against resistance, by pain on isometric abduction or external rotation (a positive "tendon sign"), or by crepitance with rotation of the partially elevated arm (a

positive "abrasion sign"). These partial defects are more likely to be associated with shoulder stiffness than are larger full thickness defects, because the larger defects in the cuff provide the equivalent of a capsular release. Non-operative management must emphasize stretching in internal rotation, cross-body adduction, and elevation. When a comfortable normal range of passive motion is reestablished, gentle progressive strengthening of the cuff muscles is instituted. An emphasis is always placed on gentle and comfortable progress of this rehabilitation program.

In many respects, the treatment of a partial cuff tear is analogous to the treatment of a partial Achilles tendon tear or tennis elbow. The functional deficits are likely to be related to tension on a partially torn tendon. Treatment requires first stretching and then gentle strengthening. Surgery is usually considered only if symptoms persist in spite of regaining normal passive motion and if the patient is prepared for an extended recovery period.

In planning surgical management for refractory problems from partial thickness tears, it must be determined if the patient's functional deficits are related to tension on a partially torn tendon as indicated by a positive tendon sign. In this instance, completion of the detachment and reattachment as for a full thickness tear may be necessary. This procedure tightens the shoulder and is *not* a suitable treatment for a contracted shoulder. Alternatively, the symptoms may be related to secondary subacromial abrasion from the slight superior instability resulting from the tendon defect as well as the associated thickening of the intervening bursa. Under these circumstances, the abrasion sign (rotating the partially elevated arm beneath the coracoacromial arch) should reproduce the patient's symptoms. In the second instance, an anterior inferior acromioplasty and bursal resection may be of benefit as long as normal shoulder flexibility has been restored to eliminate the effect of a tight posterior capsule. Anterior acromioplasty does not treat shoulder stiffness, which must be eliminated by exercises or by surgical releases.

The decision to complete a partial thick-

UNIVERSITY OF WASHINGTON SHOULDER AND ELBOW SERVICE

Rehabilitation After Rotator Cuff Surgery

You have had a surgical repair of your rotator cuff. We have attempted to make an optimal surgical repair, but the repair will remain quite weak until your body has time to complete the bonding of the tissue to bone. This may require as long as 6 months. Use of the arm before the healing is complete can cause the repair to fail. On the other hand, immobilizing the shoulder for a long period to protect the repair can cause shoulder stiffness. For these reasons, careful postoperative rehabilitation is an essential part of your surgery. There are two aspects of the rehabilitation program: preventing unwanted scar formation and protecting the repair.

Protect your repair by being careful that your arm does not participate in lifting, pushing, or pulling and that it is not raised away from the side under its own power. Unless we tell you otherwise, you may use your hand for typing or writing as long as the elbow is kept at your side. Raising the arm even a small amount places demands on your repair and should be avoided. We will tell you how long these restrictions need to be in effect. During this time you should not drive!

While your shoulder is healing, *passive* motion is necessary to prevent unwanted scar tissue formation. Passive motion means that the shoulder is moved, but not under its own power. These exercises must be comfortable for you—if you have problems doing them comfortably, let us know. Your operated shoulder is moved by your other hand while the muscles of the operated shoulder are completely relaxed. You can move your shoulder passively by standing up and bending over at the waist, allowing the operated arm to dangle down in a relaxed way. Passive motion is also easily done while you are lying on your back. Grasp the wrist of your operated shoulder with the opposite hand, and slowly lift the arm up to a vertical position and then over your head. On lowering it back down, you will need to concentrate on keeping the operated shoulder completely relaxed.

A second exercise is performed while you are lying down with both your elbows bent to a right angle. Using a cane, a dowel, or a yardstick, gently push the wrist of the operated shoulder out to the side while keeping your elbow at the side.

These passive motion exercises and precautions against active use are continued until we tell you it is time to start the next phase of exercises. Please do not change your program just because it seems time to do so. We need to supervise your program carefully. If you have any questions, please let us know.

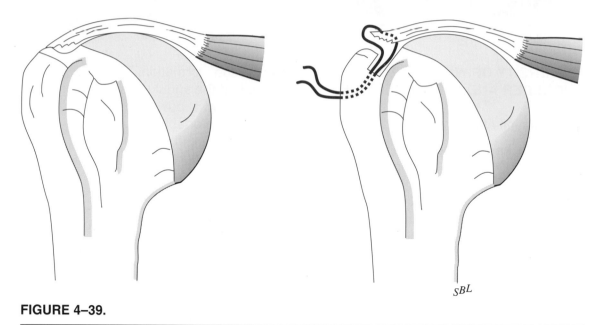

FIGURE 4–39.

Repair of a partial thickness defect by converting it to a full thickness defect and gathering the medially retracted deep fibers with suture.

ness cuff defect may be influenced by surgical findings. The thickness of the cuff can be determined at acromioplasty by inspection for superior surface defects. For deep surface or intratendinous lesions, the cuff thickness is determined by palpation, by injection of saline or dilute methylene blue solution in the joint, or by use of a depth gauge or calibrated nerve hook. A tenotomy can also be performed in the most suspicious area along the line of the tendon fibers to explore the full thickness of the tissue. If, as is usually the case, the defect is near the anterior insertion of the supraspinatus, a longitudinal tenotomy and capsulotomy are performed along the anterior aspect of the supraspinatus in the rotator interval capsule. This cut is then extended at right angles posteriorly through the partially detached cuff at its insertion to the greater tuberosity, turning back the flap of cuff until tendon of full thickness is encountered. Next, an attempt is made to retrieve and consolidate any split laminations of cuff that may have retracted medially (Fig. 4–39). These are usually on the deep articular surface where the cuff lesion begins and may have retracted medially up to 1 cm. Release of the coracohumeral ligament and rotator interval capsule from

the base of the coracoid minimizes tension on the repair, then the resulting full thickness defect is repaired in the manner previously described. The shoulder is then put through a full range of motion to verify that the acromioplasty is adequate to protect the repaired tendon from acromial abrasion.

Postoperative management is the same as for the full thickness defects.

Results of Treatment

Patients are usually pleased with the results of cuff surgery, yet it may be difficult to determine what aspect of the treatment program is responsible for the improvement. It is known that many patients with deficient cuffs are surprisingly comfortable and functional and, therefore, never undergo surgery. It is also known that the tissue encountered at surgery is not infrequently insufficient to allow a durable repair, yet the patient is improved after surgery. These observations bring up the question of the relationship of cuff integrity to the quality of the result after cuff surgery. To help answer this question, we undertook a study of 105 of our own surgical repairs of chronic rotator cuff tears in 89 patients at an average of 5 years postoperatively. The patients' ages at the time of repair averaged 60 years (ranging from 32 to 80 years). The number of patients in each age decade were as follows: 30–39: 1; 40–49: 16; 50–59: 31; 60–69: 42; 70–79: 14; and 80–89: 1. Eighty-six (82 percent) of the shoulders had no prior attempt at repair of the cuff.

In all of the surgeries, an anteroinferior acromioplasty was carried out. The involved tendon or tendons were mobilized as necessary. A bony trough was created in the humerus to reattach the mobilized tendons. The site of reattachment was usually in the sulcus adjacent to the humeral articular surface. In some instances, the trough was placed somewhat more medially if, after mobilization, the tendons did not reach their original anatomic attachment without undue tension when the arm was at the side. The cuff was protected from active use for at least 3 months postoperatively.

We correlated the functional result with the integrity of the cuff, as determined by expert ultrasonographic examination. Expert ultrasonography was selected because of its superior accuracy-to-cost ratio and practicality.

We characterized the status of the cuff at surgery and at followup in terms of the integrity of the different tendons. *Type 1A* refers to thinning or a partial thickness defect of the supraspinatus tendon. *Type 1B* refers to a full thickness defect of the supraspinatus. *Type 2* refers to a full thickness two-tendon defect involving the supraspinatus and the infraspinatus. *Type 3* refers to a full thickness defect involving three tendons: the supraspinatus, the infraspinatus, and the subscapularis.

The results are summarized in Table 4–3. No patient who had a partial thickness tear repaired had a full thickness retear. In 80 percent of shoulders with repaired full thickness supraspinatus tears, the cuff was found to be intact at followup. Only 57 percent of cuffs that had tears involving both the supraspinatus and infraspinatus were intact at an average followup of 6 years. Less than one third of the cuffs that had tears involving all three major tendons were in-

tact after repair at an average of 4 years of followup. It is evident, therefore, that the rotator cuff is more likely to develop a secondary defect after the repair of a large tear. This may be a reflection of the age of the patient, the quality of the tissue, the quantity of tissue, the effect of tendon mobilization on tendon viability, or the greater difficulty in getting healthy tendon securely implanted in bone when there is a major deficiency in the cuff.

Patients were generally satisfied with the results of surgery, even when expert ultrasonographic examination showed that the cuff was no longer intact (Table 4–4). This would indicate that patient satisfaction is not a reliable indicator of cuff integrity.

Shoulders with intact repairs at followup had the greatest range of active flexion (129 ± 20 degrees) as compared to those with large recurrent defects (71 ± 41 degrees) (Fig. 4–40). These patients also demonstrated the best function in activities of daily living. Where the cuff was not intact, the degree of functional loss was related to the size of the recurrent defect (Fig. 4–41). These results indicate that integrity by ultrasound correlates with cuff function.

Patients with intact repairs of large tears had just as good function as did those with intact repairs of small tears. We found an overall greater incidence of recurrent defects in shoulders with repeat repairs. However, shoulders with intact cuffs after repeat repairs functioned as well as did those with intact primary repairs (Fig. 4–42).

From this study we concluded that the integrity of the rotator cuff at followup (and *not* the size of the tear at the time of repair) is the major determinant of the outcome of surgical repair. An intact repair of a recurrent tear is likely to yield a result comparable with that of an intact repair of a primary tear. Likewise, intact repairs of large tears yield results comparable with intact repairs of small tears.

The chances of the repair of a large tear remaining intact, however, are not as good as those for a small tear. Older patients tended to have larger tears and to have a higher incidence of recurrent defects (Table 4–5).

Text continued on page 148

TABLE 4–3. Integrity of Cuff Repairs at Followup*

| Defect at Surgery | Primary Repairs | Repeat Repairs | Total No. of Repairs | Cuff Defect at Followup Examination | | | | | Percentage Intact | Average Years of Followup (Range) |
				None	Partial	Supraspinatus Tear	Supraspinatus and Infraspinatus Tears	Supraspinatus, Infraspinatus, and Subscapularis Tears		
All cases	86	19	105	40	28	12	14	11	65	5 (2–11)
Partial tears	5	1	6	4	2	0	0	0	100	2.7 (2–6)
Supraspinatus tears	39	10	49	23	16	3	5	2	80	5.1 (2–10.5)
Supraspinatus and subscapularis tears	25	3	28	7	9	6	5	1	57	5.9 (2–6)
Supraspinatus, infraspinatus, and subscapularis tears	17	5	22	6	1	3	4	8	32	4.1 (2–11)

*Results are grouped according to size of defect at surgery and whether the procedure was a primary repair or a revision.

144

TABLE 4–4. Average Active Motion, Comfort, and Satisfaction at Followup*

Cuff Defect at Followup	Number	Flexion (degrees)	External Rotation at Side (degrees)	External Rotation at 90 Degree Abduction	Internal Rotation	Total Painless	Total Satisfied
None	40	132	41	71	T7	37	39
Partial	28	124	38	68	T7	21	23
Supraspinatus	12	107	34	63	T8	8	12
Supraspinatus and infraspinatus	14	109	25	48	T9	10	10
Supraspinatus, infraspinatus, and subscapularis	11	71	27	61	T10	8	10
Total	105					84	94

*Results are grouped by followup cuff integrity.

TABLE 4–5. Rotator Cuff Repairs: Average Active Motion at Followup*

Defect at Surgery	Number	Age at Repair (mean ± SD)	Flexion (degrees)	External Rotation at Side (degrees)	External Rotation at 90 Degree Abduction	Internal Rotation
Partial	6	49 ± 13	126	38	68	T8
Supraspinatus	49	57 ± 8	129	40	70	T7
Supraspinatus and infraspinatus	28	64 ± 8	119	28	60	T8
Supraspinatus, infraspinatus, and subscapularis	22	64 ± 8	92	33	60	T10

*Results are grouped by defect at surgery.

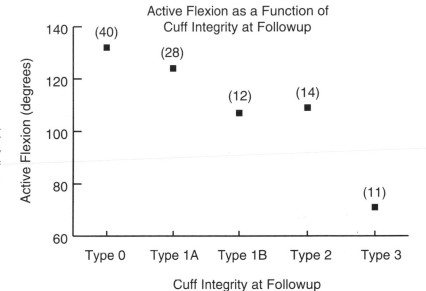

FIGURE 4–40.

Active flexion after cuff repair as a function of cuff integrity at followup. The numbers of shoulders are in parentheses.

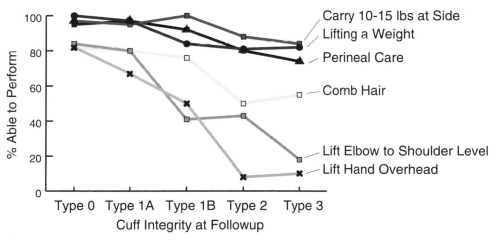

FIGURE 4–41.

The ability to perform activities of daily living as a function of cuff integrity at followup. The ordinate indicates the percentage of shoulders that were functional enough for the patient to perform the activity.

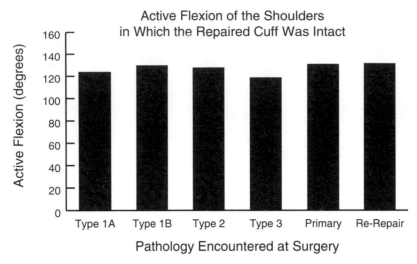

FIGURE 4–42.

Active flexion of the shoulders in which the repaired cuff remained intact was independent of the pathologic conditions encountered at surgery.

Arthrodesis

When a massive cuff defect coexists with a detached, denervated, or dysfunctional deltoid, the shoulder is without effective glenohumeral motors. Under these circumstances, a glenohumeral arthrodesis provides a salvage option. By securing the humeral head to the scapula, the scapular motors can be used to power the humerus through a limited range of humerothoracic motion. We prefer a fusion technique that preserves all remaining deltoid muscle and that uses decortication of the humerus and glenoid, 6.5-mm compression screws across the joint, and a neutralization plate from the scapular spine across the joint and down the humeral shaft.

The best candidates for this procedure are those patients with (1) permanent and severe weakness due to loss of cuff and deltoid function; (2) a good understanding of the limitations and potential complications of a shoulder fusion; (3) intact scapular motors; (4) good motivation; and (5) minimal complaints of pain.

To establish the limitations of shoulder fusions, we studied the humerothoracic motion of twelve patients who had glenohumeral arthrodeses at least 2 years prior to the time of study. Elevation in the plus 90 degree (anterior sagittal) plane averaged 47 degrees. External rotation averaged 9 degrees and internal rotation 46 degrees. These ranges of motion were similar to the scapulothoracic motion measured in normal subjects. Only one of the patients could reach his hair without bending his neck forward; only five patients could reach their perineum, six the back pocket, seven the opposite axilla, and ten the side pocket.

We studied normal *in vivo* shoulder kinematics to predict the functions that would be allowed by various positions of glenohumeral arthrodesis, assuming that the scapulothoracic motion would remain unchanged. Using the normal scapulothoracic motions, we were able to model the functional effects of fusion positions (reported in relation to the thorax). We found that activities of daily living could be performed best if the joint was fused in 15 degrees of flexion, 15 degrees of abduction, and 45 degrees of internal rotation (Fig. 4–43). This low angle of elevation and relatively high degree of internal rotation facilitated reaching the face, op-

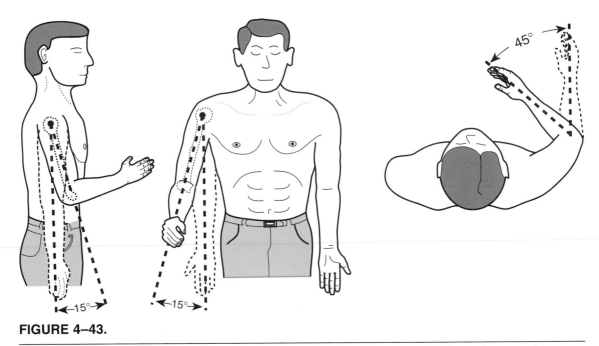

FIGURE 4–43.

Recommended arthrodesis position: 15 degrees of humerothoracic flexion *(left)*, 15 degrees of humerothoracic abduction *(middle)*, and 45 degrees of internal rotation *(right)*.

posite axilla, and perineum. However, all positions represented major compromises in normal function.

CONCLUSION

In summary, rotator cuff defects are common causes of shoulder weakness. Usually, cuff tears are associated with degenerative changes, which make the tissue susceptible to failure with low applied loads, especially those applied eccentrically. Alternatively, cuff tears can occur in stronger cuff tissue, but these injuries require the application of much greater loads. Cuff defects produce weakness of elevation and external rotation

as well as a possible loss of stability of the humerus against upward-displacing loads from the deltoid. Shoulders may be comfortable and able to carry out certain functions in the presence of significant cuff defects. Cuff repair surgery can restore the strength of the shoulder if the cuff tissue is of sufficient quantity and quality. To minimize the risk of retear, a substantial period of minimal loading needs to follow cuff repair surgery. Returning to heavy work after a cuff repair risks the integrity of the repair. Preservation of deltoid function is essential in rotator cuff surgery. If the function of both the cuff and deltoid are lost, glenohumeral arthrodesis may represent the only surgical option for salvage.

CHAPTER

5

Smoothness

There are five areas in which smoothness is required for shoulder function. Three of these are cartilage-to-cartilage articulations: the glenohumeral, acromioclavicular, and sternoclavicular joints. These joints are stabilized by joint capsules, ligaments, and intraarticular labra or menisci. The smoothness of their cartilage surfaces is at risk for congenital, metabolic, traumatic, degenerative, septic, and non-septic inflammatory joint disease. Collapse of the bone supporting the joint surface may be caused by avascular necrosis, tumor, or osteomyelitis. Labral tears or loose bodies may become interposed between the articular surfaces, causing joint roughness.

At the glenohumeral joint, different processes produce different patterns of joint surface destruction. In *degenerative joint disease,* the glenoid cartilage and subchondral bone are typically worn posteriorly, sometimes leaving intact articular cartilage anteriorly. The cartilage of the humeral head is eroded in a "Friar Tuck" pattern of central baldness, often surrounded by a rim of remaining cartilage and osteophytes. In *inflammatory arthritis,* the cartilage is usually destroyed evenly across the humeral and glenoid joint surfaces. *Cuff tear arthropathy* occurs when a chronic large rotator cuff defect subjects the uncovered humeral articular cartilage to abrasion by the undersurface of the coracoacromial arch. The erosion of the humeral articular cartilage begins superiorly rather than centrally (see Chapter 4).

Neurotrophic arthropathy arises in association with syringomyelia, diabetes, or other causes of joint denervation. The joint and subchondral bone are destroyed because of the loss of the trophic and protective effects of its nerve supply. In *capsulorrhaphy arthropathy,* prior surgery for glenohumeral instability leads to joint surface destruction. In this situation excessive anterior or posterior capsular tightening produces obligate translation, which forces the head of the humerus out of its normal concentric relationship with the glenoid fossa. The eccentric glenohumeral contact increases contact pressures and joint surface wear. Most commonly, overtightening of the anterior capsule produces obligate posterior translation, posterior glenoid wear, and central wear of the humeral articular cartilage (see Chapter 2).

The other two locations requiring smoothness are atypical articulations: the scapulothoracic motion interface and the non-articular humeroscapular motion interface. In these locations, motion occurs between tissue planes rather than at joints lined with articular cartilage. Malalignment of the sliding surfaces, surface irregularities, or thickening of interposed tissue can interfere with smooth motion at these articulations.

The *scapulothoracic motion interface* is the site of movement between the scapula and the chest wall. The deep aspect of this interface consists of the ribs and their covering musculature. The superficial aspect of the interface consists of the scapular border along with the serratus muscles (Fig. 5–1). No muscle covers the anteriorly inclined superior medial corner of the scapula. This corner is a potential site of bony contact between the scapula and the thoracic wall, especially if the normal postural relationship between the scapula and the rib cage is altered. If injury or disuse allows the scapula to ride low on the chest, for example, the superior medial corner of the scapula may "washboard" over the ribs, producing a snapping scapula (Fig. 5–2). Thinning of the interposed subscapularis and serratus muscles may yield a similar effect. Malunions of scapular or rib fractures can also present major irregularities at the scapulothoracic motion interface. Hypertrophy of the subscapular bursa or osteochondromata of the anterior surface of the scapula can also disrupt smooth gliding of the scapula on the chest wall. Problems caused by minor irregularities at this motion interface can be exacerbated by restrictions of glenohumeral motion that place greater demands on scapulothoracic motion, such as with frozen shoulder and glenohumeral arthrodesis.

Normal motion between the humerus and the scapula requires not only smoothness of the glenohumeral joint but also smoothness of the *non-articular humeroscapular motion interface.* This interface has a superficial aspect consisting of the acromion, deltoid, coracoid, coracoacromial ligament, and the

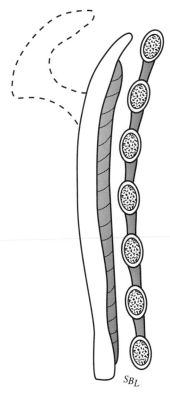

FIGURE 5–1.

Anatomy of the scapulothoracic motion interface, showing the serratus muscle covering its anterior costal surface except for a bare, anteriorly inclined superior medial angle that can catch as it slides over the ribs, particularly if the interposed muscles are small.

muscles originating from the coracoid. Its deep aspect consists of the proximal humerus, rotator cuff, and long head of the biceps. Excursions of much as 4 cm take place at this non-articular interface (see Fig. 2–21). This motion interface includes what is often referred to as the *subacromial "space."* It is evident, however, that no empty spaces exist in the intact shoulder and that the area beneath the acromion and coracoacromial ligament is occupied by bursa and cuff in contact with each other. Normal humeroscapular motion requires smoothness at this interface just as much as it depends on smoothness at the glenohumeral articulation. Loss of smoothness can result from altered relationships between the humerus and the scapula, roughness of the inner or

outer aspects of the motion interface, or interposed tissue.

Alterations in the normal postural relationships of the humerus and scapula can result from capsular imbalance or cuff deficiency. Tightness of the posterior capsule can produce superior obligate translation of the humerus on elevation in anterior scapular planes, forcing abrasive contact between the cuff and the undersurface of the coracoacromial arch (see Fig. 2–28). Instability from cuff deficiency may also allow superior translation of the humerus in relation to the scapula, creating localized abrasion of the proximal humerus beneath the unyielding acromion (see Fig. 4–26). Repeated forced contact of the cuff or proximal humerus with the undersurface of the anterior acromion

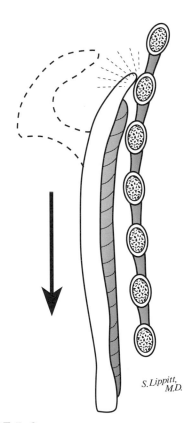

FIGURE 5–2.

Sagging, or ptosis, of the scapula allows the superior medial border of the scapula to catch on the ribs.

can produce a traction spur extending out into the coracoacromial ligament that may further compromise the smooth passage of the humerus and cuff beneath the arch. Continued subacromial abrasion may grind up the remaining interposed rotator cuff tissue. When the cuff is gone, this abrasive contact erodes the humeral articular cartilage. Destruction of the joint surface associated with the excessively superior position of the humeral head in massive cuff deficiency is known as *cuff tear arthropathy.*

Roughness of the superficial aspect of the motion interface (the undersurface of the coracoacromial arch) may result from developmental variances in the shape of the acromion or coracoid or from secondary traction spurs in the coracoacromial ligament. Roughness of the deep aspect of the interface may be compromised by complete or partial thickness cuff tears involving the upper surface of the tendon, by sutures or lumpy tendon attachments following cuff repair, by prominent tendon calcifications, or by abnormal prominence of the tuberosities. Finally, roughness at the humeroscapular interface can result from a thickened subacromial bursa or from post-traumatic or post-surgical scarring.

The concepts of smoothness and motion are closely related. If the glenohumeral joint surfaces are rough because of degenerative glenohumeral joint disease, for example, the shoulder will have a marked tendency to become stiff. Restoration of function to such a joint may require not only a resurfacing arthroplasty to restore glenohumeral smoothness but also a capsular release and tendon lengthening to restore motion. However, lack of smoothness and stiffness need not coexist. Avascular necrosis with collapse of subchondral bone deprives the shoulder of normal smoothness but is not usually associated with stiffness. Conversely, a frozen shoulder deprives a shoulder of its motion, yet joint surface roughness is not present. Because these two aspects of normal joint function are distinguishable and require separate and distinct treatment, we discuss them in two different chapters.

DIAGNOSIS

Roughness, catching, grinding, crunching, or snapping may compromise functioning of the shoulder. A good history and physical examination along with high-quality plain radiographs provide sufficient information to diagnose most functionally significant problems of shoulder roughness. Table 5–1 lists the necessary and sufficient criteria for making some of these diagnoses.

History

The history includes a description of the onset of the problem, the mechanism of any injuries, and the nature and progression of functional difficulties. Systemic or polyarticular manifestations of sepsis, degenerative joint disease, or rheumatoid arthritis may provide helpful clues. A past history of steroid medication, fracture, or working at depths may suggest the diagnosis of avascular necrosis. Past injury or surgery increases the risk of infection, scarring, or abnormal surface contours. Disuse may give rise to abnormal relative positions of the moving surfaces.

The symptoms from lack of smoothness typically occur during use of the shoulder. Often, the patient can describe certain motions that are problematic or specific maneuvers that are required to "unlock" or get past a certain sticking point. Occasionally, patients describe a sensation of apparent instability or unwanted shifting of the shoulder. The positions and circumstances that elicit the functional problem must be carefully defined in the history. The patient should also be asked about the response of the shoulder to previous treatment, including exercises, injections, physical therapy, and surgery.

The age of the patient at the time of presentation may provide valuable clues to the diagnosis (Fig. 5–3).

Physical Examination

Physical examination includes the careful observation of the patient's posture for

TABLE 5–1. Necessary and Sufficient Diagnostic Criteria for Problems of Shoulder Roughness

I. Subacromial Abrasion
  A. History
    1. Limited function with the arm in intermediate positions of elevation
  B. Physical Examination
    1. Subacromial crepitance that reproduces the function-limiting symptoms, particularly on rotation of the humerus with the arm in intermediate positions of elevation
  C. Radiographs
    1. Diagnosis is supported by primary or secondary changes on the undersurface of the coracoacromial arch, such as acromial sclerosis and a traction spur in the coracoacromial ligament
    2. Diagnosis is supported by the coexistence of incomplete thickness cuff lesion or full thickness rotator cuff tear
II. Degenerative Joint Disease (primary)
  A. History
    1. Absence of major joint trauma, previous surgery, or other known causes of secondary degenerative joint disease
    2. Age over 30 years, usually over 40 years
    3. Limited motion and function
  B. Physical Examination
    1. Limited glenohumeral motion
    2. Diagnosis is supported by bone-on-bone crepitance
  C. Radiographs
    1. Joint space narrowing
    2. Periarticular sclerosis
    3. Periarticular osteophytes
    4. Absence of other pathologic changes
    5. Diagnosis is supported by posterior glenoid erosion with posterior subluxation of the humeral head
III. Secondary Degenerative Joint Disease
  A. History
    1. Evidence of major joint trauma or other known causes of secondary degenerative joint disease
    2. Limited motion and function
  B. Physical Examination
    1. Limited glenohumeral motion
    2. Diagnosis is supported by bone-on-bone crepitance
  C. Radiographs
    1. Joint space narrowing
    2. Periarticular sclerosis
    3. Periarticular osteophytes
    4. Diagnosis is supported by radiographic evidence of previous trauma or other known causes of secondary degenerative joint disease
IV. Rheumatoid Arthritis
  A. History
    1. American Rheumatological Association criteria for rheumatoid arthritis
    2. Limited motion and function
  B. Physical Examination
    1. Limited glenohumeral motion
    2. Diagnosis is supported by findings of muscle atrophy and weakness and/or bone-on-bone crepitance
  C. Radiographs
    1. Joint space narrowing
    2. Periarticular osteopenia
    3. Diagnosis is supported by the absence of osteophytes and sclerosis
    4. Diagnosis is supported by the presence of periarticular erosions and medial erosion of the glenoid
V. Avascular Necrosis (Atraumatic)
  A. History
    1. Limited shoulder function
    2. Diagnosis is supported by the presence of risk factors, such as steroid use
  B. Physical Examination
    1. Diagnosis is supported by glenohumeral crepitance
  C. Radiographs
    1. Sclerosis within the humeral head
    2. Collapse of subchondral bone of the humeral head
    3. Absence of other pathologic changes (e.g., tumor, cuff tear arthropathy)

TABLE 5–1. Necessary and Sufficient Diagnostic Criteria for Problems of Shoulder Roughness *Continued*

VI. Capsulorrhaphy Arthropathy
    A. History
        1. Functionally significant restricted glenohumeral motion
        2. History of previous repair for glenohumeral instability
    B. Physical Examination
        1. Limited motion and function (especially external rotation)
        2. Diagnosis is supported by bone-on-bone crepitance
    C. Radiographs
        1. Joint space narrowing
        2. Periarticular sclerosis
        3. Periarticular osteophytes
        4. Diagnosis is supported by posterior glenoid erosion with posterior subluxation of the humeral head
VII. Cuff Tear Arthropathy
    A. History
        1. Limited motion and function
        2. Weakness in elevation and rotation
        3. Diagnosis is supported by previously confirmed cuff tear
    B. Physical Examination
        1. Limited glenohumeral motion
        2. Evidence of large cuff defect, such as
            a. Supraspinatus and infraspinatus atrophy
            b. Weakness of external rotation and elevation
            c. Superior position of the humeral head relative to scapula
            d. Palpable rotator cuff defect
        3. Bone-on-bone crepitance
    C. Radiographs
        1. Superior displacement of the humeral head relative to the glenoid leading to contact with coracoacromial arch
        2. Secondary degenerative changes of the glenohumeral joint
        3. Diagnosis is supported by erosion of the greater tuberosity ("femoralization" of the proximal humerus)
        4. Diagnosis is supported by a contoured coracoacromial arch and upper glenoid to produce a socket for the proximal humerus ("acetabularization")
        5. Diagnosis is supported by the collapse of the superior subchondral bone of the humeral head

asymmetric shoulder drooping and muscle atrophy. The rhythm of active rotation and elevation in different planes is observed for breaks in continuity. The patient is asked to demonstrate any maneuvers that produce roughness, catching, snapping, or locking and to localize the site of the problem by pointing with the opposite finger. Patients are usually quite able to indicate one of the five anatomic sites commonly associated with roughness.

The examiner can help distinguish scapulothoracic roughness from glenohumeral problems or from problems at the humerothoracic motion interface by selectively restricting the motion first at one site and then the other. Shrugging, protracting, and retracting the scapula while the examiner disallows glenohumeral motion permits independent assessment of the smoothness of the scapulothoracic motion interface. Palpation for the site of roughness may localize the problem to the superior medial border of the

spine of the scapula. Alternatively, rotating and elevating the arm while the examiner stabilizes the clavicle, acromion, and scapular spine on the chest wall allows independent evaluation of the glenohumeral joint and the humeroscapular motion interface. Roughness in the subacromial area of the non-articular humeroscapular motion interface is usually manifested on rotation of the arm near 90 degrees of humerothoracic elevation, a position in which the capsule is normally lax. Crepitance on this maneuver, which reproduces the patient's complaint, constitutes a positive subacromial "abrasion sign." Roughness between the subscapularis insertion and the short head of the biceps is evident on rotation of the arm at the side while the biceps is isometrically tightened. Crepitance at the glenohumeral joint is often best palpated posteriorly just beneath the angle of the acromion. It may be accentuated by pressing the humerus toward the glenoid while the joint is rotated. Symptoms from

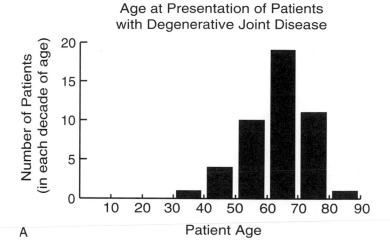

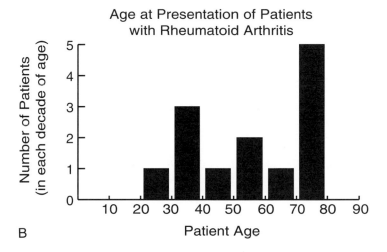

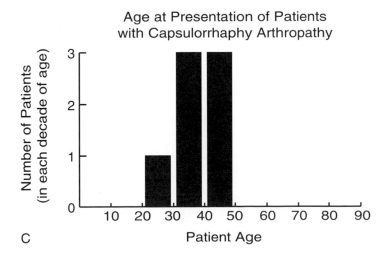

FIGURE 5–3.

Distribution of the age at presentation for patients with the following conditions: *A*, Degenerative joint disease; *B*, Rheumatoid arthritis; *C*, Capsulorrhaphy arthropathy;

Illustration continued on following page

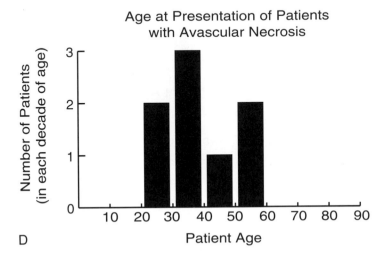

Age at Presentation of Patients with Avascular Necrosis

D

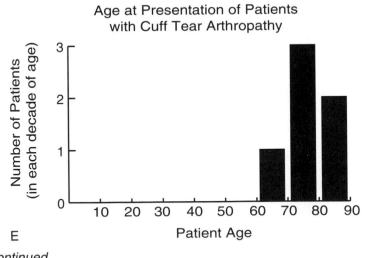

Age at Presentation of Patients with Cuff Tear Arthropathy

E

FIGURE 5–3 *Continued*

D, Avascular necrosis; and *E*, Cuff tear arthropathy.

the sternoclavicular or acromioclavicular joints are usually easy to localize on physical examination.

The tenor of the noise, as well as its location, gives a clue to its etiology. For example, a snapping scapula usually produces a low-pitched clunking, similar to the noise produced when two sets of knuckles are rubbed against each other. Subacromial abrasion usually produces a higher-pitched crepitance, like the sound of wadding up a piece of paper. Dry, bone-on-bone grating is typical of roughness of the glenohumeral articular cartilage, producing a grating like sandpaper on wood.

Because shoulder roughness may be accompanied by shoulder stiffness and weakness, the range of glenohumeral and scapulothoracic motion and the strength of the shoulder motors should be recorded as described in Chapters 2 and 4.

Radiographs

The history and physical examination should point to the likely cause and the functional significance of the roughness. The clinical examination suggests which radiographs may be helpful. Thus, the radiographic evaluation is customized to the patient's clinical presentation rather than ordered as part of a routine.

Scapulothoracic roughness should be evaluated by an anteroposterior view in the plane of the scapula and by a lateral view in the plane of the scapula (Fig. 5–4) to reveal osteochondromata or malunited fractures of the scapula or ribs. CT scanning can help localize the sites of specific entities but is of minimal value in evaluating a snapping scapula resulting from abnormal posture.

A coned-down view of the acromioclavicular joint and an axillary radiograph provide a good two-plane evaluation of this articulation.

Sternoclavicular roughness can be best evaluated with a CT scan.

The glenohumeral joint is radiographed using an anteroposterior view in the plane of the scapula and a true axillary view. If the arm is placed in the "centered position" (Fig. 5–5), the middle of the humeral articular surface is in the middle of the glenoid fossa. An anteroposterior view and an axillary view taken with the arm in this centered position provide excellent opportunities to evaluate the thickness of the cartilage space

(A)

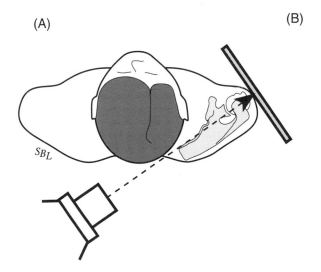

(B)

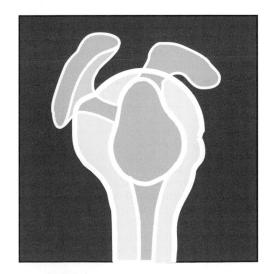

FIGURE 5–4.

Radiographic technique for scapular lateral view. *A,* In this view, the cassette is placed at the anterolateral humerus at right angles to the plane of the scapula. The radiographic beam is parallel to the scapular spine and aimed at the humeral head from medial to lateral. *B,* A representation of the resulting scapular lateral radiograph.

(A)

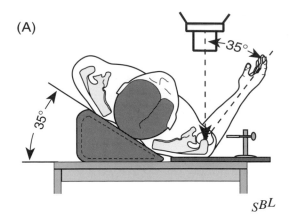

(B)

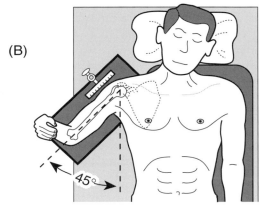

(C)

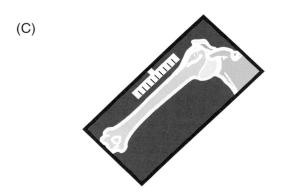

FIGURE 5–5.

Anteroposterior radiograph in the "centered position." The humerus is positioned in neutral rotation with respect to the thorax and abducted 45 degrees. The anteroposterior radiograph in the plane of the scapula is obtained by positioning the scapula flat on the cassette and aiming the beam at the joint. The beam makes a 35-degree angle with the forearm, and the thorax makes a 35-degree angle with the cassette. A centimeter marker held adjacent to the lateral humerus helps correct for radiographic magnification. The final radiographic appearance is as shown in *C*.

between the subchondral bone of the humerus and that of the glenoid, to assess the regularity of the subchondral bone, and to evaluate any translation of the head of the humerus relative to the glenoid. The anteroposterior radiograph taken in the scapular plane with the arm in the centered position places the humeral neck in maximal profile, which is required for accurate use of a humeral prosthesis template.

Fortuitously, the anatomy of the proximal humerus and the relationship of the scapula on the chest wall make it possible to obtain radiographs that reveal simultaneously the profile of the proximal humerus and the glenoid. Because this view centers the head of the humerus on the glenoid, it also is the projection most likely to reveal the thinning of the central aspect of the humeral articular cartilage typical of degenerative joint disease (the Friar Tuck pattern), whereas radiographs with the arm in other positions may indicate the presence of a thicker layer of cartilage at the periphery of the head.

The relevant anatomy is straightforward. The plane of the scapula makes a 35 degree angle with the plane of the thorax. The humeral neck is in 35 degrees of retroversion with respect to the forearm of the flexed elbow. The humeral neck is also at 45 degrees with the long axis of the humeral shaft. Thus, if the forearm of the flexed elbow is perpendicular to the plane of the thorax and if the humerus is abducted 45 degrees, the center of the humeral head is pointed at the center of the glenoid. With the arm in this position, an anteroposterior radiograph in the plane of the scapula will reveal the desired relationships (see Fig. 5–5).

In degenerative joint disease, these radiographs typically show narrowing of the cartilage space between the humeral head and the glenoid, sclerosis, osteophyte formation, and a posterior wear pattern in which the humeral head is posteriorly subluxated in association with erosion of the posterior half of the glenoid. In avascular necrosis, the predominant radiographic finding is collapse of the subchondral bone of the head of the humerus. In advanced rheumatoid arthritis, the predominant findings usually include loss of the cartilage space between the humerus and the glenoid, erosions at the margins of the humeral articular surfaces, medial erosion of the glenoid, and generalized osteopenia; these changes are often symmetric, affecting both glenohumeral joints.

The bony anatomy of the humeroscapular motion interface can be seen on the anteroposterior view in the plane of the scapula, the lateral view of the scapula, and the axillary view. These radiographs may reveal a narrowed radiographic acromiohumeral interval, sclerosis of the undersurface of the acromion, acromial anomalies, traction spurs in the coracoacromial ligament, and malunited or non-united fractures of the acromion. These views may demonstrate other potential causes of roughness in the non-articular humeroscapular motion interface, such as anomalies of the proximal humerus, malunited tuberosity fractures, and functionally significant calcium deposits in the cuff tendons. We have not found the shape of the acromion itself to be useful for separating those shoulders having subacromial roughness from those that do not.

Imaging of the rotator cuff is only carried out if it will affect management of the patient. If the patient meets our criteria for exploration of the subacromial space, as described later, we will usually avoid cuff imaging because we will be able to evaluate the cuff directly at surgery and will have obtained preoperatively the patient's permission to perform any indicated cuff surgery.

Functional Effects of Loss of Smoothness

Using the Simple Shoulder Test (SST; see Chapter 1), we collected data on the functional effects of some common causes of shoulder roughness when patients presented for evaluation (Fig. 5–6).

GENERAL PRINCIPLES OF TREATMENT

Because shoulder roughness is usually of insidious onset, there is usually a good opportunity to try non-operative management. Unless the diagnostic evaluation dictates otherwise, the patient is reassured that crepitus and occasional catching do not mandate surgical intervention. For many of the causes of shoulder roughness, a general exercise program to optimize shoulder mechanics is appropriate (see Patient Information 5–1). This program is designed to minimize shoulder stiffness and to optimize posture and strength.

Roughness at the Scapulothoracic Motion Interface

Rarely, roughness in the scapulothoracic motion interface is caused by an anatomic abnormality such as a malunited fracture or an osteochondroma on the anterior undersurface of the scapula. These unusual causes can often be diagnosed on a lateral radiograph of the scapula. Most commonly, scapulothoracic crepitus, or "snapping scapula," is caused by altered scapulothoracic posture and mechanics. Using a skeleton, the clinician can demonstrate to the patient how drooping of the scapula produces contact between the superior medial angle of the scapula and the rib cage. Thus, the primary treatment of this condition is reassurance, restoration of normal posture, and strengthening of the serratus anterior, subscapularis, trapezius, and rhomboids. It is essential that the patient avoid voluntary or habitual scapulothoracic snapping.

More aggressive treatment is considered only in the rare patient who has functionally significant, involuntary, non-vocationally related scapulothoracic snapping that has failed to respond to a prolonged, non-operative management program. Refractory cases of snapping scapula may respond to local injection, to bursal resection, or to resection of the superior medial angle of the scapula. Because these procedures do not treat the primary problem of altered scapulothoracic posture, failure to achieve improved shoulder function is not infrequent. Complications of surgery can be related to failure to reattach securely the muscles inserting on the superior medial angle of the scapula, to injury to the nerve to the lower trapezius, to leaving residual prominent edges of the scapula, and to scarring in the scapulothoracic motion interface.

Text continued on page 176

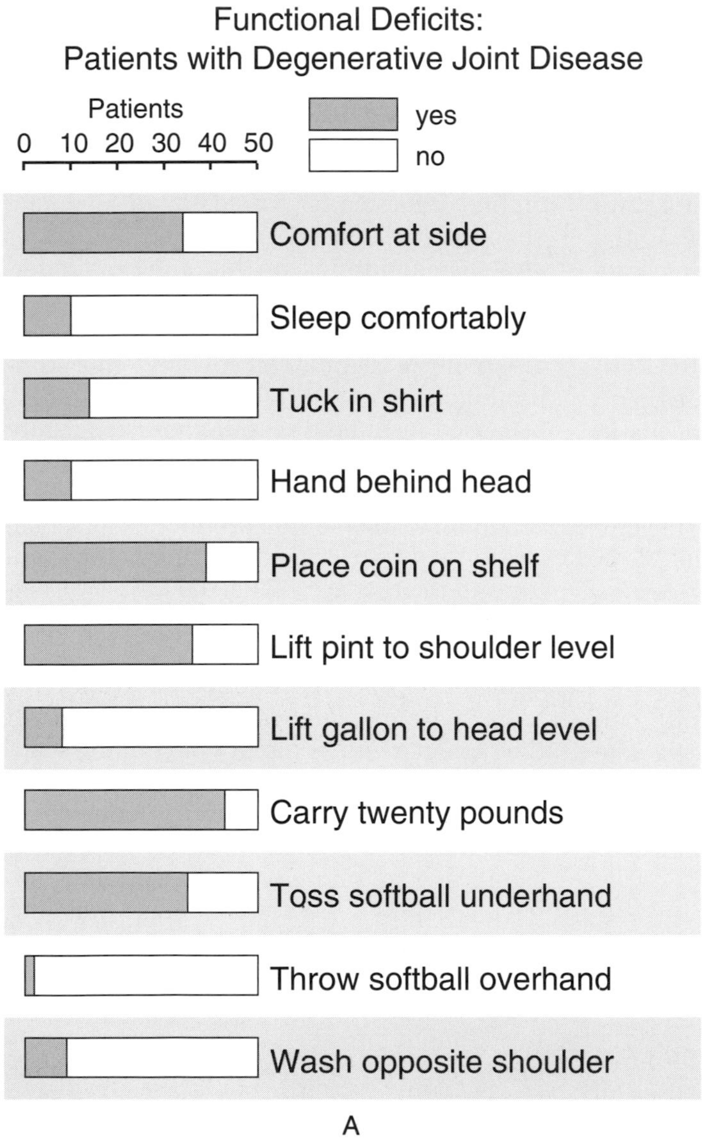

Functional Deficits:
Patients with Degenerative Joint Disease

Patients | yes
0 10 20 30 40 50 | no

Comfort at side

Sleep comfortably

Tuck in shirt

Hand behind head

Place coin on shelf

Lift pint to shoulder level

Lift gallon to head level

Carry twenty pounds

Toss softball underhand

Throw softball overhand

Wash opposite shoulder

A

FIGURE 5–6.

The functional deficits of patients with conditions of shoulder roughness indicated by the Simple Shoulder Test results at the time of presentation. *A*, Degenerative joint disease.

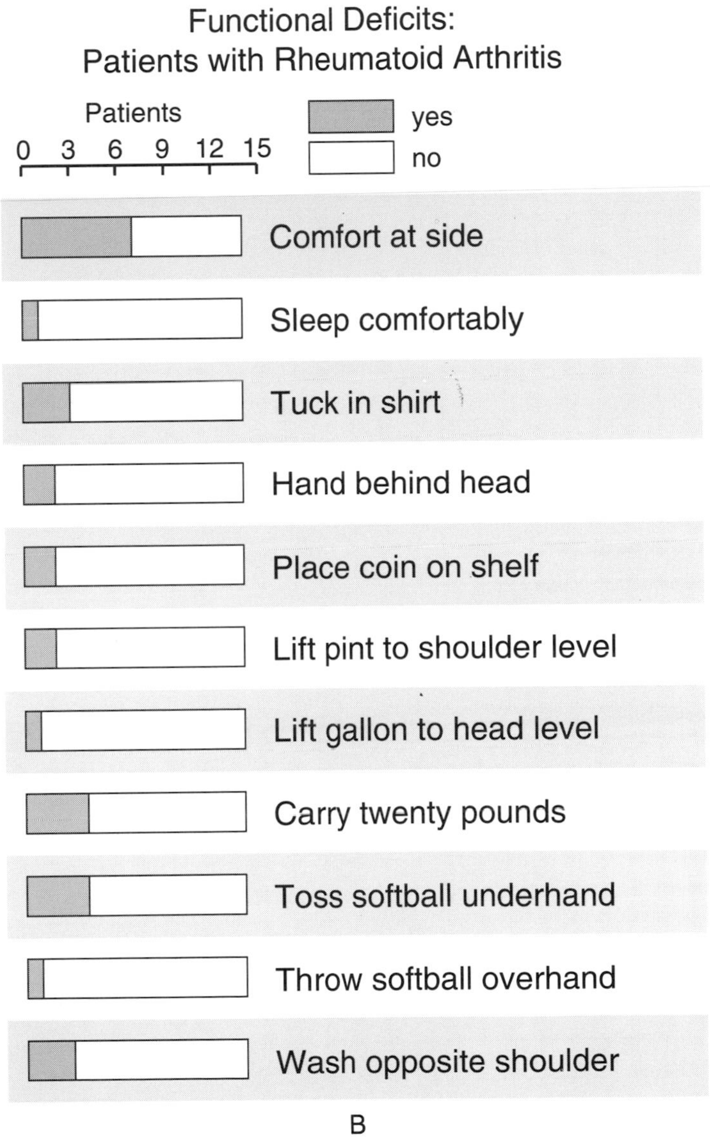

FIGURE 5–6 *Continued*

B, Rheumatoid arthritis.

Functional Deficits:
Patients with Rheumatoid Arthritis

Patients

0 3 6 9 12 15

yes

no

Comfort at side

Sleep comfortably

Tuck in shirt

Hand behind head

Place coin on shelf

Lift pint to shoulder level

Lift gallon to head level

Carry twenty pounds

Toss softball underhand

Throw softball overhand

Wash opposite shoulder

B

Illustration continued on following page

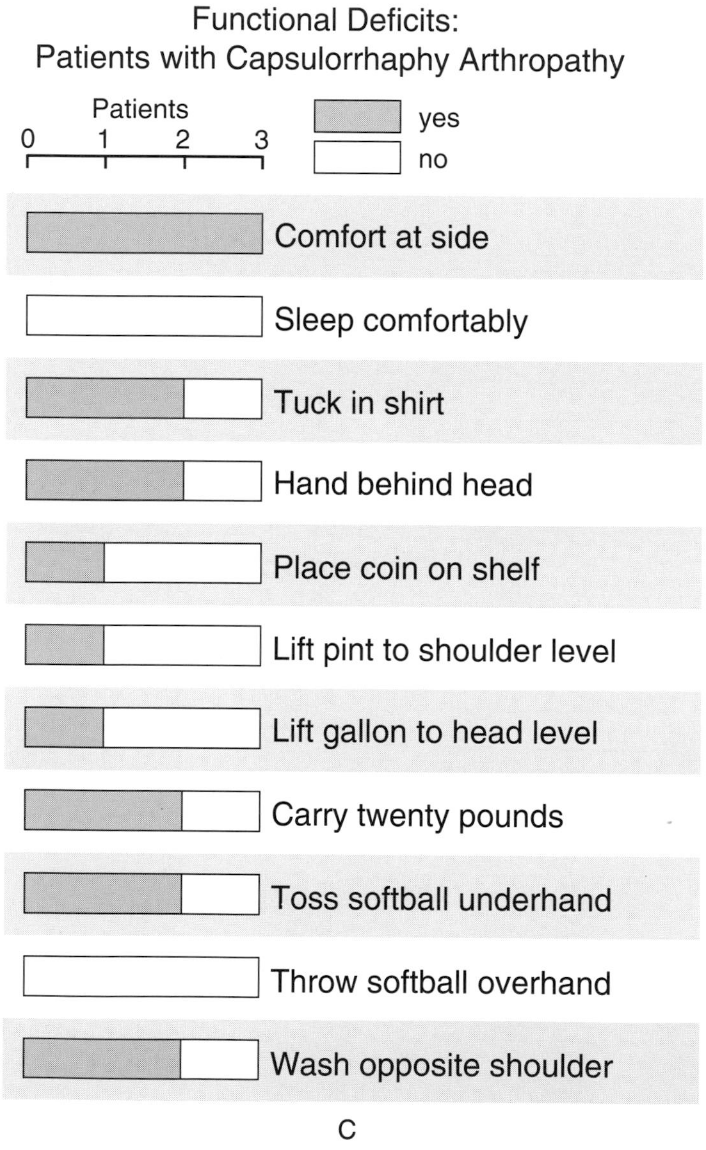

Functional Deficits:
Patients with Capsulorrhaphy Arthropathy

Patients

0   1   2   3

□ yes
□ no

Comfort at side

Sleep comfortably

Tuck in shirt

Hand behind head

Place coin on shelf

Lift pint to shoulder level

Lift gallon to head level

Carry twenty pounds

Toss softball underhand

Throw softball overhand

Wash opposite shoulder

C

FIGURE 5–6 *Continued*

C, Capsulorrhaphy arthropathy.

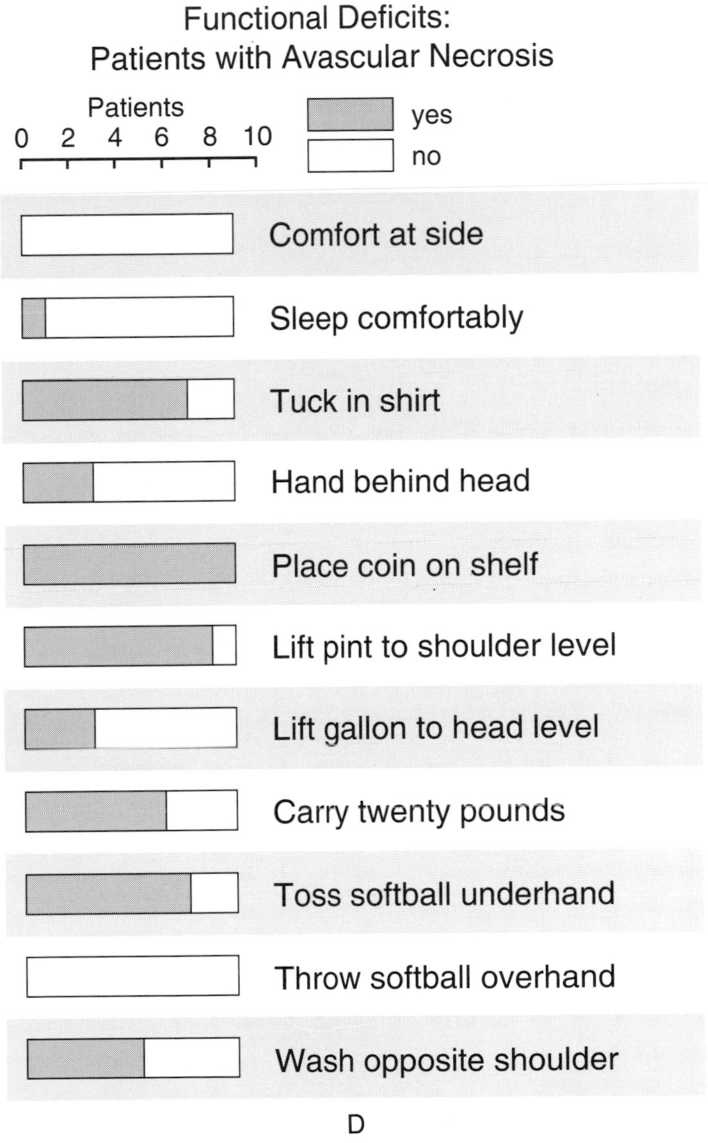

FIGURE 5–6 *Continued*

D, Avascular necrosis.

Functional Deficits:
Patients with Avascular Necrosis

Patients
0 2 4 6 8 10

yes
no

Comfort at side

Sleep comfortably

Tuck in shirt

Hand behind head

Place coin on shelf

Lift pint to shoulder level

Lift gallon to head level

Carry twenty pounds

Toss softball underhand

Throw softball overhand

Wash opposite shoulder

D

Illustration continued on following page

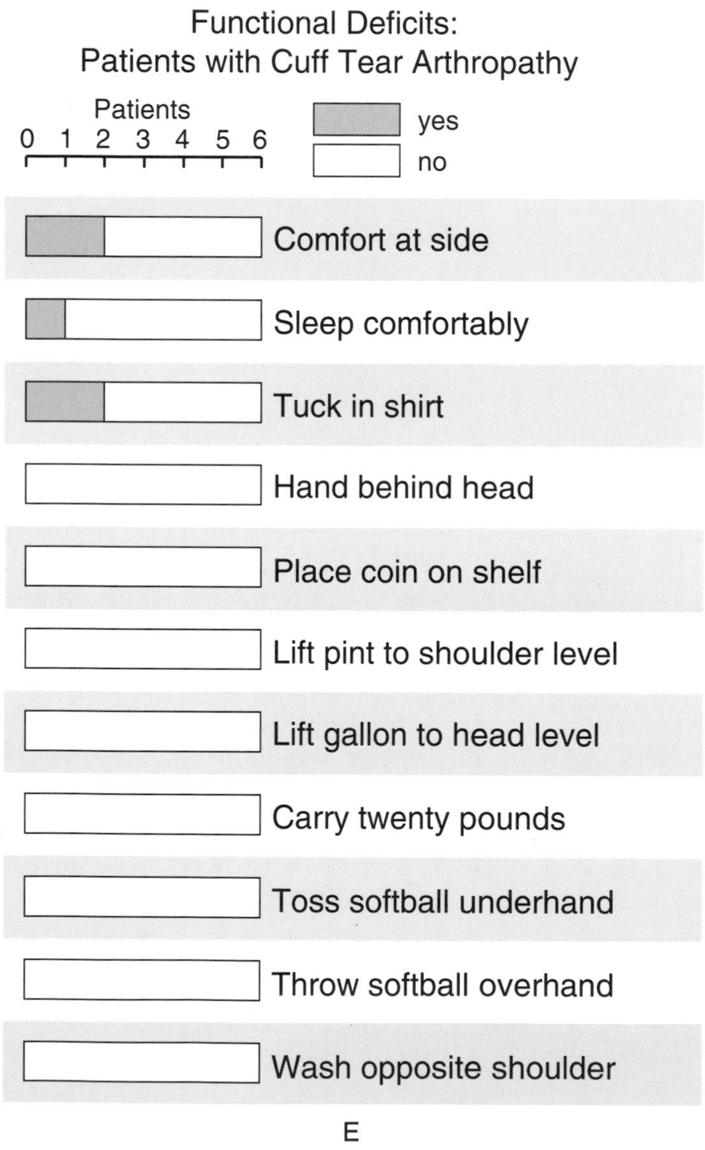

Functional Deficits:
Patients with Cuff Tear Arthropathy

Patients
0 1 2 3 4 5 6

yes
no

Comfort at side

Sleep comfortably

Tuck in shirt

Hand behind head

Place coin on shelf

Lift pint to shoulder level

Lift gallon to head level

Carry twenty pounds

Toss softball underhand

Throw softball overhand

Wash opposite shoulder

E

FIGURE 5–6 *Continued*

E, Cuff tear arthropathy.

PATIENT INFORMATION 5–1

UNIVERSITY OF WASHINGTON SHOULDER AND ELBOW SERVICE

Home Exercise Program for the Rough Shoulder

Shoulders can lose their normal smoothness of motion for a wide variety of reasons. In many situations the roughness is related to tightness of the soft tissues around the joint, to abnormal posture, or to shoulder weakness. Normally, the shoulder is flexible, allowing the shoulder to maintain its usually large range of motion. Should tissues become thickened or scarred, they lose their normal resilience, suppleness, strength, and smoothness. Even if you have had an injury, or if there is some arthritis in your shoulder, it is likely that you can benefit from a simple home program to optimize your shoulder's comfort and function.

There are three components to the home program for rough shoulders. The first is a series of stretching exercises, the second involves posture and strengthening, and the third relates to regular participation in a fitness program.

STRETCHING. Your opposite arm is a great therapist for your rough shoulder. Your "therapist arm" is always available to apply a gentle stretch in any direction of tightness. Each of these gentle stretches needs to be held up to a count of 100. The basic program includes four directions of stretching

1. Overhead reach of the arm.
2. External rotation of the arm at the side.
3. Reaching up the back.
4. Reaching across the body.

If other directions of stiffness are identified, they can be stretched with a similar approach. An important principle of the stretching exercises is to allow your muscles to relax so that the stretch can be applied to the soft tissues without muscle interference. Tissues of a tight shoulder do not like to be stretched suddenly, roughly, or with a lot of force. Thus, the strategy is to apply a gentle stretch so that, at most, minimal soreness results. Any soreness should go away within 15 minutes after you stop the exercises.

Overhead reach is stretched by helping to lift your stiff arm up as high as it will go. Lie flat on your back; relax, and grasp the wrist of the tight shoulder with your opposite hand. Using the power in your opposite arm, bring the stiff arm up as far as it is comfortable. Start holding it for 10 seconds and then work up to a count of 100. Breathe slowly and deeply while the arm is moved. Repeat this stretch three times, trying to help the arm up a little higher each time (Fig. 5–7).

An alternative method of stretching to overhead reach is to use the "progressive forward lean." Sit so that a table, shelf, armchair back, or other fixed object supports your arm in a comfortable amount of elevation in overhead reach. Then, by leaning forward, allow the fixed object to apply a gentle, upward-directed force on the arm for a count of 100. The advantage of this method is that it does not require the help of the other arm and it can be sustained for several minutes (Fig. 5–8).

External rotation is stretched by turning the stiff arm out to the side while your elbow stays close to your body. Lie on your back, holding a cane, yardstick, broom handle, or umbrella in both hands. Bend both elbows to a right angle. Use steady, gentle force from your normal arm to rotate the hand of the stiff shoulder out away from your body, keeping your elbow at your side. Continue the rotation as far as it will go comfortably. Work up to holding it there for a count of 100. Repeat this exercise three times (Fig. 5–9).

An alternative method of stretching in

167

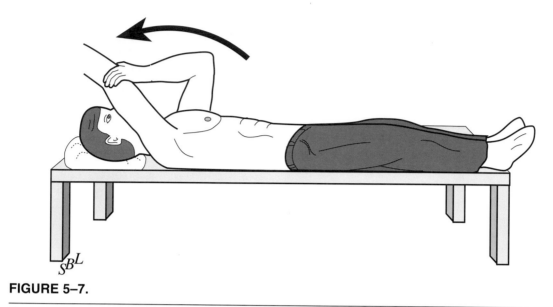

FIGURE 5–7.

Stretching in overhead reach using the opposite arm as the "therapist."

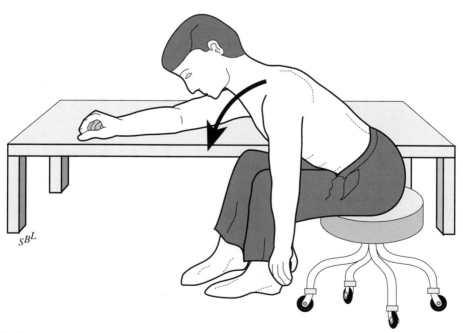

FIGURE 5–8.

Stretching in overhead reach using the progressive forward lean to apply a gentle force to the arm.

168

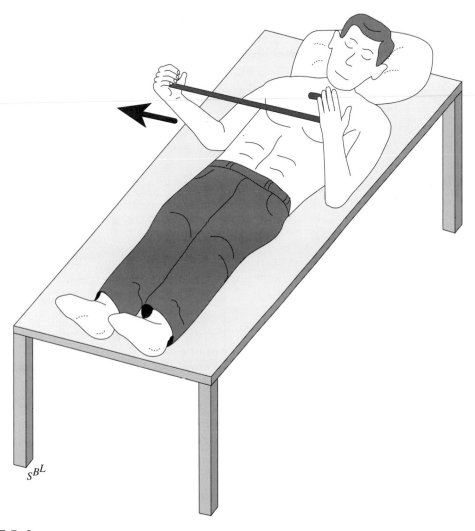

FIGURE 5–9.

Stretching in external rotation using the opposite hand as the "therapist."

external rotation is to hold onto a fixed object and gently turn your body away while holding your elbow at the side. The advantage of this method is that it does not require the help of the other arm and it can be sustained for several minutes (Fig. 5–10).

Internal rotation is stretched by reaching up your back. Grasp a towel behind your back in both hands. Gently pull the hand of the stiff shoulder up your back. Work up to holding the maximum comfortable stretch for a count of 100. Repeat the exercise three times (Fig. 5–11).

An alternative method of stretching in internal rotation is to hold onto a fixed object behind you with your hand as high up

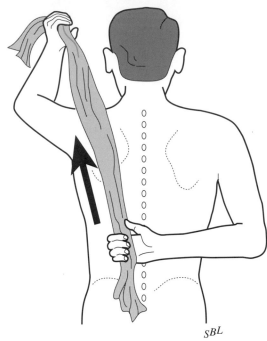

FIGURE 5–11.

Stretching in internal rotation using a towel to apply a gentle stretching force.

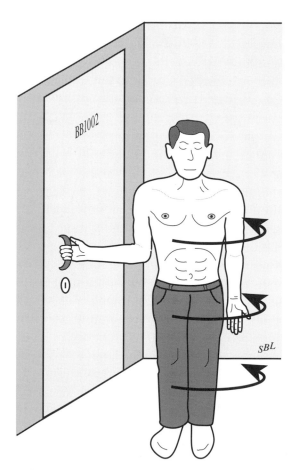

FIGURE 5–10.

Stretching in external rotation by turning the body away from a fixed object to apply a gentle stretching force.

your back as it will easily reach. Then, by bending your knees, a gentle stretching force can be applied and sustained for a count of 100.

Cross-body reach is stretched by reaching across your chest so that your elbow approaches your opposite shoulder. Grasp the elbow of the stiff shoulder in your opposite hand, and pull it toward the opposite shoulder. Work up to holding the maximum comfortable stretch for a count of 100. Repeat the exercise three times (Fig. 5–12).

You should carry out this shoulder-stretching sequence three times a day. As much as possible, these sessions should be performed after the shoulder has been relaxed by a hot shower, bath, or aerobic exercise. For each stretch, make a note of the maximum range obtained with each session. Try to establish a new "bench mark" each time, so that you can see your progress each time.

170

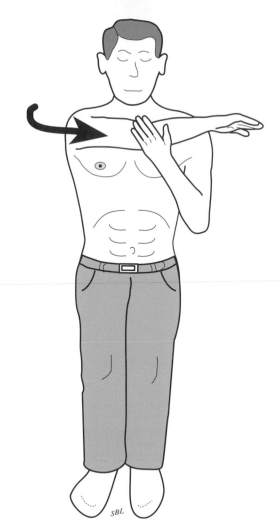

FIGURE 5–12.

Stretching in cross-body reach using the opposite arm as the "therapist."

POSTURE AND STRENGTHENING. Shoulders require good muscle strength and posture. The rotator cuff muscles are important shoulder muscles because they hold the ball properly aligned in the socket. They are strengthened by working against resistance in rotation internally (toward the body) and externally (away from the body). It is important that your shoulder have both strength and endurance of internal and external rotation. This means that you need to carry out at least five exercise sessions each day, each tak-

ing only about 5 minutes. Internal rotation is strengthened by holding the elbow close to the side and trying to rotate the arm inward against resistance. This resistance can be isometric (unmoving), such as the opposite hand, a wall, or another fixed object. You can also use dynamic exercises against rubber tubing, weights and pulleys, or free weights while you lie on your side (Fig. 5–13). External rotation is strengthened by holding the elbow at the side and trying to rotate the arm outward against either isometric or dynamic resistance (Fig. 5–14).

A second important group of muscles, the scapular muscles, are those that control the posture of your shoulder blade on the chest wall. The purpose of these exercises is to strengthen these scapular muscles and to eliminate bad habits or posture that your shoulder may have developed. The largest and most important muscle groups are those that move your shoulder blade forward (the serratus and pectoralis) and those that lift the shoulder blade (the trapezius, levator scapulae, and rhomboids). The first group of muscles is strengthened by a bench press–type exercise performed while you lie on your back holding a weight bar alone. At first, only the bar is used while you concentrate on powering the shoulder blade upward. When you lift your shoulder blade off the bed or table, we call this the "press plus." The "plus" is important for training the shoulder blade muscles. Once you can control the bar alone for twenty repetitions, add weight to the bar progressively up to about half your body weight. Never use a weight heavier than what you can control for twenty repetitions. Once you feel confident in the shoulder, you can start doing a one hand press using a 1 lb weight and building up to 20 percent of your body weight (Fig. 5–15).

The second muscle group helps strengthen your shoulder during lifting at the side. Start with a simple shoulder

(A)

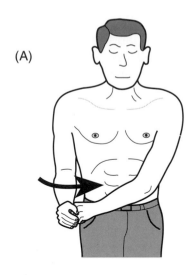

(B)

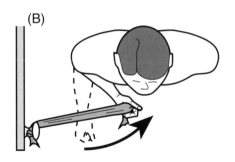

FIGURE 5–13.

Internal rotation can be strengthened with isometrics *(A)*, rubber tubing *(B)*, or free weights *(C)*.

(C)

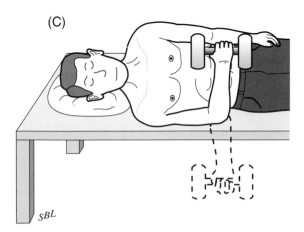

SBL

172

(A)

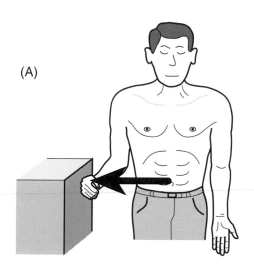

(B)

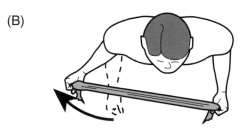

FIGURE 5–14.

External rotation strengthening using isometrics *(A)*, rubber tubing *(B)*, or free weights *(C)*.

(C)

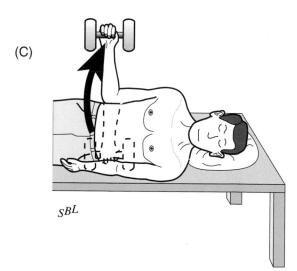

SBL

173

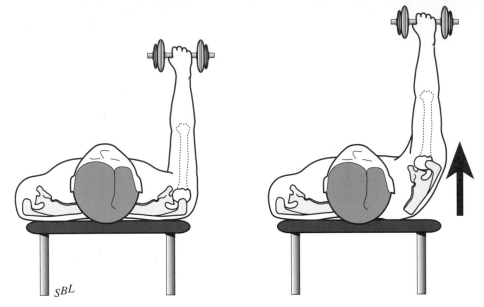

FIGURE 5–15.

In the press plus, the arm is pushed upward until the shoulder blade is lifted off the table or bed.

shrug, lifting the point of your shoulder as high as it will go twenty times. Once the shoulder shrug becomes easy, add weight 1 lb at a time, keeping the number of repetitions at twenty. With each shrug, concentrate on lifting the tip of the shoulder (Fig. 5–16).

As you gain strength and coordination, try to carry out progressively more of your usual activities, concentrating on using smooth motions. Try to avoid actions that make your shoulder pop, snap, or catch. Swimming, rowing, and using cross-country ski simulators are all good exercises for developing strength, coordination, and endurance. They also have the advantage of exercising both shoulders at the same time.

FITNESS PROGRAM. Regular fitness exercise helps keep your joints supple. This "lubricating" effect is optimized if you perform a half-hour of aerobic exercise each day. This exercise may take a variety of forms, including brisk walking, jogging, riding a stationary or mobile bicycle, rowing, climbing stairs, or using a cross-coun-

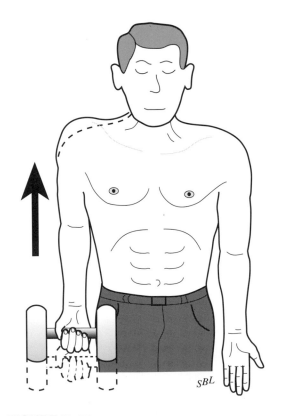

FIGURE 5–16.

The shoulder shrug exercise: lift the tip of the shoulder toward the ear while holding the elbow straight.

174

try ski simulator. If you have concerns about your ability to carry out such an exercise program, you should consult your general physician. It is not important that these exercises be carried out vigorously; it is only important that, in addition to the stretching and strengthening program, a half-hour of your day be devoted toward some form of aerobic exercise.

What if you have already "had therapy?" Our repeated observation is that many patients who have not responded to formal therapy sessions can still improve their shoulder function using a home program in which they are in charge. Remember that your shoulder problem has been present for quite a while. Improvement in your range of motion, strength, smoothness, and comfort may not be noticeable until 6 weeks of persistence with the program.

We have found that medication is not very helpful in managing rough shoulders. Mild analgesics (such as aspirin, ibuprofen, and acetaminophen) may be used in conjunction with this program, if desired. Narcotic medications, "muscle relaxants," and sleeping pills have not proved helpful to our patients.

We encourage you to use your shoulder actively within the range of comfort. For example, if you can do some water exercises or swimming without aggravating the shoulder, please do so. On the other hand, activities that produce shoulder pain should be avoided.

We hope this program is easy for you to understand and carry out. If you have any problems or questions, please let us know.

Roughness at the Non-articular Humeroscapular Motion Interface

Crepitus on moving the humerus with respect to the deltoid and the coracoacromial arch is quite common and often of little functional significance; some form of subacromial roughness can be found in most adult shoulders. Occasionally, patients demonstrate compromised smoothness of various aspects of the humeroscapular motion interface after injury or surgery, for example, roughness at the site of surgical reattachment of the subscapularis as it passes beneath the coracoid muscles on rotation.

In patients with functionally significant roughness of the non-articular humeroscapular motion interface, the aim of non-operative management is to restore normal kinematics. The first goal is flexibility, eliminating adhesions or posterior capsular tightness that may cause obligate anterosuperior humeral translation and subacromial abrasion (see Fig. 2–28). As flexibility is improved, attention is also directed at optimizing the normal stabilizing effect of the rotator cuff musculature by strengthening exercises, emphasizing internal and external rotation strength and endurance.

If a persistent and proper rehabilitation effort fails to restore functional humeroscapular smoothness, consideration may be given to a surgical approach to the problem. Surgical smoothing is likely to be of functional benefit only if the patient's functional problem can be clearly localized. This procedure is not appropriate for shoulder pain that is poorly defined, cuff strain, partial thickness cuff tears, or shoulder stiffness. If stiffness is not resolved preoperatively, subacromial surgery is likely to make the shoulder function worse. We have found that surgical treatment of subacromial roughness is most likely to be successful in a well-motivated patient older than 40 years of age whose problem has been refractory to a good home program effort and who has a positive "abrasion" sign (rotation of the arm elevated to the horizontal position reproduces the crepitance that the patient recognizes as the primary problem in his or her shoulder).

Before this surgery the patient needs to understand what the procedure may or may not accomplish. Patient Information 5–2 outlines the information that may be provided to the patient.

Surgical Approach to Roughness at the Non-articular Humeroscapular Motion Interface

The surgical approach to roughness in the humeroscapular motion interface must be guided by the location of the problem. A shoulder having roughness after previous surgery is generally approached through the previous incision because this provides best access to the postoperative scar. Prior to the incision, the passive motion of the shoulder is verified under anesthesia. If tightness is identified, the approach may need to be modified to allow appropriate releases, as described in Chapter 2.

Previously unoperated shoulders with positive subacromial abrasion signs are approached through an anterosuperior acromioplasty approach. The incision is in the skin lines, crossing the anterior corner of the acromion and ending just lateral to the coracoid process. The deltoid muscle is split in line with its fibers through the middle of the tendons, separating its anterior and middle thirds, preserving the continuity of the tendinous fibers of origin with the muscle (see Fig. 4–32). The subdeltoid bursa on the deep surface of this muscle is entered. Thickened bursa is resected to help smooth the space and to allow inspection of the subjacent rotator cuff. An evaluation of the integrity of the cuff is made at this time. If a cuff defect is present, its reparability is assessed. As emphasized in Chapter 4, a traditional acromioplasty with resection of a substantial amount of the anterior inferior acromion and the coracoacromial ligament must be avoided in the presence of a large irreparable rotator cuff defect. This is because the coracoacromial arch provides needed secondary stability when the primary stabilizing function of the cuff is rendered ineffectual. Thus, when substantial roughness of the non-articular humeroscapular motion interface exists in the presence of an irreparable

PATIENT INFORMATION 5–2

UNIVERSITY OF WASHINGTON SHOULDER AND ELBOW SERVICE

Surgery for Subacromial Roughness

One of the important aspects of shoulder function is the smooth sliding of the upper arm bone (humerus) and the tendons attached to it (the rotator cuff) beneath an arch made of bone and ligaments. This smooth sliding may be interrupted by changes in the mechanics of the joint, by shoulder tightness, by muscle weakness, or by changes in the bone structure. In most instances, much of the function of the shoulder can be regained if you carry out a quality stretching and strengthening exercise program. These exercises are described in a separate information sheet (see Patient Information 5–1).

For shoulders in which a diligent course of quality exercises does not restore a satisfactory level of function, a surgical approach to the area of roughness may be considered. In this surgery, the area between the bone on top of the shoulder and the upper end of the arm bone is smoothed by removing any thickened tissue and prominent bone. Immediately after this procedure, it is essential to perform motion exercises to reestablish full motion and to prevent scar tissue from forming in the area. It is often necessary to open the deltoid muscle to gain access to the affected area. In these instances, it is important to avoid active use of the arm away from your side for 6 weeks after the operation, until this muscle heals.

The procedure is not expected to restore the shoulder to heavy work or to high-level athletics, but it should improve the shoulder's ability to perform activities of daily living, light work, and recreation. Maximal improvement after this procedure may take 6 to 12 months and will require home exercises on your part that are identical to those we recommended before surgery.

The potential complications of this surgery include infection, injury to the nerve to the deltoid muscle, fracture of the bone on top of the shoulder, stiffness, weakness, instability, pain, and the need for a repeat operation. At the time of surgery, other abnormalities may be encountered that need attention, such as a defect in the rotator cuff, bony abnormalities, and calcium deposits. Unless you tell us otherwise, we will do our best to manage whatever abnormalities we encounter.

This procedure is not an emergency. If you have questions concerning it or your underlying surgical condition, please ask us about it before we proceed.

cuff defect, emphasis must be placed on smoothing the contacting surfaces rather than "decompression." Rough edges of the acromion, hypertrophic bursal tissue, prominent tuberosities, previously placed sutures, scar, and irregular edges of cuff tissue are removed to leave the smoothest possible non-articular humeroscapular motion interface. We perform this smoothing sequentially, putting the arm through a complete range of elevation and rotation, identifying bony contact points and then smoothing them down with a burr or rongeur. This process is continued until smoothness and lack of acromiohumeral contact can be verified in all humeroscapular positions. Smoothness of the motion between the anterior aspect of the subscapularis and the deep surface of the muscles originating from the coracoid process must be verified as well.

If the rotator cuff is intact or reparable with good-quality durable tissue, a standard acromioplasty is performed with resection of the anterior undersurface of the acromion and coracoacromial ligament (see Fig. 4–34). Again, the potential areas of contact are examined repeatedly in different positions to ensure that adequate smoothness of the undersurface of the coracoacromial arch and the superficial surface of the rotator cuff and humerus has been achieved. Major cuff defects are repaired securely after appropriate releases so that the cuff is under physiologic tension with the arm at the side. Because the primary goal of the procedure is to regain smooth motion, any repair must be sufficiently strong to allow immediate postoperative passive ranging of the shoulder. Again, before closing, the shoulder is put through a complete range of motion to verify smoothness of the non-articular humeroscapular motion interface, in both the subacromial and coracoid areas.

The deltoid is repaired securely (see Fig. 4–33) so that immediate postoperative motion can be established. We hypothesize that immediate postoperative passive motion induces the undifferentiated cells in the surgical site to generate a smooth new motion interface rather than irregular and adherent opposing surfaces. For this reason we use immediate postoperative continuous passive

motion in the post anesthesia care unit and continue it until the patient can carry out his or her mobilization program without assistance.

At present, "failed acromioplasty" is a common condition among patients referred to our shoulder service. Postacromioplasty complaints often include (1) no improvement, (2) increased pain, (3) loss of anterior deltoid strength, (4) increased stiffness, and (5) anterosuperior instability. These failed open or arthroscopic acromioplasties were usually performed for a preoperative diagnosis listed as "impingement syndrome." However, a careful history often suggests other diagnoses, such as a partially frozen shoulder, cuff strain, partial cuff tears, and non-specific shoulder pain. Thus, these failures seem to be the result of (1) performing an acromioplasty for non-specific shoulder symptoms; (2) performing an acromioplasty in the presence of shoulder stiffness; (3) failing to institute immediate postoperative motion, allowing for subacromial scarring; (4) failing to manage rotator cuff pathologic changes; (5) failing to ensure a strong deltoid reattachment to the acromion; or (6) performing a technically poor acromioplasty in which either an excessive amount of acromion was removed, the acromion was transected, or an irregular undersurface of the acromion was left as a new and persisting cause of roughness in the non-articular humeroscapular motion interface.

Roughness at the Glenohumeral Joint

Roughness of the glenohumeral joint surface is commonly accompanied by stiffness related to contracture and adhesions involving the glenohumeral capsule, the cuff muscles, and the non-articular humeroscapular motion interface. Weakness of the cuff muscles results from disuse or fiber failure. Finally, instability patterns may also complicate glenohumeral roughness, such as the posterior subluxation characteristic of degenerative joint disease and capsulorrhaphy arthropathy or the superior subluxation characteristic of cuff tear arthropathy. Thus, the management of glenohumeral roughness provides an opportunity to combine all available knowledge about the shoulder in formulating the best treatment plan for the patient. Ultimately, surgery offers the opportunity to optimize capsular laxity and muscle mechanics, as well as joint surface smoothness, size, shape, and orientation.

In the early stages of glenohumeral roughness, the mechanics of the shoulder can be optimized by patient-conducted gentle range of motion and strengthening exercises described earlier in this chapter. It is important that vigorous torques and forces not be applied in an attempt to regain motion because of the concern for causing obligate translation and accelerated wear.

Surgery is considered for well-informed, well-motivated, cooperative, healthy patients with functionally significant glenohumeral roughness that is not responsive to the home exercise program. Four procedures can be considered.

Glenohumeral arthrodesis is usually reserved for attempts at salvaging septic arthritis or complex deficiencies of the joint surface associated with permanent loss of the cuff and deltoid (see Chapter 4). The remaining procedures include *non-prosthetic arthroplasty, humeral hemiarthroplasty,* and *glenohumeral arthroplasty.*

Non-prosthetic arthroplasty is considered for the uncommon young shoulder demonstrating early glenohumeral joint surface roughness. Even though such a shoulder may have a tight anterior capsule and glenohumeral osteophytes, it may also have substantial remaining articular cartilage and no posterior subluxation of the head on the glenoid. In this circumstance, a capsular release and thorough osteophyte resection anteriorly, inferiorly, and posteriorly may help restore smoothness and motion. The technique of soft tissue release is essentially the same as that described in Chapter 2 for frozen shoulder. Postoperative management is the same as for prosthetic arthroplasty.

Prosthetic humeral hemiarthroplasty is considered in four circumstances: (1) if the humeral joint surface is rough, but the cartilaginous surface of the glenoid is intact; (2) if there is insufficient bone to support a glenoid component (for example, after severe medial erosion of the glenoid in rheumatoid arthritis); (3) if there is fixed upward displacement of the humeral head in relation to the glenoid in association with massive cuff deficiency; and (4) if extraordinary demands will be placed on the shoulder that would increase the risk of glenoid component complications (such as motion disorders and paralysis of the lower extremities).

Glenohumeral prosthetic arthroplasty is considered in patients who understand the risks and limitations of this procedure and who have sufficient bone stock, stability, and muscle control.

Capsular release, subscapularis lengthening, and freeing of the non-articular humeroscapular motion interface are usually incorporated in each of these three types of arthroplasty. The technical demands of these procedures are high because of the critical interplay between the pathoanatomy, the amount of bone resected, the soft tissue balancing, the size and positioning of the components, and the quality of the bone and soft tissues.

Contraindications to arthroplasty include an active or recent shoulder infection and major loss of deltoid function. Other factors lessen the chances of a good result: a history of remote infection, defects in the rotator cuff, compromise of the deltoid, tuberosity non-union or malunion, poor quality of tissues, history of smoking or narcotic use, previous shoulder surgery, previous shoulder trauma, neurotrophic arthropathy, unrealistic patient expectations, and poor patient motivation.

Patients who are well informed and motivated prior to shoulder reconstruction are more likely to obtain an optimal result. The realistic goals of glenohumeral arthroplasty for a given shoulder should be discussed with the patient. Prosthetic arthroplasty is not recommended for patients who intend to return to occupational or recreational activities that apply sudden impact or heavy loads to the joint. Such persons should be counseled to delay the procedure, consider an alternative reconstructive operation, or alter their lifestyle to accommodate more appropriately a prosthetic arthroplasty.

Patient Information 5–3 details some of

PATIENT INFORMATION 5–3

UNIVERSITY OF WASHINGTON SHOULDER AND ELBOW SERVICE

Surgery for Joint Surface Roughness

Like all of the major joints of the body, the shoulder is subject to loss of the smooth cartilage that normally provides a smooth bearing surface for movement. Under selected circumstances, severe loss of joint surface smoothness can be improved by an artificial joint surface replacement. This procedure is a major one and is undertaken only when joint surface roughness leads to severe loss of function. The quality of the result is determined by the underlying condition of the joint, the surgical technique, and your rehabilitative effort.

The procedure cannot make your shoulder normal. After this procedure, you should avoid heavy use of the shoulder. However, gentle repetitive activities such as swimming are often well tolerated. The tendons and muscles about the shoulder are weakened from prolonged disuse; thus, slow, gentle rehabilitation is needed. We have found that the most successful approach to rehabilitation is for us to teach you some simple postoperative exercises and for you to take the responsibility for doing them on a daily schedule. This program is continued for a long time after surgery: it may take 1 to 2 years before your shoulder has achieved maximal improvement from the procedure.

The alternatives to this surgery include having no surgery, a release of the tight tissues without joint replacement, cutting out the joint, and fusing the joint. We may need to alter our plan based on the findings at surgery: sometimes we do not proceed with any joint replacement, and at other times we undertake only a partial joint replacement. At surgery, muscles and other tissues about the shoulder are cut, tightened, and loosened to balance the joint. The bone is cut and shaped to fit the artificial parts of metal and plastic. Bone cement may be used. After surgery, a drain will remove excess fluids from around the shoulder. A motion machine may move the shoulder for the first few days. The risks of this procedure include infection, injury to nerves and blood vessels about the shoulder, fracture, stiffness of the joint, instability of the joint, loosening of the artificial parts, failure of the rotator cuff, pain, and the need for revision surgery. Blood transfusion is often necessary. Usually, we can arrange for you to donate blood several weeks before your operation and return your own blood to you at the time of surgery.

Shoulder arthroplasty is not an emergency. You should be in the best possible condition for this procedure. Any smoking should be stopped 2 months before the procedure. Any heart, lung, kidney, bladder, tooth, or gum problems should be managed before surgery. Any infection may be a reason to delay the operation. Please be sure we know everything about your health, including your allergies and any medications or drugs you are taking, because some of these (even aspirin) may affect the way your blood clots.

Immediately after this procedure, your arm may be less useful than it is now. This will require special planning to manage the activities of daily living during the period of recovery. You should not plan on driving for 6 weeks after your surgery.

We hope this information is helpful. Please be sure we answer all of your questions before surgery.

the information to be shared with patients as they consider prosthetic arthroplasty.

Mechanics of Glenohumeral Arthroplasty

Glenohumeral arthroplasty provides the opportunity to employ all of our understanding of glenohumeral mechanics: many of the important variables are under the surgeon's control with this procedure. It provides an opportunity to synthesize some of the key elements of motion, stability, strength, and smoothness and to point out how these considerations relate to the conduct of the surgical procedure.

Motion. The motion of a shoulder arthroplasty is dependent on reestablishing

1. Normal excursion at the humeroscapular motion interface.
2. Sufficient humeral articular surface so that the tuberosities do not abut against the glenoid.
3. Appropriate position of the joint surfaces.
4. Freedom from excessive capsular tightness by surgical releases sufficient to accommodate the intraarticular aspects of the components.

Freedom of motion at the humeroscapular motion interface must be reestablished as a part of the arthroplasty procedure. Normally, approximately 4 cm of excursion takes place in portions of this interface. Adhesions, or "spot welds," across this interface can impede the necessary excursion and seriously compromise the range of shoulder motion, even if the intraarticular aspect of the arthroplasty is perfectly balanced.

The relative geometry of the articular surfaces can also affect the range of glenohumeral motion. If the humeral articular surface ends at the bone of the humerus, the motion that can be accomplished before the humeral bone contacts the glenoid is equal to the difference between the angle subtended by the humeral and the glenoid articular surfaces (Fig. 5–17). For example, if the humeral articular surface ends at the bone, and if the superoinferior glenoid and humeral joint surface arcs are equal, no angular

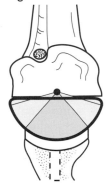
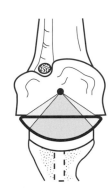

Large Head Size Large Arc of Motion   Smaller Head Size Smaller Arc of Motion

FIGURE 5–17.

The arc of motion that can be accomplished at the glenohumeral joint before running out of humeral articular surface is determined by the difference between the angles subtended by the humeral and the glenoid articular surfaces in the direction of motion. Thus, although a smaller humeral head component may increase capsular laxity, its smaller surface arc may actually diminish the glenohumeral motion allowed before the bone of the humerus contacts the glenoid.

elevation of the humerus relative to the scapula is possible before contact occurs between the humerus and the glenoid. These considerations indicate that humeral components with a small subtended arc may limit the range of motion, even though their small size might be thought to be advantageous by increasing capsular laxity.

The glenohumeral capsule is normally lax through most of the functional range of shoulder motion. As the joint approaches the limit of its range, the tension in the capsule and its ligaments increases sharply, serving to check the range of rotation (see Fig. 3–25). In many conditions requiring shoulder arthroplasty, the capsule and ligaments are contracted and therefore excessively limit the range of rotation. Shoulder arthroplasty tends to further tighten the capsule because the degenerated humeral head is replaced by a larger one, and because a glenoid component is added to the surface of the glenoid bone, consuming more space than the degenerated cartilage it replaces. Thus, the components "stuff" the joint. Unless sufficient capsular releases have been performed to accommodate this stuffing, the joint is "overstuffed" so that the motion is restricted.

To investigate this phenomenon, we measured in eight cadaver shoulders the range of motion that could be achieved with a fixed torque (1500 Newton/mm) (1) in the anatomic shoulder; (2) in the shoulder with an anatomic-sized humeral head replacement and a 4-mm–thick glenoid component (4 mm of overstuffing); and (3) in the shoulder with the same glenoid along with humeral component with a 5-mm–longer neck (9 mm total of overstuffing). No capsular releases were performed. The ranges of maximal elevation, internal rotation at zero degrees of elevation, external rotation in 50 degrees of elevation, and external rotation at zero degrees of elevation are shown for each preparation in Figure 5–18. In this model, the insertion of arthroplasty components diminished the range of joint motion in proportion to the size of the intraarticular aspect of the components. The effect was remarkably consistent: the range of each of the four motions was reduced between 3 and 4 degrees for each millimeter of overstuffing.

In arthroplastic surgery, the amount of stuffing can be estimated by adding the thickness of the glenoid component to the difference between the amount of intraartic-

ular humerus replaced and the amount of humerus resected. To be comparable, the measurement of the amount of humeral head resected and the measurement of the amount of intraarticular humeral prosthesis added must both be made from the cut surface of humeral neck to the articular surface. In modular humeral components, the amount of bone replaced must include the thickness of the collar and the exposed part of the Morse taper stem as well as the head itself (Fig. 5–19). The increment in stuffing can be predicted using templates with correction for magnification and proper preoperative radiographs (see Fig. 5–5).

It is of interest that stuffing not only decreases the range of motion but also increases the stiffness of the shoulder (i.e., the torque necessary to achieve a specified position). The overstuffed joint requires additional muscle force to achieve certain positions. This was demonstrated in the cadaver study described previously. Figure 5–20 shows the torque required to achieve 60 degrees of elevation in an anterior plane at right angles to the scapula (the plus 90 degree scapular plane). The required torque is almost three times higher for the joint overstuffed with 9 mm of intraarticular component.

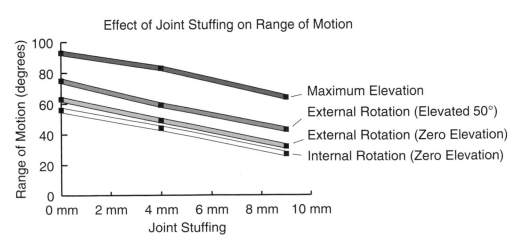

FIGURE 5–18.

The effect of joint stuffing on the range of motion. This graph compares the ranges of four humeroscapular motions that could be achieved with an applied torque of 1500 Newton/mm for (1) an anatomic joint, (2) an anatomic humeral arthroplasty with a 4-mm–thick glenoid component, and (3) an arthroplasty with a 4-mm–thick glenoid and a 5-mm oversized humeral neck (total overstuffing is 9 mm). Note the sequential loss of each of the motions with increasing degrees of stuffing.

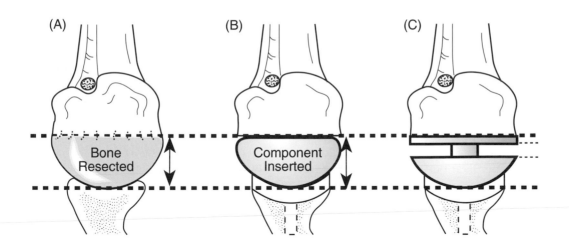

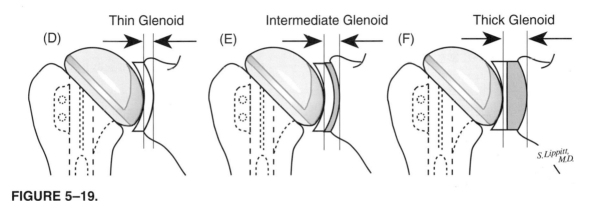

FIGURE 5–19.

A to C, The amount of humeral stuffing is measured by comparing the amount of humerus resected *(A)* to the amount of intraarticular humeral prosthesis added *(B).* In modular systems, the amount of prosthesis added needs to include the collar and the exposed part of the Morse taper as well as the prosthetic head *(C). C to F,* The amount of glenoid stuffing is determined by the distance between the bone surface and the prosthetic articular surface. This distance is greater in proportion to the thickness of the glenoid components.

FIGURE 5–20.

Comparison of the average torque necessary to achieve 60 degrees of elevation in the plus 90 degree scapular plane for the anatomic shoulder, an anatomic shoulder arthroplasty with 4 mm of glenoid stuffing, and an arthroplasty with 4 mm of glenoid and 5 mm of humeral overstuffing (total stuffing is 9 mm). The required torque is almost three times higher for the joint overstuffed with 9 mm of component than for the anatomic joint.

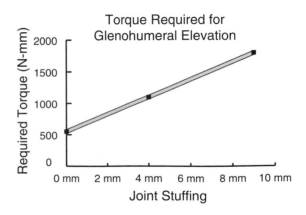

The amount of stuffing from the glenoid component is related primarily to its thickness along with less significant effects related to the amount of glenoid reaming, the presence or absence of cement between the component and bone, and the use of bone grafts. The thickness of currently available glenoid components varies from 3 to more than 15 mm. Thicker glenoid polyethylene may help manage contact stresses and may have superior wear properties. Metal-backed glenoid components affect load transfer and offer opportunities for screw fixation and tissue ingrowth. However, both thicker polyethylene and metal backing contribute to joint stuffing, which becomes particularly problematic in shoulders that remain tight even after soft tissue releases (see Fig. 5–19).

The amount of stuffing from the humeral component is determined by both the geometry of the component and the position in which it is placed. The size of the intraarticular aspect of the humeral component is related to the radius of curvature, the arc subtended by the articular surface, and the distance between the humeral neck cut and the articular surface of the prosthesis (which includes any collar or neck on the component [see Fig. 5–19]). The position of the component also has a major effect on the degree to which it stuffs the joint. A component inserted into varus disproportionately stuffs the joint when the arm is at the side. This outcome is more likely when the stem of the prosthesis does not fit the humeral canal snugly. A component inserted excessively high tightens the capsule as the arm is elevated (similar to a mechanical cam) and limits the range of elevation (Fig. 5–21).

Some humeral prostheses are designed to fit the humeral canal snugly. Under these circumstances, the canal rather than the neck cut becomes the primary determinant of the medial-lateral, anteroposterior and varus-valgus position of the component. In fact, with a snug canal fit, only 2 degrees of freedom of the humeral component with respect to the humeral bone remain: component height and component version. Canal-fitting components usually are inserted after reaming of the canal to the necessary depth and to a diameter judged safe and snug by the surgeon. We refer to the axis of this reamed proximal humeral canal as the "orthopaedic axis" of the humerus. The significance of this axis is that it defines much of the positional geometry of a humeral component press fit into it.

Using this axis as a reference, we measured several geometric parameters of ten cadaver humeri ranging in age from 37 to 78 years (mean 60 years). The anatomic humeral parameters measured for each specimen included the following (Fig. 5–22):

1. The surgically determined reamed diameter (DC) of the humeral canal (the diameter of the largest reamer that could be reasonably placed down the canal).
2. The diameter of curvature of the humeral head articular surface, including articular cartilage (DH) (twice the head radius).
3. The effective humeral neck length (ENL), defined as the distance between the center of the humeral head and the orthopaedic axis.
4. The subtended angle of the humeral joint surface (AH), defined as the angle between the lines connecting the anterior and posterior extents of the articular cartilage to the orthopaedic axis.
5. The offset of the center of the humeral head (OH), defined as the perpendicular distance between the orthopaedic axis and a line connecting the midpoint of the articular surface and the center of the humeral head.

The data from this study are summarized in Table 5–2. It is these relationships that must be duplicated if a canal-fitting prosthesis is to replicate the location of the humeral joint surface. This is of particular relevance in hemiarthroplasty, when it is desirable to match the position and the radius of curvature of the biologic humeral articular surface. For the group of cadaver humeri studied, anatomic replacement with a canal-fitting prosthesis would have required stem diameters ranging from 8 to 14 mm, a distance between the center of the head and the center of the canal (the effective neck length) averaging just over 1 cm, and head diameters of curvature ranging from 39 to 51 mm. Some of these head diameters are sub-

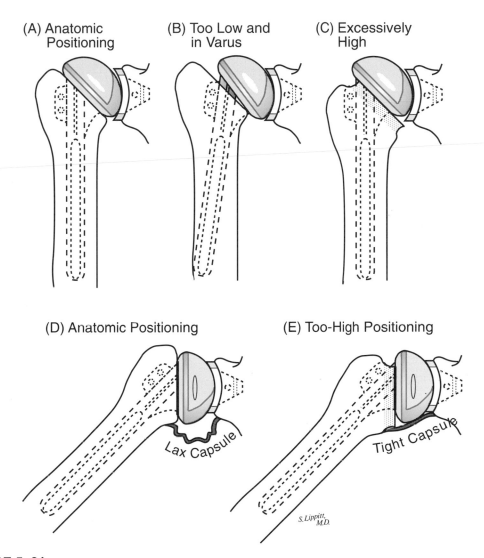

FIGURE 5–21.

The position of the humeral component is an important determinant of the amount of stuffing. *A,* Anatomic positioning of the humeral component. *B,* A component placed low and in varus will disproportionately stuff the shoulder while the arm is at the side as well as make the tuberosity proud. *C,* A component placed excessively high. *D,* Normal anatomic relationships on humeral elevation. *E,* A humeral component that is too high causes tightening of the capsule as the humerus is elevated.

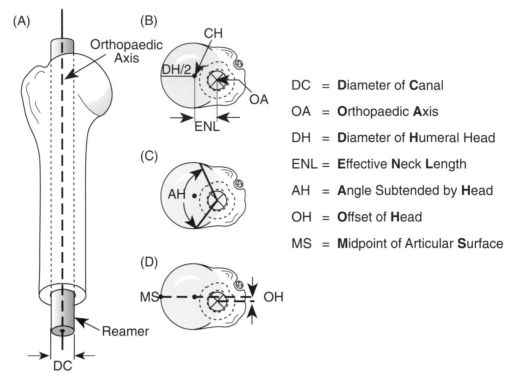

DC = **D**iameter of **C**anal

OA = **O**rthopaedic **A**xis

DH = **D**iameter of **H**umeral Head

ENL = **E**ffective **N**eck **L**ength

AH = **A**ngle Subtended by **H**ead

OH = **O**ffset of **H**ead

MS = **M**idpoint of Articular **S**urface

FIGURE 5–22.

A, The humeral medullary canal is reamed to a diameter (DC) defining the orthopaedic axis (OA). *B,* The diameter of curvature of the humeral articular surface is DH (radius is DH/2). The effective neck length (ENL) is the distance between the center of the humeral head (CH) and the orthopaedic axis (OA). *C,* The angle based at the orthopaedic axis and subtended by the humeral articular surface is AH. *D,* The offset of the center of the humeral head (OH) is defined as the perpendicular distance between the orthopaedic axis (OA) and a line connecting the midpoint of the articular surface (MS) and the center of the humeral head (CH).

TABLE 5–2. Geometric Characterization of Ten Anatomic Humeri

Humerus No.	Canal Diameter (DC) (mm)	Head Diameter (DH) (mm)	Neck Length (ENL) (mm)	Joint Surface Arc (AH) (degrees)	Head Offset* (OH) (mm)
1	8	46	13	116	3
2	10	39	11	115	1
3	10	40	12	120	4
4	10	40	11	110	−3
5	12	44	11	105	3
6	12	48	14	119	2
7	12	48	11	112	4
8	12	46	9	113	1
9	12	39	10	104	0
10	14	51	7	115	0
Range	8–14	39–51	7–14	104–120	(−3)–4
Mean	11	44	11	113	2
SD	1.7	4.1	2.1	5.3	2.2

*Posterior offset of the head has a positive sign; anterior offset has a negative sign.

stantially smaller than those available in many currently available component systems; a substantial range of prosthetic head diameters of curvature is required to match this anatomic variability. The angles subtended by the anatomic head articular surfaces were 15 percent larger than those of most current prostheses. Because the humerus rotates around the center of the humeral head, a smaller radius of curvature coupled with a larger subtended articular surface angle provides a larger rotational range of motion for a specified excursion of capsule and cuff tendons (Fig. 5–23).

For canal-fitting components, changes in humeral version must take place about the orthopaedic axis. The effect on soft tissue tension resulting from changes in version is determined by the effective neck length. If the center of curvature of the head lies on the orthopaedic axis, the effective neck length will be zero and changes in version will not alter the distance between the soft tissue attachments on the humerus and the

glenoid (Fig. 5–24). When the center of curvature of the head is at some distance from the orthopaedic axis, the effects of changes in version are related to the effective neck length and the amount of change in version. For the anatomic humerus, the effective neck length is relatively small (mean of 11 mm); thus, changes in version have much less effect than in the hip where the effective neck length is an order of magnitude larger. Furthermore, with a humeral neck osteotomy made at the appropriate location just inside the cuff insertion, a significant change in the angle of humeral version cannot be accomplished without jeopardizing the tuberosity and cuff insertion. On these bases, we suspect that the effectiveness of changes in version in adjusting soft tissue tension is relatively small.

Stability. The stability of a shoulder arthroplasty is dependent on reestablishing

1. *Capsular ligaments* that are neither too short (in which case obligate translation

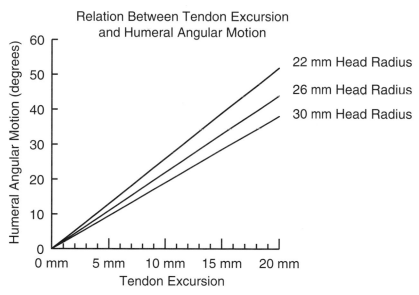

FIGURE 5–23.

The relationship between the radius of curvature of the humeral articular surface (R) and the angular motion (θ) associated with a specified excursion of the rotator cuff (E).

$$\theta = 57 \text{ degrees} \times E/R$$

Thus, humeral heads with smaller radii require less tendon excursion to produce a given angular displacement.

(A)

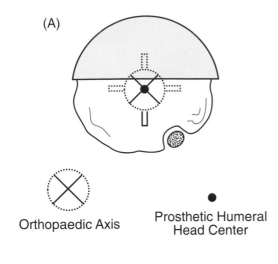

Orthopaedic Axis — Prosthetic Humeral Head Center

(B)

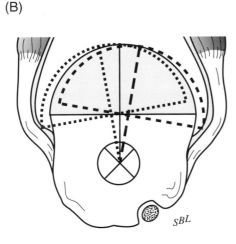

SBL

FIGURE 5–24.

The effect of changing the humeral version in a canal-fitting prosthesis is determined by the effective neck length of the prosthesis (the distance between the orthopaedic axis and the center of curvature of the head) and the amount of change in the version. *A,* If the effective neck length is zero, no amount of change in version will affect the distance between the tuberosities and the glenoid that the soft tissues must span. *B,* For anatomic humeri, the effective neck length is small (average 11 mm). If the humeral neck cut is made just inside the cuff insertion to the tuberosities, little angular change of the humeral component can be accomplished without jeopardizing the integrity of the cuff insertion. Thus, in a canal-fitting humeral component, changes in version do not have a major effect on soft tissue balance.

may occur at the limits of motion) nor too long (in which case the joint may overrotate beyond the positions in which the muscles can stabilize the head in the socket).

2. *Compression* by repairing, balancing, and rehabilitating the cuff muscles.
3. *Full surface contact* through the useful range of the joint.
4. *Balance* of the net humeral joint reaction force by ensuring that the glenoid component is properly oriented with respect to the scapula.
5. *The glenoid concavity* with a glenoid prosthesis, if the biologic glenoid is destroyed. The glenoid component needs to be firmly supported by the subjacent bone.

As discussed in Chapter 3, laxity (translation on examination of the joint) is not the same as instability (the inability to hold the head centered in the glenoid). Translation in the midranges of motion where most functions are carried out is an important property of normal glenohumeral joints. As a rule of thumb during arthroplasty, we strive for translation of 15 mm on the posterior drawer test to help ensure that the joint has not been overstuffed. The effect of overstuffing on translation is seen in Figure 5–25, from our cadaver study of shoulder arthroplasty. The average translations on all three laxity tests (anterior drawer, posterior drawer, and sulcus) were 15 to 16 mm in the anatomic preparations for these eight shoulders when no capsular release was performed. Increased

FIGURE 5–25.

The effect of overstuffing on three directions of translation in eight cadaver shoulders of mean age 73 ± 8.5 years. The intact shoulders demonstrated 15 mm of translational laxity. Overstuffing by 9 mm decreased this normal joint laxity by approximately 50 percent in all directions.

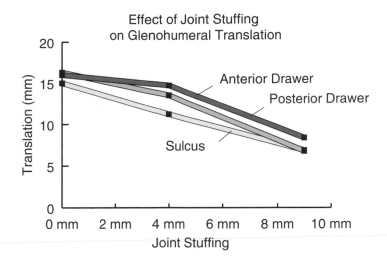

degrees of stuffing progressively compromised this normal joint laxity. Overstuffing of 9 mm reduced the normal laxity in all directions by almost 50 percent.

If normal capsular laxity is not present, instability may result from obligate translation. This may appear counterintuitive: a too-tight joint can be unstable. Yet as is demonstrated in Figures 2–27 and 2–28, tightness of the anterior capsule can force the humeral head out of the back of the joint on external rotation, and tightness of the posterior capsule can force the humeral head out of the front of the joint on elevation in anterior scapular planes. In our cadaver study we found that only half as much motion could be achieved before obligate translation occurred in the overstuffed shoulder in comparison with the anatomic shoulder (Table 5–3).

When the humeral and glenoid prosthetic joint surfaces are conforming (identical radii of curvature), any amount of translation will result in rim loading, causing extremely high contact pressures with resulting polyethylene wear and cold flow (see Fig. 5–28). Prosthetic glenoid rim destruction is a frequent feature of the glenoid components we have retrieved from failed shoulder arthroplasties. Rim contact from unwanted translation also predisposes to glenoid component loosening by the "rocking horse" mechanism (Fig. 5–26). Thus, it appears that normal ligamentous laxity is a desired characteristic after shoulder arthroplasty; the surgeon must strive to provide this laxity through capsular releases and by avoiding excessively large prosthetic components, which would overstuff the joint.

Stability of the arthroplasty is also related to strong muscle forces that are balanced so that the net humeral joint reaction force passes through the glenoid fossa. Loss of the coordinated strength of the cuff muscles through disuse, denervation, tendon failure, iatrogenic damage, or tuberosity non-union

TABLE 5–3. Range of Angular Motion Before Onset of Obligate Translation*

	Anatomic Shoulder (degrees)	Joint Overstuffed 9 mm (degrees)
Elevation in the plus 90 degree scapular plane	60	30
External rotation of the arm elevated 50 degrees	60	32

*Values represent the maximal elevation achieved with no more than 2 mm of obligate translation.

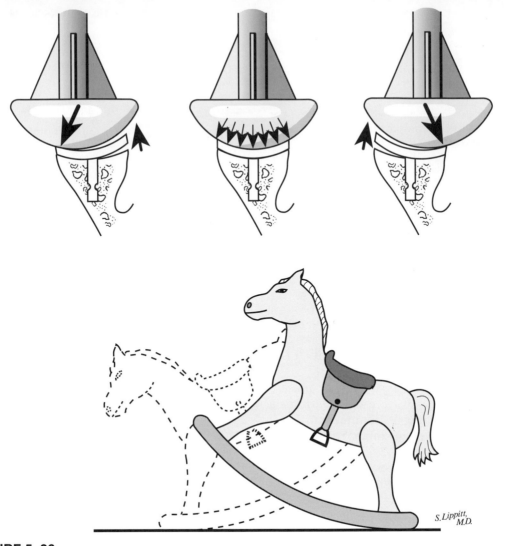

FIGURE 5–26.

"Rocking horse" loosening of the glenoid component results when translation of the head on the glenoid produces eccentric forces on the component from glenoid rim loading.

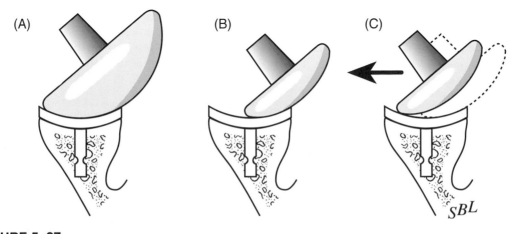

(A)   (B)   (C)

FIGURE 5–27.

The effect of humeral contact area on translational stability. Full surface contact provides maximal joint stability (A). When full surface contact is lacking because of a small humeral joint surface angle (B), the humeral component can be translated in the direction of the empty part of the glenoid (C).

190

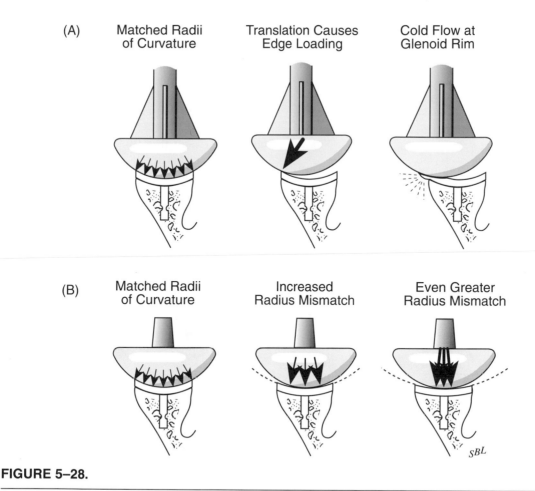

(A) Matched Radii of Curvature | Translation Causes Edge Loading | Cold Flow at Glenoid Rim

(B) Matched Radii of Curvature | Increased Radius Mismatch | Even Greater Radius Mismatch

FIGURE 5–28.

A, When the joint surfaces of the glenoid and humeral components have identical radii of curvature, any amount of translation (however small) causes rim loading. Rim loading in turn results in high contact pressures, rim wear, and cold flow. *B,* When the radius of curvature of the glenoid component surface is larger than that of the humerus, there is an increase in joint pressure (load per unit area) related to the degree of mismatch.

or malunion can render a shoulder unstable in spite of appropriate position and orientation of the joint surfaces. In cuff tear arthropathy, chronic massive cuff deficiency deprives the joint of normal compression, allowing upward instability of the humerus in relation to the glenoid. In this situation, the cuff is frequently not reconstructable. If the humerus has been chronically subluxated in a superior direction with loss of the superior glenoid concavity, it is unlikely that cuff reconstruction can restore normal stability through compression. Under these circumstances, insertion of a glenoid component risks problems related to the abnormal humeral position: glenoid rim contact, rim wear, and rocking horse loosening.

Stability of the arthroplasty is further related to the ability of the articulation to offer full surface contact through a wide range of motion. Humeral components that subtend a small surface angle allow only a small range of full surface contact. When the joint is positioned out of the range of full surface contact, the humeral head can be translated in the direction where contact is lacking (Fig. 5–27).

ACTIVITY

Holding a humeral and glenoid component in your hands, verify that the components are stable while they are in full surface contact. However, when the humerus is rotated so that the edge of the humeral articular surface lies within the glenoid fossa, the humerus can be translated toward the empty part of the glenoid.

Balancing the net humeral joint reaction force is one of the major mechanisms by which the prosthetic arthroplasty is stabilized. Proper balance requires that the glenoid be properly oriented with respect to the scapula. Excessive posterior inclination of the prosthetic joint surface is an important cause of postoperative posterior instability. When a portion of the glenoid cartilage remains intact, the subchondral bone beneath it may be used as a guide to the normal orientation of the glenoid face. This feature is useful in capsulorrhaphy arthropathy and in degenerative joint disease, in which glenoid wear may be confined to the posterior half of the fossa. In rheumatoid arthritis, the glenoid version is usually unchanged because the erosion takes place symmetrically in a medial direction.

A simple cadaver study demonstrated a practical method for normalizing the glenoid orientation in the general case. We took a group of ten normal cadaver scapulae and located the center of the face of the glenoid. We then inserted a drill perpendicular to the face starting at the glenoid center. In each instance, the drill emerged from the anterior glenoid neck at the lateral aspect of the subscapularis fossa at a point midway between the upper and lower crura of the scapula (Fig. 5–29). We refer to this spot in the subscapular fossa as the *centering point*. This point is easily palpated at arthroplasty surgery after an anterior capsular release has been performed. It is unaffected by arthritis. The line connecting it to the center of the glenoid face is the normalized glenoid center line (see Fig. 3–1). Orienting the prosthetic glenoid to this normalized glenoid center line enables the surgeon to correct pathologic glenoid version, which is frequently encountered in degenerative joint disease and other conditions requiring shoulder arthroplasty.

ACTIVITY

Take a group of normal cadaver scapulae and drill holes perpendicular to the center of the glenoid articular surface, observing the spot where the drill exits the anterior glenoid neck.

Concavity compression is another major mechanism by which shoulder arthroplasties are stabilized in functional positions. A humeral hemiarthroplasty can be stabilized by muscular compression if the glenoid concavity is intact. In degenerative joint disease and in capsulorrhaphy arthropathy, how-

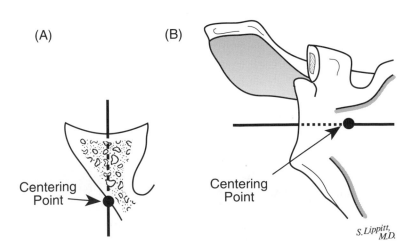

(A)　(B)

Centering Point →

Centering Point

S. Lippitt, M.D.

FIGURE 5–29.

The normal glenoid center line passes perpendicular to the center of the glenoid articular surface and exits the glenoid neck at the "centering point" between the upper and lower crura of the scapula in the lateral aspect of the subscapularis fossa.

ever, the posterior half of the glenoid concavity is usually eroded away, depriving the shoulder of the concavity necessary for stability. Thus, even if excellent articular cartilage exists on the anterior half of the glenoid, a humeral hemiarthroplasty cannot be stable without this posterior glenoid lip.

Humeral hemiarthroplasty may be stabilized in cuff tear arthropathy, even though the superior lip of the glenoid is eroded away by superior humeral subluxation. In this situation, the prosthetic humeral head is captured by an acetabular-like socket consisting of the acromion, the coracoacromial ligament, the coracoid, and the eroded upper glenoid. In performing a special hemiarthroplasty under these circumstances, it is vital that the surgeon not compromise this socket by sacrificing the anterior acromion or the coracoacromial ligament; otherwise, the humeral head is likely to be destabilized in an anterosuperior direction.

Glenohumeral arthroplasty provides the surgeon the opportunity to control the depth of the prosthetic glenoid concavity. As shown in Figure 3–15, the depth of the glenoid concavity is related to dimensions of the face of the glenoid (superoinferior and anteroposterior breadth) and to the radius of curvature. For a given radius of joint surface curvature, larger components are deeper than smaller ones. For a given glenoid size, components with a smaller radius of curvature are deeper than those with larger radii of joint surface curvature.

If the glenoid and humeral radii of curvature are equal, the head will be held precisely in the center by concavity compression; no translation can occur unless the humeral head is allowed to lift out of the fossa (the glenoidogram would show a tight V) (Fig. 5–30; see also Fig. 3–13). Although this tight conformity provides excellent stability, it has the potential disadvantage that displacing loads applied to the humerus will be transmitted fully to the glenoid and thence to the glenoid-bone interface. In the biologic glenoid, the compliance of the articular cartilage and glenoid labrum provides shock absorption for transverse displacing loads. Because polyethylene is much stiffer than cartilage and labrum, this shock absorption is not present in prosthetic glenoid arthroplasty. Thus, glenoid fixation is at risk for substantial peak loads when the glenoid and humeral joint surfaces are totally conforming.

Some degree of shock absorption can be provided by a slight mismatch between the humeral and glenoid diameters of curvature,

FIGURE 5–30.

The path that the center of the humeral head takes during translation relative to the glenoid (the "glenoidogram" path). A, Conforming surfaces yield a tight V on the glenoidogram. B, When the glenoid diameter of curvature is slightly larger than that of the humerus, the glenoidogram yields a U shape. The diameter of the central part of the U is equal to the difference between the diameter of curvature of the glenoid and that of the humerus.

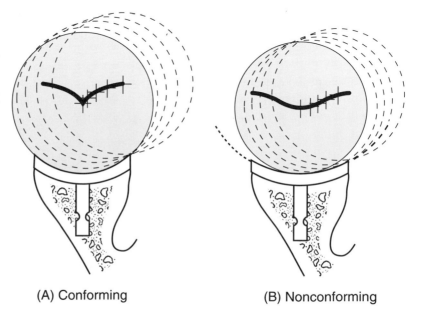

(A) Conforming   (B) Nonconforming

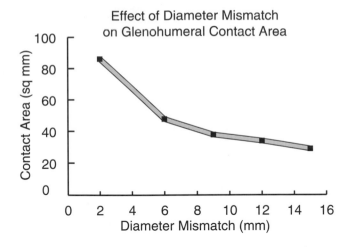

FIGURE 5–31.

Results of a finite element model analysis of a polyethylene glenoid showing the effect of diameter mismatch on the contact area. Even a slight amount of diameter mismatch dramatically reduces the contact area. Increasing the mismatch further reduces the contact area.

that of the glenoid being slightly larger. This allows some translation before the humeral head must lift out of the fossa (the glenoidogram becomes more a U than a tight V; see Fig. 5–30). This too is a compromise, however, in that the degree of mismatch decreases the contact area and increases the contact pressures with potential risk of polyethylene failure. In a finite element model using conventional polyethylene, we predicted the surface area of contact with a load of typical body weight 625 Newtons (140 lb). Figure 5–31 shows the dramatic drop in contact area with increasing degrees of diameter mismatch. This drop in contact area has a corresponding effect on the contact stresses. Figure 5–32 shows that for loads of 625 Newtons, the contact stress exceeds the predicted yield stress for conventional poly-

ethylene when the diameter mismatch is greater than 6 mm.

For the glenoid to stabilize the humeral head against transverse loads, it must be well supported by the bone beneath it. Our clinical observations suggest that a primary mechanism of glenoid loosening is via the rocking horse mechanism when eccentric loads are applied (see Fig. 5–26). In a series of ten cadaver glenoids, we studied the effect of glenoid bone preparation on the stability of a 3-mm–thick, non-clinical glenoid component with a diameter of curvature of 60 mm. To emphasize the effect of glenoid surface preparation, the component was secured to the bony glenoid with only a single, flexible, uncemented central peg. The component was loaded with an eccentric force of 200 Newtons applied at an angle of 14

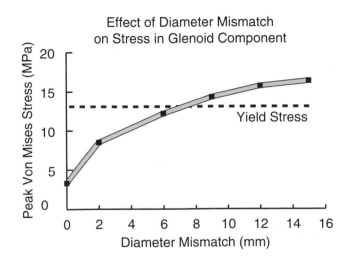

FIGURE 5–32.

Results of a finite element model analysis of the effect of diameter mismatch on the peak contact stresses (pressure-modified Von Mises stress) in a polyethylene glenoid component. The applied compressive load is 625 Newtons (approximately one body weight). The predicted yield stress for the component is shown. A load of one body weight with diameter mismatch in excess of 6 mm is predicted to exceed the yield stress of ordinary polyethylene.

degrees with the glenoid center line. While the component was loaded, we measured the wobble of the component with respect to the bone and the warp, or deformation, of the component using displacement transducers. The stability of the component was measured sequentially after three different glenoid preparations: (1) curettage of the articular cartilage, (2) meticulous burring of the bone by hand to fit the back of the component, and (3) preparation using a reamer with a diameter of curvature of 60 mm centered in a hole along the glenoid center line. We found that spherical reaming dramatically diminished both the wobble and the warp of the glenoid component with eccentric loading in comparison with the other two methods of bone preparation (Fig. 5–33). We presume that an even greater increment in stability would accrue with the use of careful reaming in a deformed bony glenoid, such as that found in degenerative joint disease. This study demonstrates that precise contouring of the bone to fit the back of the glenoid component provides excellent support of the prosthesis, even without fixation using multiple pegs, keels, cement, screws, or tissue ingrowth. We conclude that spherical reaming along the anatomic glenoid center line has two important advantages: (1) it normalizes glenoid version, and (2) it provides ''bone back'' support of the glenoid component with the opportunity for optimal stability and load transfer without the need for metal backing.

Strength. The strength of the shoulder after arthroplasty is dependent on reestablishing integrity, strength, and coordination of the muscles controlling the glenohumeral and scapulothoracic articulations.

The amount of stuffing of the joint sets the resting length of the cuff muscles and, to a lesser extent, that of the deltoid. If the components are too small, the cuff will be slack at rest and thus place the muscles at the low end of the ideal length-tension relationship. If the joint is overstuffed, the cuff muscles may be at the high end of their length-tension curve. The distance between the effective cuff insertion and the humeral head center establishes the moment arm for the cuff.

The deltoid is the most important motor of the shoulder arthroplasty. The integrity of its origin, insertion, and nerve supply must be maintained. This is most easily accomplished by gently approaching the joint through the deltopectoral interval and by identifying and protecting the axillary nerve both anteromedially as it crosses the subscapularis and inferior capsule and laterally as it exits the quadrangular space and winds around the tuberosities on the deep surface of the deltoid. Rehabilitation of the deltoid is critical to the active motion following arthroplasty.

The rotator cuff mechanism is in jeopardy in shoulder arthroplasty for several reasons. The suprascapular nerve, which supplies the supraspinatus and infraspinatus, is at risk during surgical releases as it courses medial to the coracoid and then down the back of the glenoid 1 cm medial to the glenoid lip. The cuff tendons are at risk during surgery because the humeral cut must come close to their insertion to the tuberosities superiorly and posteriorly. A humeral cut made in excessive retroversion is likely to detach the cuff posteriorly, and a cut made too low on the humerus is likely to detach the cuff superiorly (Fig. 5–34). Overstuffing the joint places the cuff under tension when the arm is adducted or rotated (Fig. 5–35). Most shoulder arthroplasties are performed in older persons in whom the quality of the cuff tissue may be compromised not only from age-related changes but also from disuse enforced by chronic glenohumeral roughness. Shoulder arthroplasty may quickly restore motion and smoothness to the joint, placing new and substantial demands on the disused cuff tissue. Thus, the rehabilitation program and the patient's activities after arthroplasty must *gradually* increment the loads on the cuff, allowing the tissue the opportunity to toughen over time.

If a cuff defect exists at the time of the arthroplasty, a cuff repair to bone should be carried out if the quantity and quality of the cuff tissue are sufficient to allow a durable repair under physiologic tension with the arm at the side. If the tuberosities are nonunited, or if a tuberosity osteotomy is performed, secure fixation is required to restore cuff function. Under these circumstances,

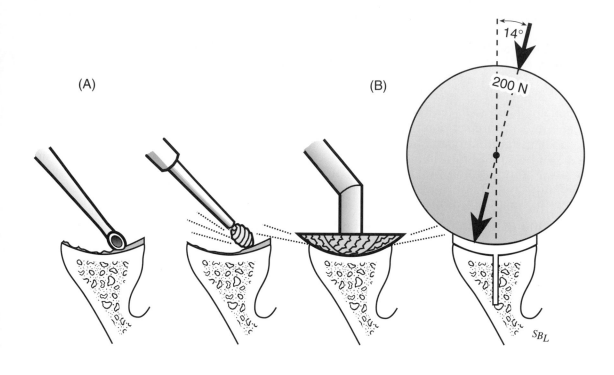

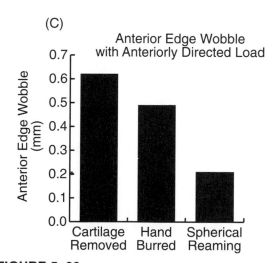

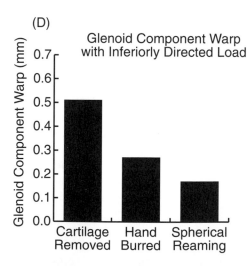

FIGURE 5–33.

The effect of glenoid-bone preparation on component stability. *A*, Three methods of bone preparation were compared: curettage, hand burring, and spherical reaming. *B*, Loads of 200 Newtons were applied through a metal ball at an angle of 14 degrees with respect to the glenoid center line. The glenoid was fixed only with a single uncemented flexible central peg. Displacement transducers measured the change in position of the edges of the glenoid component. *C* and *D*, Data on the stability of a glenoid component with three different types of glenoid surface preparation. Spherical reaming of the glenoid along the glenoid center line significantly reduced the wobble *(C)* and warp *(D)* of the glenoid component and thus provided more glenoid component stability than did curettage or hand burring.

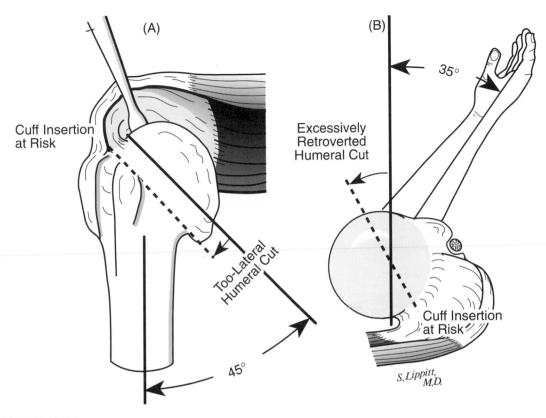

FIGURE 5-34.

A, A cut that is too lateral risks detaching the cuff insertion superiorly. *B*, A humeral cut made in excessive retroversion risks detaching the cuff posteriorly.

the rehabilitation program after arthroplasty is changed dramatically to allow for secure healing of the cuff mechanism to the humerus.

Smoothness. The smoothness of the shoulder arthroplasty is dependent on reestablishing smooth joint surfaces and smoothness of the non-articular humeroscapular motion interface.

Providing joint smoothness is a primary objective of shoulder arthroplasty. In the presence of an intact glenoid fossa covered with good articular cartilage, a humeral hemiarthroplasty should suffice. The articular cartilage may be assessed by preoperative radiographs and at surgery by observation and palpation and by listening to the sound when it is struck with a small blunt elevator. Thin cartilage or bare bone causes the elevator to ring, whereas normal cartilage yields only a dull "thunk."

In glenohumeral arthroplasty, joint smoothness is provided by the metal on polyethylene articulation. Care must be taken to ensure the absence of non-articular contact between humeral bone and the prosthetic glenoid. Inferior or posterior humeral osteophytes can present a particular problem in this regard.

In hemiarthroplasty for cuff tear arthropathy, the undersurface of the "acetabularized" coracoacromial arch is usually polished smooth with a consistent diameter of curvature. The prosthetic humeral articular surface and the tuberosities must provide a smooth congruent surface to mate with this arch. Achieving this goal requires attention to the selection and positioning of the prosthetic humeral joint surface so that it replicates that of the joint surface that is excised. The tuberosities are sculpted so that they are congruent with the prosthetic joint surface. We hypothesize that the large smooth joint

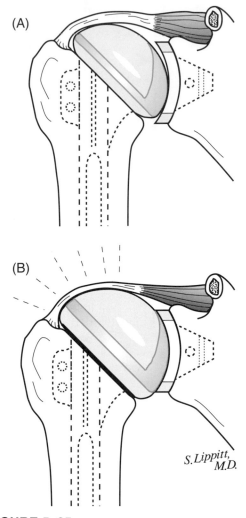

(A)

(B)

S.Lippitt, M.D.

FIGURE 5–35.

As compared with the normal joint *(A)*, an over-stuffed joint places excessive tension on the cuff when the shoulder is adducted *(B)*.

contact area achieved in this procedure decreases joint contact pressures and is thus responsible for its success in restoring comfort and function in the difficult problem of cuff tear arthropathy.

The arthroplasty must also establish smoothness at the non-articular humeroscapular motion interface. Scar, adhesions, and hypertrophic bursa must be excised. The sites of reattachment of the rotator cuff, including the subscapularis, must slide smoothly against the outer aspect of the motion interface. Immediate postoperative motion may be helpful in preventing the reformation of scar and adhesions in this motion interface.

Surgical Procedure

The characteristic pathologic processes of the disease help guide the surgical approach. Prosthetic humeral hemiarthroplasty without a glenoid component offers the opportunity to restore the normal convexity of the proximal humeral articular surface, provided that the glenoid surface is essentially normal. This situation most commonly arises in atraumatic avascular necrosis or in fractures involving the humeral head. When performing a hemiarthroplasty, the goal is to restore the humeral articular surface to its normal location and configuration. Because the glenoid is not replaced, the size, radius, and orientation of the prosthetic humeral joint surface must duplicate that of the biologic humeral head. Templating standardized radiographs is an essential step in preoperative planning.

In degenerative joint disease, the glenoid face is typically flattened and often eroded posteriorly from chronic posterior subluxation (Fig. 5–36). The glenoid may be distorted by peripheral osteophytes masking the location of the anatomic fossa. The humeral head may be flattened in a corresponding manner and effectively enlarged by the proliferation of "goat's beard" osteophytes from the anterior, inferior and posterior articular rim. Intraarticular loose bodies may lie hidden in the subcoracoid or axillary recesses. Anterior capsular and subscapularis contractures are common in degenerative joint disease.

In the rheumatoid shoulder, the soft tissues and the osteopenic bone are often fragile and susceptible to disruption or fracture at and following surgery. Usually, the glenoid face has been concentrically eroded in a medial direction (Fig. 5–37), occasionally to an extent that precludes placement of a glenoid component. The humeral head and glenoid are often small, with a corresponding reduction in joint volume. The rotator cuff may be torn or attenuated. In juvenile rheumatoid arthritis, the diminutive osseous morphology may require smaller or even custom-made components.

Shoulders affected by capsulorrhaphy arthropathy present additional challenges, such as neurovascular scarring from pre-

(A) (B)

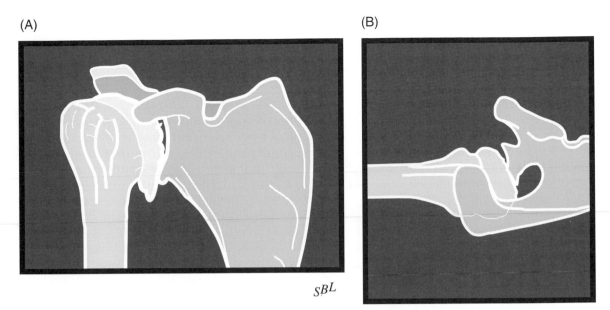

SBL

FIGURE 5–36.

Glenohumeral degenerative joint disease. *A*, Anteroposterior view showing typical "goat's beard" osteophyte enlarging the apparent superoinferior dimension of the head. *B*, Axillary view showing posterior subluxation and posterior rim wear.

FIGURE 5–37.

Axillary view of glenohumeral rheumatoid arthritis showing medial erosion of the glenoid bone stock.

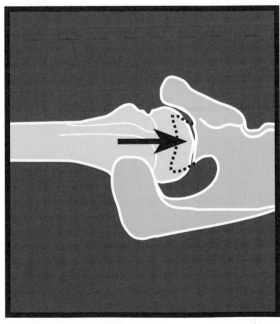

S. Lippitt, M.D.

vious surgery, soft tissue contractures, bone deficiencies, implants from previous surgery, changes of glenoid version, and an increased potential for glenohumeral instability after the arthroplasty (Fig. 5–38). Occasionally, tendon autografts or allografts are required to replace deficient anterior soft tissue structures.

Scar tissue, altered neurovascular relationships, and skeletal or soft tissue deficiencies or deformities may exist in posttraumatic arthritis. These factors complicate surgical exposure, protection of nerves and blood vessels, soft tissue balancing, bone preparation, and implant positioning. Malunions or non-unions of the humeral shaft, surgical neck, tuberosities, or glenoid substantially increase the difficulty of the bony reconstruction.

A series of high-quality standardized radiographs are helpful in preoperative planning. If the arm is placed in the "centered position," the necessary information can be obtained from an anteroposterior

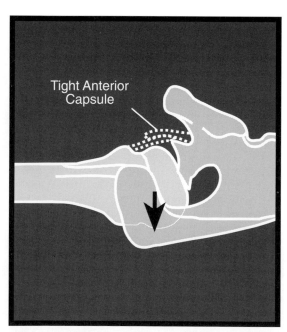

FIGURE 5–38.

Axillary view of capsulorrhaphy arthropathy, in which an excessively tight anterior capsular repair forces the head of the humerus posteriorly. This effect is accentuated by forced external rotation. Note also the typical posterior glenoid erosion.

view in the plane of the scapula and an axillary view (see Fig. 5–5). These radiographs should reveal the amount, quality, and orientation of the glenoid bone as well as the size and configuration of the humerus down to where the tip of the humeral prosthesis will rest. Using templates is helpful for selecting the components that will best replace the damaged joint surfaces. Drawing the cuts and the implants on the preoperative radiographs helps the surgeon determine where the humeral and glenoid components should be positioned and whether any particular problems in their placement can be anticipated. Is there significant glenoid erosion or altered version? Are there potentially confusing glenoid osteophytes? Is there enough bone to support a glenoid component? What is the diameter of the humeral joint surface? Is the humeral canal straight? What size is it? What is the position of the tuberosities in relation to the canal and the joint surface? How much humeral bone will need to be excised? Are there other major abnormalities of bony structure that could change the procedure? In press fit components, will the medullary space accommodate the size and shape of the stem and the body of the prosthesis without risk of fracture?

Component Selection

Some general principles must be considered in prosthetic component selection. The glenoid component should be as thin as its strength and wear properties allow to conserve the limited joint volume. This consideration favors the use of all polyethylene components in most instances because metal-backed components take up more room in the joint. The superoinferior and anteroposterior size of the component should be the maximum that can be supported by the glenoid bone.

The glenoid component system should facilitate the attainment of proper orientation with respect to the glenoid center line and a good geometric match with the glenoid bone. The glenoid fixation system should be one in which the geometry is defined precisely to avoid the uncertainty of freehand sculpting. This precision is enhanced by a glenoid reamer keyed to the normalized glenoid center line. The use of a drill guide to establish precise geometry for multiple glenoid fixation pegs may provide better fixation with minimal sacrifice of glenoid bone stock and requires minimal amounts of cement with minimal risk of heat necrosis. Fixation anterior and posterior to the vertical axis of the glenoid component helps prevent "lift off" during eccentric loading. As presented earlier in this chapter, there are theoretical advantages of a small degree in undersizing of the humeral diameter of curvature with respect to that of the glenoid. The relative clinical advantages of different degrees of humeroglenoid diameter mismatch are yet to be determined.

Multiple considerations affect the choice of the humeral component as well. Good fit and fill of the humerus can often provide secure fixation without cement, but press fitting does increase the risk of humeral fracture. Whether the medullary canal needs to be sealed to prevent entry of polyethylene debris remains a theoretical consideration. The humeral head needs to provide the appropriate diameter of curvature in both humeral and glenohumeral arthroplasty. In humeral hemiarthroplasty, the diameter of curvature should match that of the biologic articular surface. In glenohumeral arthroplasty, the diameter of curvature should be appropriate for the glenoid component selected. The arc subtended by the humeral articular surface should be maximized rather than having part of this arc sacrificed to a non-articular humeral neck (Fig. 5–39). Canal-fitting prostheses allow less flexibility in positioning: the reamed canal largely controls the medial-lateral, anteroposterior, and varus-valgus degrees of freedom. Thus, the surgeon needs to ensure that the selected prosthesis will provide the appropriate effective neck length and component height to establish the desired position of the articular surface. Ideally, the humeral prosthesis should restore the joint surface to its anatomic location.

Technique of Glenohumeral Arthroplasty

Glenohumeral arthroplasty provides the surgeon with the opportunity to use all the principles related to the restoration of motion, strength, stability, and smoothness. All adhesions and contractures must be released, and the smoothness of the non-articular humeroscapular motion interface must be reestablished. Obligate translation is avoided by appropriate capsular releases.

FIGURE 5–39.

A, Ideally, the humeral component provides a maximal articular surface area. *B,* Significant portions of the intraarticular space can be consumed by non-articular aspects of a modular prosthesis.

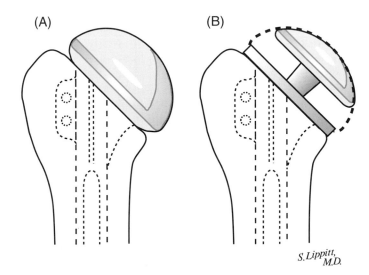

Strength is optimized by placing the muscle-tendon units under proper tension. Stability is achieved by normalizing joint surface orientation and providing the appropriate geometry for the concavity compression stabilization and balance mechanisms. Smoothness is provided by the prosthetic joint surfaces and by immediate postoperative motion.

Surgical Approach

After a brachial plexus block or general anesthetic, the patient is placed in the beach chair position with the thorax up at an angle of 30 degrees. The shoulder is just off the edge of the operating table so it can be moved freely through an entire range of motion. The anesthesiologist is positioned at the side of the neck on the opposite side from the shoulder being operated on. A careful double skin preparation includes the entire arm and forequarter, anteriorly and posteriorly. Draping allows access to the entire scapula, clavicle, and humerus.

Skin Incision. This is made over the deltopectoral groove along a line connecting the midpoint of the clavicle to the midpoint of the lateral humerus and crossing over the coracoid process (Fig. 5–40). This incision avoids the axilla, protects the neurovascular supply to the deltoid, and provides direct access to the deltopectoral interval without requiring skin flaps. Gelpi retractors placed in the subcutaneous tissue help provide hemostasis as the incision is carried to the level of the deltopectoral fascia. The deltopectoral interval is developed medial to the cephalic vein, preserving its major tributaries from the deltoid muscle. Incising the clavipectoral fascia at the lateral edge of the conjoined tendon up to, but not through, the coracoacromial ligament provides entry to the non-articular humeroscapular motion interface. The axillary nerve is identified as it courses across the inferior border of the subscapularis.

The subscapularis is the one tendon incised in performing a glenohumeral arthroplasty. Restoring the excursion of this ten-

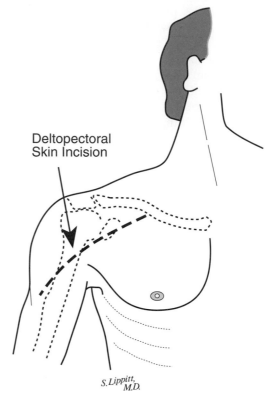

FIGURE 5–40.

Anterior deltopectoral skin incision extending along a line from the midpoint of the clavicle to the midpoint of the lateral humerus (deltoid tubercle). Note that this line of incision crosses the coracoid tip.

don as well as its firm reattachment to the humerus is critical to the restoration of the range, stability, and strength of the shoulder. Our routine is to incise the subscapularis tendon as close to the bicipital groove as possible to gain maximal length of quality tendon; no subscapularis tendon is left on the lesser tuberosity. The anterior glenohumeral capsule is incised from its attachment to the glenoid and is left attached to the deep surface of the tendon to reinforce it (Fig. 5–41). A 360 degree release of the subscapularis tendon is then performed (Fig. 5–42), ensuring that it moves freely with respect to the glenoid, the coracoid, the coracoid muscles, the axillary nerve, and the inferior capsule. Additional subscapularis length is gained at the time of closure by reattaching it with sutures placed in the anterior humeral neck rather than the lesser

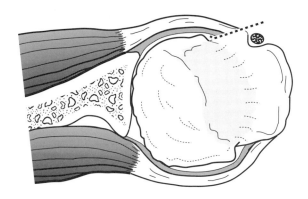

FIGURE 5–41.

The subscapularis incision. The subscapularis and the subjacent capsule are incised directly from the lesser tuberosity, striving for maximal length of the tendon.

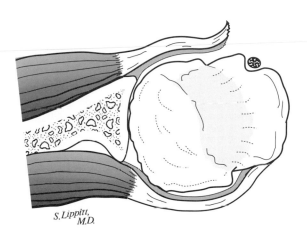

S. Lippitt, M.D.

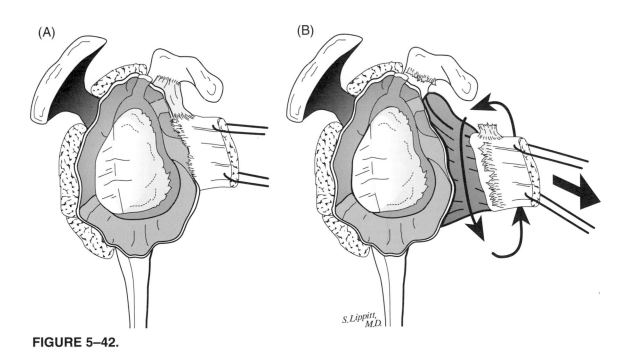

S. Lippitt, M.D.

FIGURE 5–42.

Mobilization of the subscapularis tendon. A, Attachment of the subscapularis tendon and capsule to the coracoid and glenoid. B, A complete 360-degree release about the subscapularis tendon optimizes muscular excursion and functionally increases the length of the subscapularis.

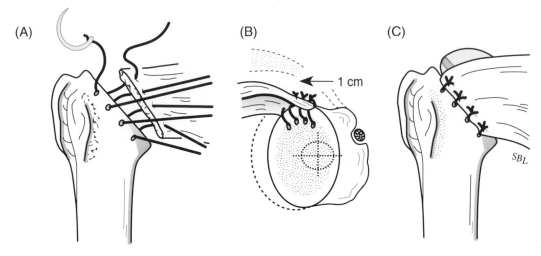

FIGURE 5–43.

The subscapularis is closed to the neck of the humerus rather than to the lesser tuberosity from which it was originally incised. This results in an effective lengthening of the tendon.

tuberosity (Fig. 5–43). If still more length is needed, an inside-out coronal plane Z-plasty can be performed, using the capsule to extend the tendon (Fig. 5–44). Each centimeter of subscapularis lengthening provides approximately 20 degrees of increased external rotation.

The capsule remaining on the anterior glenoid is excised along with any residual labrum. With a finger protecting the axillary nerve, the inferior capsule is incised from the glenoid, exposing the origin of the long head of the triceps (Fig. 5–45). Occasionally, if triceps contracture impedes motion, the

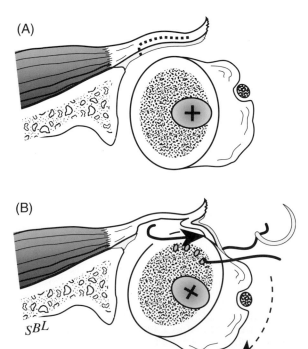

FIGURE 5–44.

The inside-out Z-plasty. *A*, Additional length of the subscapularis tendon can be gained by splitting the capsule from the tendon medially, leaving their connection laterally. *B*, The medial end of the split capsule is reflected and attached to the humeral neck.

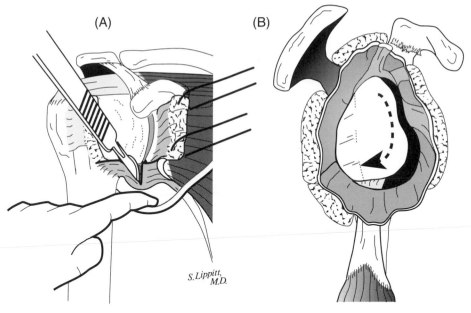

S.Lippitt, M.D.

FIGURE 5–45.

A, Division of the anteroinferior capsular attachments to the glenoid under direct vision while axillary nerve is protected and retracted. *B,* Capsular release to the 6 o'clock position on the glenoid exposes the origin of the long head of the triceps, which may require release as well.

triceps origin may need to be released in a manner similar to the adductor release in hip arthroplasty. If the posterior capsule is tight, it can be released later under direct vision after the humeral head has been excised. Posterior capsular release should not be performed if there is preoperative evidence of posterior subluxation.

Humeral Preparation. The humeral head is dislocated anteriorly by *gentle* external rotation and slight extension of the arm. Special care is exercised in elderly patients and in those with rheumatoid arthritis or other causes of fragile bone. Any resistance to this maneuver indicates the need for additional soft tissue release. Posterior humeral head osteophytes can impede the dislocation maneuver by impinging on the glenoid as the humerus is externally rotated. This phenomenon is suggested if the glenohumeral joint opens anteriorly like a book as the humerus is externally rotated. Often, in this situation, the humeral head along with the osteophytes can be safely and gently lifted into the joint with a flat elevator used as a "shoe

horn," inserted while the humerus is internally rotated (Fig. 5–46). A malunited greater tuberosity or large osteophytes may require osteotomy. By incorporating the movements of external rotation, anterior subluxation, and extension of the arm, the articular surface of the humerus is brought into view.

The humeral osteotomy requires attention to detail. In degenerative joint disease, the apparent articular surface does not provide an accurate indication of the plane of humeral head resection. Failure to account for the apparent elongation of the articular surface by inferior osteophytes results in an inordinately vertical (varus) resection level (Fig. 5–47). An excessively inferior or retroverted plane of resection jeopardizes the greater tuberosity and the insertion of the rotator cuff. To avoid these pitfalls, the humeral cut is based on readily identifiable landmarks. The ideal cut plane passes just inside the supraspinatus insertion to the tuberosity, at an angle of 45 degrees with the long axis of the shaft, and in 35 degrees of retroversion as judged by the external rota-

(A)

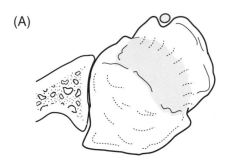

(B)

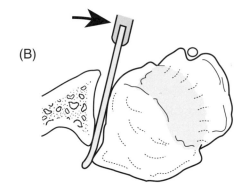

FIGURE 5–46.

Large posterior humeral osteophytes can form a barrier to external rotation and dislocation of the humeral head at arthroplasty surgery *(A)*. Reduction of large posterior osteophytes onto the glenoid face can usually be accomplished by placing a smooth retractor through the joint while the humerus is in internal rotation *(B)* and then gently externally rotating the humerus *(C)*.

(C)

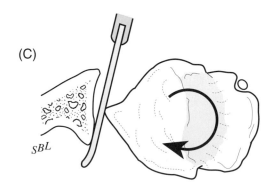

SBL

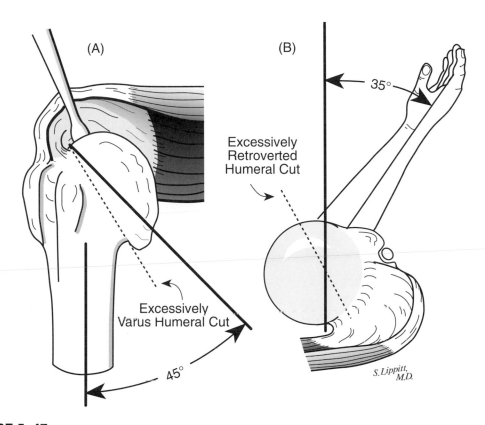

FIGURE 5–47.

Humeral osteotomy planes. *A,* The preferred osteotomy plane passes just inside the insertion of the rotator cuff to the greater tuberosity and proceeds at a 45-degree angle with respect to the long axis of the humeral shaft. If the osteotomy is incorrectly oriented such that it emerges at the margin of the osteophytes *(dotted line)*, the resulting cut will be in excessive varus. *B,* Humeral osteotomy also requires careful attention to version. An excessively retroverted cut *(dotted line)* compromises the cuff insertion.

tion of the forearm with the elbow flexed to a right angle. Cutting the head under direct vision with an osteotome while protecting the cuff with a blunt elevator facilitates verification of the plane and safety of the cut. Throughout the osteotomy, the cuff insertions and the biceps tendon are protected and observed as the osteotome passes by.

At this point the surgeon has an opportunity to judge the laxity of the joint. By placing the arm in 45 degrees of elevation and by using a finger to push the humeral neck laterally, the surgeon can get an idea of the joint volume remaining for the glenoid and humeral head component. This step is helpful in determining the need for further soft tissue balancing. If the capsule is so tight that even the smallest head will not fit, more release is required. Cutting away more neck

is not an option because the humeral cut is already at the cuff insertion.

The medullary canal of the humerus is reamed, starting at a point lateral on the cut surface just behind the bicipital groove. Starting with a small-diameter reamer, reaming is continued up to the diameter appropriate to the component, using a slight valgus bias and while protecting the biceps and cuff. Slots are made in the tuberosity to accommodate the fins of the component. The slot for the lateral fin should be just posterior to the bicipital groove (Fig. 5–48). In the presence of dense bone, failure to achieve adequate depth of these slots may result in the component being pushed into a varus orientation by contact between the fin and the bone of tuberosity. A trial component body is inserted so that the prosthetic neck

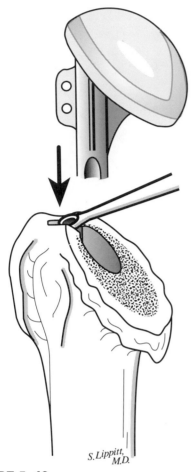

FIGURE 5–48.

Before implantation of the trial component, a slot is curetted in the tuberosity just posterior to the bicipital groove to accommodate the fin of the trial component.

is centered on the neck of the bony humerus, being neither too high (where the component will lead to excessive tension on the superior cuff), nor too low (where it will lead to subacromial abrasion of the tuberosities on elevation of the arm). The trial component is used as a guide to the excision of the osteophytes all around the humeral neck (Fig. 5–49). The rotator cuff, axillary nerve, and glenoid are protected during osteophyte excision.

While the trial humeral head is in place, the surgeon can verify that there is sufficient subscapularis length to allow 40 degrees of external rotation and adequate posterior laxity as indicated by 70 degrees of internal rotation of the arm elevated to 90 degrees in the coronal plane ("scarecrow" position) and 15 mm of translation on the posterior drawer test. If the joint is too tight with the trial head component alone, it will be even tighter after the glenoid is inserted. If necessary, additional capsular releases are performed at this stage to achieve the desired laxity. Additional posterior capsular release may be accomplished by incising the capsule at the glenoid rim while the capsule is held in tension by a proximal humeral retractor (Fig. 5–50). Care is taken to protect the axillary nerve below and the cuff behind.

With the trial humeral component removed and the proximal humerus displaced medially into the joint, the rotator cuff is

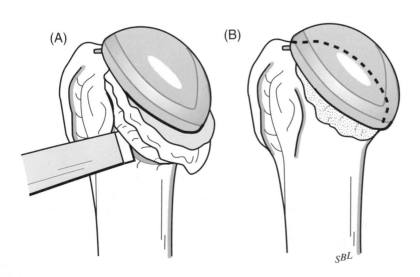

FIGURE 5–49.

A, Trial prosthetic head seated against osteotomy where it can serve as a guide for resecting any anterior, inferior, and posterior osteophytes that extend beyond its extrapolated articular surface. B, Osteophytes resected from the anterior, inferior, and posterior humeral neck. Posterior osteophytes must be removed with great care to protect rotator cuff insertion.

FIGURE 5–50.

If necessary, the sequential posterior release is accomplished by incising the capsule at the glenoid rim (release at the humerus would jeopardize the cuff insertion). During this release, the capsule is tensed by twisting the humeral retractor. Care is taken to protect the axillary nerve below and the cuff behind.

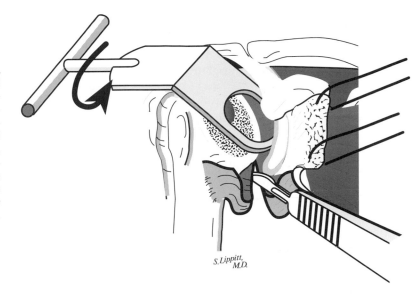

palpated to establish its integrity. If a reparable defect involving quality cuff tissue is identified, the retracted tendon is mobilized so it can reach the tuberosity without undue tension with the arthroplasty components in place. Sutures are placed in the edges of torn cuff tendon and through drill holes in the tuberosities for later tying after the components have been implanted (Fig. 5–51). Shorter humeral head components may facilitate cuff repair without undue tension. Cuff repair in association with shoulder arthroplasty tightens the joint and slows the rehabilitation. Thus, the surgeon must ensure that the repair is strong and durable. Suturing of poor-quality tendon or attempting repairs when insufficient tissue is present is not advised.

Tuberosity non-unions should be identified and mobilized at this point. Severe tuberosity malunions should be osteotomized; however, this should not be performed lightly: gaining tuberosity union can be difficult in the presence of a metal humeral component, diminished bone stock, and soft tissue contractions.

Preparation of the Glenoid. Accurate preparation of the glenoid bone requires the excellent surgical exposure provided after humeral head and osteophyte excision and capsular release. A flat retractor is placed behind the posterior glenoid lip to push the

head of the humerus posteriorly. When the resected surface of the humeral neck is flat against the back of the retractor (the arm externally rotated 35 degrees), the humerus can be pushed posteriorly with minimal force. In degenerative joint disease, this pos-

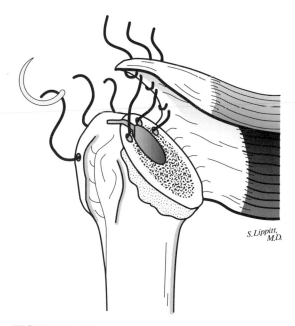

FIGURE 5–51.

Repair of a rotator cuff tear. If tissue is adequate for repair, drill holes are placed in the tuberosities for cuff attachment before the insertion of the humeral component.

terior displacement of the humerus is often facilitated by the fact that the humeral head has been chronically subluxated in the posterior direction. Initially, the glenoid exposure in degenerative joint disease may appear to be poor because the eroded glenoid appears to face excessively posteriorly. The exposure is often better than it initially seems, however, because the preparation of the glenoid surface will be along the normalized glenoid center line.

The goals of the glenoid part of the arthroplasty are (1) normalized glenoid orientation, (2) direct support of the component by precisely contoured bone, (3) secure fixation, and (4) avoidance of overstuffing.

We define glenoid orientation in terms of the glenoid center line, that is, the line perpendicular to the center of the normally oriented glenoid face. The shoulder arthroplasty surgeon should practice verifying the landmarks for a normal glenoid center line by drilling holes perpendicular to the midpoint on the glenoid face of normal cadaver scapulae and observing their exit in a consistent spot just medial to the anterior scapular neck, that is, the centering point. This spot lies between the upper and lower crura of the body of the scapula as they approach the neck. After the capsular releases have been performed at surgery, this centering point can be palpated at the lateral extent of the subscapularis fossa.

Because the location of this centering point is unaffected by arthritis, it is of great value in normalizing the orientation of a distorted glenoid face. It is particularly useful in correcting the posterior facing of the glenoid face that commonly results from posterior erosion in degenerative joint disease.

An index finger identifies the centering point on the anterior scapular neck (Fig. 5–52) while a hole is drilled from the center of the glenoid face toward it. Thus, the glenoid center line is defined from anatomic landmarks that are independent of the direction in which the pathologic glenoid appears to be facing. The orientation of the glenoid face is normalized using a spherical reamer with a guiding peg inserted along the glenoid center line drill hole (Fig. 5–53). In degenerative joint disease, this usually requires removal of more glenoid bone anteriorly than posteriorly because of the pathologic posterior erosion of the glenoid bone typical of this condition. During the reaming process, the amount of remaining bone supporting the anterior glenoid margin can be monitored under direct vision to ensure that adequate bone stock remains to support the component. Ideally, reaming is continued until the entire bony glenoid face is spheri-

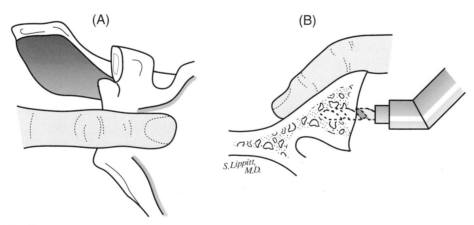

(A)   (B)

S. Lippitt, M.D.

FIGURE 5–52.

Use of the glenoid centering point to help orient the hole for glenoid fixation. *A,* The index finger is inserted anterior to the glenoid so that its tip palpates the centering point in the sulcus bounded by the thick upper and lower crura of the scapula and the flare of the glenoid vault. *B,* This centering point serves as a useful guide for drilling along the normal glenoid center line, particularly when the anatomic structure is distorted by eccentric glenoid wear. The normal glenoid center line connects the center of the glenoid face with the centering point.

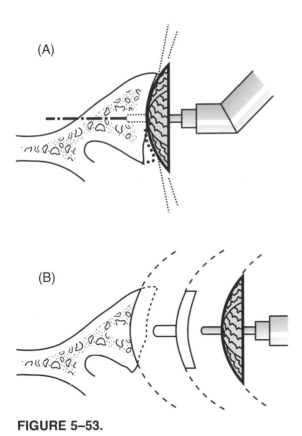

FIGURE 5–53.

A, Reaming along the drilled glenoid center line. The objective is to normalize the glenoid orientation and to contour the glenoid face to match the back of glenoid component. *B,* Accurate contouring of the glenoid face improves the quality of bony support for the glenoid component.

cally symmetric about the glenoid center line. Sufficient reaming is indicated if a smooth back trial glenoid slips easily around on the prepared surface while maintaining congruent contact with the prepared bone (the "Ivory Soap" sign). Rarely, if significant posterior bony support cannot be obtained without removing excessive anterior glenoid bone, a bone graft can be considered posteriorly (Fig. 5–54). In rheumatoid arthritis, minimal reaming is necessary and caution is needed—rheumatoid bone is soft and reams quickly.

Once the reaming is completed, the glenoid center line hole can be used to orient precisely a drill guide for making additional fixation holes as required by the particular glenoid component design. Each hole is checked to determine if it is competent or if it extends through the bone.

A glenoid component is selected that covers the prepared glenoid face with minimal overhang. A bigger component provides more stability and more component-to-bone load transfer. The quality of the glenoid bone preparation is checked by inserting the glenoid trial and ensuring that it does not rock even when the surgeon's finger applies an eccentric load to the rim.

After water spray irrigation, the holes can be cleaned and dried with a spray of sterile CO_2 gas. A small amount of cement is added to the holes, and the component pressed into position. If the back of the glenoid component matches the prepared bony face, there is no advantage in an interposed layer of cement, which could fail and displace, leaving the glenoid component relatively unsupported. Contact between precisely contoured bone and polyethylene provides an optimal load transfer mechanism. Fixation is checked, and the absence of residual cement bits in the posterior shoulder is verified.

In certain circumstances it may be advisa-

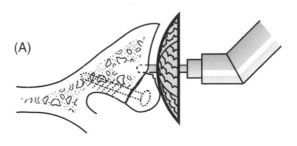

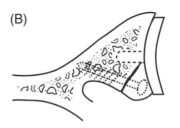

FIGURE 5–54.

Posterior glenoid bone grafting. When there is a major defect of the posterior glenoid, humeral head or iliac bone graft can be used to replace a deficient glenoid lip. If the fixation screw is recessed, the bone graft can be contoured and reamed for balanced support of glenoid component.

ble not to insert a glenoid component in spite of major abnormalities of the glenoid articular surface. One is the condition known as cuff tear arthropathy, for which the surgical approach is described in some detail later. Other conditions in which a glenoid is not inserted include situations when there is insufficient bone to support the component or where there is insufficient room within the soft tissue envelope of the shoulder to accommodate even the thinnest prosthetic glenoid. Glenoid component replacement may be inadvisable after a previously failed glenoid replacement. In this situation, the bone of the glenoid vault is compromised, and the chances of obtaining durable fixation of another component are greatly reduced. Finally, when there is a previous history of infection that has been clinically silent for a number of years, performing a cementless humeral hemiarthroplasty without a glenoid component may be a less risky approach than a full glenohumeral arthroplasty. In these situations it may also be advisable to perform a non-prosthetic glenoidplasty. Here the glenoid bone is prepared exactly as described earlier, using the glenoid center line and a concentric reamer of a diameter slightly larger than the diameter of the humeral head component's articular surface. However, a prosthetic glenoid is not inserted. This approach provides the advantages of normalization of the glenoid orientation and concavity without the risk of implantation of a glenoid component.

Insertion of the Humeral Body. Prior to the insertion of the body, the surgeon places at least five sutures of No. 2 non-absorbable suture in secure bone at the anterior humeral neck for later attachment of the subscapularis tendon. In a modular arthroplasty, the humeral body alone is inserted into the prepared canal at this point. If the tuberosities are intact, and if a good canal fit is obtained, no cement is required. Otherwise, cement may offer needed control of rotation and component height. The prosthetic humeral body is inserted so that its neck is centered on the anatomic humeral neck and the articular surface is correctly oriented. Proper orientation of the humeral component is more difficult than is com-

monly realized. An excessively prominent humeral component overstuffs the joint and compromises its range of motion. An excessively high component tightens the soft tissues in abduction. An excessively low component leaves the tuberosities prominent where they may impinge on the undersurface of the acromion. A varus orientation places the component in an excessively medial position, tightening the joint by increasing the distance between the scapula and the tuberosities.

Soft Tissue Balancing. Balancing of the soft tissues must be completed before the definitive humeral component is inserted. A shoulder arthroplasty with balanced soft tissues should allow (1) 70 degrees of internal rotation of the arm elevated 90 degrees in the coronal plane, (2) 15 mm of posterior subluxation of the humeral head on the posterior drawer test, (3) 140 degrees of elevation, and (4) 40 degrees of external rotation of the unelevated arm with the subscapularis approximated. A tighter shoulder not only has limited range of motion but may also foster obligate translation at the extremes of motion with resultant rim loading, risking glenoid loosening and component deformation.

We have found the following strategies useful in optimizing soft tissue balance:

1. Adjust the posterior soft tissue tension with graduated posterior soft tissue releases as necessary.
2. If the posterior soft tissues are too tight in spite of complete capsular releases, use a component with a shorter head and neck.
3. If the posterior soft tissues are too loose, try a component with a longer head and neck.
4. If there is excessive posterior instability (more than 15 mm of posterior translation or complete posterior dislocation) that cannot be managed by increased head size, the shoulder should be inspected for the sectioning of the rotator cuff attachments during the humeral head osteotomy or for excessive retroversion of the glenoid component. If disruption of the cuff has occurred, cuff repair should be carried out before the humeral prosthesis

is fixed into position. Rarely, it may be necessary to tighten the posterior capsule by suture imbrication inside the joint prior to final humeral head component placement.

It is important to remember that with a humeral prosthesis that fits snugly in the medullary canal, changes in version of the component are not likely to have a major effect in adjusting soft tissue tension or stability.

The prosthetic articulation is observed for appropriate joint surface relationships and to ensure the absence of impingement of the medial neck and shaft of the humerus on the glenoid component. It also important to check for tuberosity abutment against the glenoid at the extremes of allowed motion. No part of the bony humerus should touch the glenoid component in any allowed position of the joint.

Prior to closure the wound is thoroughly inspected for debris. The joint is put through a full range of motion to verify smoothness and lack of unwanted contact. The wound is drained. The subscapularis is repaired securely to the humeral neck so that the unelevated arm can be externally rotated by 40 degrees. If the subscapularis excessively limits the range of external rotation in spite of the 360 degree release of the tendon and the advancement from the lesser tuberosity to the neck, the inside-out Z-plasty is performed in which the capsule is used to lengthen the subscapularis tendon (see Fig. 5–44). The wound is closed in layers. Simple interrupted skin sutures are preferred when substantial drainage is anticipated or when wound healing may be impaired (such as in a patient receiving corticosteroids or with thin rheumatoid skin).

Postoperative Care

Because primary goals of arthroplasty surgery are to provide motion and smoothness, immediate postoperative passive motion is important. The immediate postoperative program is essentially the same as that used after the open release of a frozen shoulder. We use a simple motor-driven adjustable cam and pulley system that puts the shoulder through a 90 degree arc of flexion and a 45 degree arc of rotation (see Fig. 2–38). This system is used for at least 24 of the first 48 postoperative hours. The patient is taught to use the opposite arm for assisted elevation and external rotation. A "motivation" chart is maintained on the wall of the patient's hospital room displaying progress toward the discharge goals of 140 degrees of elevation and 40 degrees of rotation (see Fig. 2–44). Grip and external rotation isometrics are started immediately. Unless a rotator cuff repair has been performed, the patient is encouraged to use the shoulder as comfort permits for active elevation and activities of daily living. If rotator cuff repairs or osteotomies have been performed, active motion and isometric cuff strengthening are delayed until healing has occurred.

The details of the standard program are shown in Patient Information 5–4.

The Impact of Shoulder Arthroplasty on Shoulder Function in Degenerative Joint Disease

Figure 5-55 shows the preoperative SST results for patients having glenohumeral arthroplasty for degenerative joint disease, as well as the SST responses from patients 6, 12, and 18 months after their surgical procedure. Such data not only indicate the increment of shoulder function but also reflect the time necessary to regain the various functions of the SST.

Arthroplasty in Rheumatoid Arthritis

The basic principles of shoulder arthroplasty in rheumatoid arthritis are similar to those in degenerative arthritis, but some important differences exist. Rheumatoid tissues are much more fragile. The bone is more prone to fracture, and the muscle and tendons are more prone to tear. Thus, from the outset, extreme care must be taken to preserve bone and soft tissue integrity. We

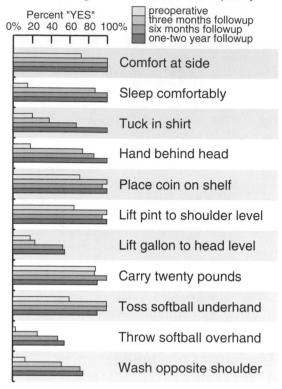

SST Data Before Surgery and Sequentially Following Total Shoulder Arthroplasty

Percent "YES"
0% 20 40 60 80 100%

- preoperative
- three months followup
- six months followup
- one-two year followup

Comfort at side
Sleep comfortably
Tuck in shirt
Hand behind head
Place coin on shelf
Lift pint to shoulder level
Lift gallon to head level
Carry twenty pounds
Toss softball underhand
Throw softball overhand
Wash opposite shoulder

FIGURE 5–55.

The Simple Shoulder Test data before and at 6, 12, and 18 months after glenohumeral arthroplasty for degenerative joint disease. These data show the characteristic severity of functional compromise prior to arthroplasty and the typical restoration of function after surgery.

refer to these requirements for extraordinary gentleness as "rheumatoid rules."

Because rheumatoid arthritis is an erosive and destructive disease, tissue deficiencies of the bone and rotator cuff are more likely than in degenerative joint disease. Thus, the soft tissues anteriorly may be insufficient to allow for a subscapularis lengthening. The glenoid bone may be so eroded that there is insufficient stock to support a glenoid component. The rotator cuff may be partially or totally deficient. Thus, in the preoperative evaluation and in discussion with the patient concerning the possible outcomes of surgery, all of these factors need to be considered.

The standard preoperative scapular anteroposterior and axillary radiographs are required to evaluate the humeral and glenoid bone stock. In rheumatoid arthritis the glenoid erosion is usually medial (rather than posterior, as in degenerative joint disease). For this reason, only minimal glenoid reaming may be necessary to achieve an excellent quality fit to the back of the glenoid component. The potential fragility of the bone and soft tissues makes it particularly important that the joint not be overstuffed and that adequate soft tissue laxity be present for immediate postoperative motion. This is particularly a challenge in diminutive patients with juvenile rheumatoid arthritis. In some instances there may be insufficient joint volume to permit the insertion of a glenoid component in spite of complete soft tissue releases.

Arthroplasty in Post-Traumatic Arthritis

In post-traumatic arthritis, the challenges may be even greater. The anatomic structure is likely to be distorted by previous fracture and surgery. The non-articular humeroscapular motion interface is likely to be scarred, obscuring important neurologic structures, such as the axillary nerve. The tuberosities,

Text continued on page 219

UNIVERSITY OF WASHINGTON SHOULDER AND ELBOW SERVICE

Rehabilitation and After-Care of the Shoulder Arthroplasty

The goal of shoulder arthroplasty is to restore function to an impaired shoulder. Good shoulder function requires motion, stability, strength, and smoothness. During the operation we seek to optimize your shoulder's motion and stability by balancing the soft tissues around your joint and releasing adhesions and contractures. The smoothness of your joint is improved by the implantation of highly polished artificial joint surfaces. The stage is now set for you to continue the improvement in motion and stability and to develop some strength in your reconstructed shoulder with a simple, but vitally important, series of exercises.

EARLY MOTION. Early on after your operation, the highest priority is maintaining the gains in motion achieved by your surgery. Because the muscles in the operated shoulder are expected to be weak after surgery, we have to depend on other means to maintain the motion during the first critical weeks. We often use a passive motion machine immediately after surgery to move the arm gently through an arc of motion even while you are recovering from your anesthetic.

You will maintain and improve your shoulder reach using a routine that includes the following three basic maneuvers.

1. *The Warm-Up.*
Bend over, letting the operated arm dangle comfortably in front of you, and move it in gentle circles in a clockwise and counterclockwise direction with your hand pointing forward and with your hand pointing back. This is predominantly to loosen up the shoulder and to relax it.

2. *Assisted Overhead Reach in the Supine Position.*
Lie on your back in a relaxed position. Grasp the wrist of the operated arm with your other hand. While relaxing the operated arm, use your unoperated arm to pull the wrist up toward the ceiling and then beyond the vertical position above your head. This exercise should be performed slowly, again with emphasis on relaxing the muscles in the operated shoulder and on comfort. When you get the arm to the position where things seem to get tight, try to relax the muscles even further to allow a few more degrees of motion. When you get to the maximum amount of elevation, hold the arm there for a count of twenty, again while trying to maximize muscle relaxation (see Fig. 5–7).

3. *The Pulley.*
A pulley is mounted on a door with handles for both hands. Sit in a chair facing the door. Place one handle in the hand of the operated shoulder while it is relaxed at your side. Using the unoperated hand to pull down on the other handle, gently raise the operated shoulder to a horizontal and then toward a vertical position. Again, this exercise is performed with total relaxation of the operated arm. When the arm appears to stop because of stiffness, you should concentrate on relaxing the operated arm, trying to get even greater degrees of elevation. When you finally reach the apparent maximum in elevation, hold it for a count of twenty while optimizing the relaxation.

It is essential that these range of motion exercises be performed at least five times a day. Maintaining the range of motion gained at surgery is one of the essential ingredients in restoring the function to your shoulder. There is no one more qualified to do that than you. Devise a system for registering your progress in these motion exercises. For example, mark a spot on the bedpost that you can reach while lying on your back, or mark the height on the door that you can reach with the pulley. Keeping track of your progress on a daily basis will make sure that you are moving forward and provide you with well-deserved positive feedback.

Your goal for overhead reach is 140 degrees. We will help you keep track of your progress toward this goal.

Other motion exercises are important to your rehabilitation. We have indicated the exercises you should do with a check preceding the descriptions below. Please do the indicated exercises five times each day.

☐ *External Rotation.* External rotation refers to the movement of the forearm out away from the body with the elbow kept at the side. Bend your elbow to a right angle and then use a cane, yardstick, or a wooden dowel to push the hand of the operated arm out to the side, using the opposite arm for power (see Fig. 5–9). Again, the emphasis is placed on relaxation of the operated arm. Gains in motion are accomplished by relaxation of the operated arm rather than by power applied by the opposite arm. We defined the range of external rotation in terms of degrees. Zero degrees is the position in which the forearm points straight forward; 90 degrees is the position in which the forearm is rotated all the way out so that it lies flat on the bed or the floor. Your goal for external rotation is 40 degrees.

☐ *Internal Rotation.* Internal rotation is accomplished by reaching with the hand of the operated arm up the back. You should assist your operated arm by reaching up behind you with the opposite hand to grasp the wrist of the operated arm and gently draw it up your back or by using a towel (see Fig. 5–11). Note how high up your back you can reach with your thumb.

Again, these exercises are carried out with maximal relaxation of your operated arm. Your goal for internal rotation is to reach the small of your back.

☐ *Cross-Body Movement.* In this exercise, you reach across the front of your chest (see Fig. 5–12). Again you use the opposite hand to grasp the elbow of the operated arm and gently draw it across your chest toward the other shoulder.

ACTIVITIES WITH THE OPERATED ARM. Comfortable activities with the operated arm are encouraged after surgery. We have determined that the activities checked below are appropriate for you at this time:

☐ Working on your grip by squeezing play putty, foam, or a tennis ball.

☐ Raising your hand to your face to eat and wash.

☐ Writing, keyboarding, sewing, and answering the telephone.

☐ Swinging the arm in a relaxed way at your side while walking.

GENERAL AEROBIC EXERCISES. Often, your shoulder condition, your surgery, and the immediate postoperative recovery have slowed your general activities. Immediately after surgery is the time to begin a gentle conditioning program, which can include walking, using a stationary bicycle or a stair climber, or a combination of other gentle, general exercises. Ideally, this kind of exercise should be performed at least a half-hour every day. Overall conditioning will have a direct positive effect on the recovery of your shoulder.

STRENGTHENING. Strengthening of the shoulder after arthroplasty is a vital step in the restoration of function. However, strengthening exercises early after the operation are not nearly as important as es-

216

tablishing motion. Therefore, we institute strengthening exercises only after you can achieve excellent motion and shoulder comfort. After your prolonged shoulder arthritis and your shoulder replacement, your muscles are expected to be weak and sore. In many instances, a period of time for muscle healing is required before strengthening can be started. Please be sure that you do not do any strengthening exercises that are painful: this is *not* a "no pain, no gain" situation. If you have any questions about the advisability of these strengthening exercises, wait until you have checked with us.

Strengthening concerns primarily the muscles that raise the arm: the anterior deltoid and the rotator cuff muscles. These muscles are strengthened by simple exercises indicated below. You should be carrying out only the exercises we have indicated below with a check in the appropriate box.

☐ *Supine Press.* This exercise has a series of stages. It is important that you achieve twenty comfortable repetitions at each stage before advancing to the next stage.

Stage 1. Hands together. Lie on your back holding a cane, a yardstick, or dowel across your chest with two hands together. Push up toward the ceiling.

Stage 2. Hands apart. Hold the cane, yardstick, or dowel 3 feet apart and push from across your chest up toward the ceiling.

Stage 3. Hand alone. Push with the hand of the operated shoulder from a position alongside the shoulder up toward the ceiling.

Stage 4. Hand alone with 1 lb weight. Same as stage 3 except holding a 1-lb weight in the hand of the operated shoulder.

Stage 5. Progressive tilt. Perform the hand alone exercise using a 1-lb weight, with your back in an increasingly vertical position (using a lawn chair or recliner) until the exercise can be performed twenty times in the full sitting position.

☐ *External Rotation.* Hold your arms with the elbows at the side and at a right angle. Externally rotate the arms against the resistance of rubber tubing held in each hand. Use only a strength of rubber tubing that allows twenty comfortable repetitions, increasing the strength of the tubing as the strength of the arm increases.

ACTIVITIES. In general, activities of the shoulder can be increased as the comfort, range of motion, and strength of the motion allow. It is essential that these activities be added gradually and progressively so that there is no risk of straining your muscles. A sudden increase in activity or abrupt jerky or forceful activities will jeopardize the comfort and function of your shoulder.

☐ *Water Exercises.* Water exercises are often well tolerated by the shoulder after arthroplasty. Gentle movements of the arm in shoulder-deep water, progressing slowly to swimming the breast stroke and then the crawl, are helpful in restoring strength, coordination, and endurance to the shoulder.

☐ *Driving.* Driving is not advised after shoulder replacement until two conditions are met: (1) it has been at least 6 weeks after the operation, and (2) the shoulder is comfortable enough and strong enough so that when you are standing, you can raise it to the horizontal position straight out in front of you twenty times. Using these criteria, we avoid placing the shoulder, passengers, other drivers, and pedestrians at risk from a shoulder that cannot perform in emergency circumstances.

To review, our goal is to teach *you* how to successfully rehabilitate *your* shoulder. This requires the early gaining of excellent range of motion and the slow but progressive addition of strength, coordination, and endurance. Frequent, gentle exercises have been proven much more effective than irregular, forceful efforts. The goal is a smooth progression in activities without any episodes of soreness from overdoing it. Make sure that each stage of exercises can be performed comfortably and with the required number of repetitions before advancing to the next stage. If soreness does develop, strengthening exercises are stopped, but the range of motion exercises must be continued so that stiffness does not result. Nothing must interfere with the regular five-times-a-day conduct of the range of motion program.

Many years of shoulder disability cannot be reversed without persistent work over time on range of motion, strength, and coordination. The shoulder requires 2 years of rehabilitative exercises to reach maximal function after a shoulder replacement. If you are willing to commit to such a rehabilitative effort, you will achieve maximum benefit from your shoulder arthroplasty. If you have any questions about this program, please be sure to ask us.

TABLE 5–4. Increment in Function After Special Hemiarthroplasty for Cuff Tear Arthropathy

	Preoperative	Postoperative
Active elevation	71 degrees	115 degrees
External rotation	30 degrees	41 degrees
Internal rotation (segment)	L5	L1
Perineal care	2/10 patients	9/10 patients
Reach opposite axilla	3/10 patients	10/10 patients
Comb hair	2/10 patients	8/10 patients
Sleep on side	2/10 patients	9/10 patients
Use above shoulder level	0/10 patients	6/10 patients

the humeral shaft, and the glenoid may be non-united or malunited.

As a first step, the motion interface must be carefully freed, and the axillary nerve identified both as it crosses the subscapularis and as it courses laterally on the deep surface of the deltoid. Case-by-case judgments must be made concerning the need for osteotomy to try to restore more normal anatomic relationships, recognizing that additional healing and postoperative protection may be required. Again, the goal is restoration of anatomic relationships, firm fixation of components, soft tissue balance, stability, and smooth gliding in the non-articular humeroscapular motion interface.

Arthroplasty in Rotator Cuff Tear Arthropathy

In rotator cuff tear arthropathy, there are several unique challenges for regaining glenohumeral smoothness. The humeral head is subluxated in a superior position so that it is articulating with the coracoacromial arch. The rotator cuff is almost never amenable to a strong repair, and the glenoid is eroded superiorly, so that an acetabular-like structure is formed in continuity with the coracoacromial arch. Under these circumstances, the surgeon must make a judgment as to whether the glenohumeral relationships can be normalized and maintained by a durable cuff reconstruction or whether one should accept the altered joint relationship that uses the "acetabulum" for secondary stability in the absence of primary stability from the rotator cuff. We often select

the latter course, performing a "special hemiarthroplasty," in which the articular surface of the proximal humerus is resurfaced with a component matching the preoperative humeral joint surface size and position. The tuberosities are smoothed so that they are congruous with the humeral articular surface. This allows for the proximal humerus to match the "acetabulum," and to articulate smoothly within it. It is important to avoid using oversized humeral components, because they overstuff the joint, do not match the concavity of the "acetabulum" and restrict joint motion. In a special hemiarthroplasty, the patient is spared the necessity of protecting a rotator cuff repair, so that immediate passive and active exercises can be instituted after surgery. The patient is also spared the risk of glenoid loosening from the rocking horse mechanism.

The ideal patient for this procedure has a normal deltoid muscle, a concentric coracoacromial "acetabulum," concentric erosion of the upper glenoid fossa, a "femoralized" upper humerus with rounding off of the greater tuberosity, an irreparable rotator cuff defect, no previous surgical compromise of the acromion or coracoacromial ligament, good patient motivation, and realistic expectations.

In a series of ten patients having special hemiarthroplasty for rotator cuff tear arthropathy, the range of active motion and function were substantially improved by this procedure (Table 5–4). These results may not be as good as those for total glenohumeral arthroplasty because the patients lack the benefit of both prosthetic glenoid smoothness as well as the function of their rotator cuff.

CHAPTER

6

Synthesis: Practice Guidelines

This chapter proposes practice guidelines for the important and treatable mechanical problems of the shoulder covered in previous chapters. The increasing demands for cost-effective health care delivery create a need for such practice guidelines to help systematize the approach to common medical conditions. These protocols suggest approaches to evaluation and management that can improve efficiency and reduce unnecessary expenditures. This chapter provides a practical synthesis of much of the information in the preceding chapters, which should be consulted for further detail.

INITIAL CLINICAL EVALUATION OF THE PATIENT WITH A CHRONIC SHOULDER PROBLEM

The purpose of the initial evaluation is to determine if the patient's problem includes one or more of the major mechanical characteristics discussed in this text: stiffness, instability, weakness, or roughness. This evaluation proceeds along the following steps:

1. The patient and family complete the Patient Information Form (see Chapter 1) before coming to the office.
2. The physician and office staff review the Patient Information Form to preplan the office visit, noting the patient's age and functional self-assessment as well as any historical, physical, and socioeconomic factors that may bear on the patient's evaluation and management.
3. At the time of the visit, the physician and patient explore the information on the Patient Information Form, seeking to differentiate mechanical from non-mechanical problems.

Mechanical problems are typically

1. Recognizable as mechanical in nature by the patient.
2. Related to certain activities or positions.
3. Reproducible.
4. Able to be localized by the patient.

Non-mechanical problems are typically

1. Not related to activity or position.
2. More difficult for the patient to localize.

In addition, these non-mechanical problems may

3. Be accompanied by heat, swelling, redness, and tenderness.
4. Have a neurologic pattern, with radiation from the neck to locations distal to the deltoid tubercle.
5. Have aggravation by neck positions rather than shoulder positions.

If the problem is non-mechanical, it needs further evaluation. Evaluation and management of non-mechanical problems are not discussed in this text.

INTERMEDIATE CLINICAL EVALUATION OF THE PATIENT WITH A MECHANICAL SHOULDER PROBLEM

The physician uses a directed history to help identify the relative contributions of stiffness, instability, weakness, and roughness, as follows:

Stiffness—The patient notes an inability to achieve full range of motion or functional positions.

Instability—The patient notes that the shoulder shifts, or "goes out," during activities.

Weakness—The patient notes insufficient strength or endurance to carry out activities.

Roughness—The patient notes the shoulder grinds or catches.

A variety of causes may produce each of the four types of mechanical shoulder problems. Usually these problems can be evaluated with a basic shoulder evaluation consisting of a good history, a good physical examination, and a few good-quality plain radiographs.

I. Shoulder Stiffness

The basic evaluation seeks to resolve the problem into one of three principal categories: frozen shoulder, post-traumatic or post-surgical stiff shoulder, and stiffness associated with glenohumeral roughness (see Chapter 2).

A. History
  1. Frozen shoulder
     a. Age typically 40 to 65 years at presentation
     b. Onset usually spontaneous
     c. Limited shoulder motion in all directions
     d. Functional problems frequently include difficulty sleeping on the affected side, placing the hand behind the head with the arm out to the side, throwing, and washing the back of the opposite shoulder
     e. May be preceded by a period of shoulder disuse
     f. Diabetes may be a predisposing factor
  2. Post-traumatic or post-surgical stiff shoulder
     a. Age at presentation varies widely (ranging from 20 to 65 years)
     b. Onset related to previous major injury or surgery
     c. Limited range of motion
  3. Stiffness plus glenohumeral roughness
     a. Usually older than 50 years of age
     b. Onset usually gradual
     c. Limited range of motion
     d. Possible history of "catching" on shoulder movement

B. Physical: humerothoracic, humeroscapular, and scapulothoracic ranges are noted for both shoulders
  1. Frozen shoulder: glenohumeral range of motion limited in all directions
  2. Post-traumatic or post-surgical stiff shoulder: glenohumeral range may be limited globally or only in specific directions. Note previous incisions and relation of previous injury or surgery to directions of motion limitation
  3. Stiffness plus glenohumeral roughness: roughness on motion within a limited range of motion

C. Radiographs: an anteroposterior view in plane of scapula and proper axillary view are obtained with the arm in the centered position (see Fig. 5–5) to help evaluate the smoothness of the glenohumeral joint surface

  1. Frozen shoulder: radiographs show no evidence of joint surface abnormality
  2. Post-traumatic or post-surgical stiff shoulder: radiographs may show evidence of previous injury or surgery
  3. Stiffness plus glenohumeral roughness: radiographs show narrowing and roughness of joint surfaces

II. Glenohumeral Instability

The basic evaluation seeks to categorize the problem into the traumatic or atraumatic type (see Chapter 3).

A. History
  1. Traumatic instability
     a. Age typically 15 to 40 years at presentation
     b. Onset most commonly related to a *major* extension and external rotation force applied to the arm elevated in the coronal plane
     c. Recurrent episodes of apprehension or unwanted translation occur in consistent positions, most frequently when the elevated arm is extended and externally rotated
     d. Diagnosis supported by previous radiographs showing glenohumeral dislocation
     e. Functional problems are often primarily with activities such as throwing or using the arm in posterior planes
  2. Atraumatic instability
     a. Age typically 15 to 35 years at presentation
     b. Onset is usually insidious, in the absence of trauma sufficient to tear stabilizing structures
     c. Recurrent episodes of unwanted translation occurring in a variety of positions, frequently with the arm at the side or when the arm is internally rotated and elevated in anterior planes
     d. Unwanted translations reduce spontaneously
     e. Patient able to demonstrate instability voluntarily

f. Functional difficulties commonly include difficulty sleeping and difficulty raising 8 lb anteriorly with arm straight

B. Physical examination

1. Traumatic instability

a. Reproduction of the patient's primary symptoms of apprehension or unwanted translation on placing the relaxed arm in the position of injury (usually elevated, extended, and externally rotated)

b. An anterior labral avulsion is suggested by crepitance or grinding with translation on the anterior drawer test

2. Atraumatic instability

a. Patient's symptoms are reproduced by translating the glenohumeral joint in various directions

b. Diminished resistance to translation in multiple directions

c. Sometimes associated with increased ligamentous laxity of both shoulders and other articulations as well

C. Radiographs: an anteroposterior view in the plane of the scapula and proper axillary view

1. Traumatic instability: diagnosis supported by radiographs showing a characteristic defect of the posterior lateral humeral head or characteristic calcification or damage of the anterior inferior glenoid lip

2. Atraumatic instability: absence of traumatic lesions

III. Weakness

The basic evaluation seeks to identify treatable rotator cuff pathologic conditions and to distinguish them from neurologic causes of weakness (see Chapter 4).

A. History

1. Incomplete thickness rotator cuff lesion

a. Age typically 30 to 55 years at presentation

b. Onset in younger patients related to injury applying unexpected eccentric load to elevated arm

c. Often related to work or sport

d. Functional difficulty in active elevation against resistance

2. Complete thickness rotator cuff tear

a. Age typically 45 to 75 years at presentation

b. Onset in younger patients related to injury applying major eccentric load to humerus

c. Onset in older patients may be insidious and apparently atraumatic

d. Significant weakness, especially on elevation of the arm in anterior planes

e. Functional problems often include difficulty sleeping, difficulty lifting 8 lb to shoulder level, and difficulty throwing

3. Neurologic causes of weakness (two important examples)

a. Brachial neuritis: several weeks of severe pain followed by weakness, often in distribution of suprascapular, long thoracic, or axillary nerve

b. Cervical radiculopathy: symptoms aggravated by neck position with radiation down the arm distal to the deltoid insertion; may have sensory or motor deficits

B. Physical examination

1. Incomplete thickness rotator cuff lesion

a. Positive tendon signs

i. Weakness of isometric elevation of arm at 90 degrees in the plus 45 degree thoracic plane

ii. Weakness of isometric external rotation (if tear involves the infraspinatus)

iii. Weakness of isometric internal rotation (if tear involves the subscapularis)

b. May have mild atrophy of supraspinatus and possibly infraspinatus

c. May have abrasion sign (crepitance on passive rotation of arm elevated to 90 degree position) if tear involves superior surface of tendon

2. Complete thickness rotator cuff tear
   a. Positive tendon signs
      i. Weakness of isometric elevation of arm at 90 degrees in the plus 45 degree thoracic plane
      ii. Weakness of isometric external rotation
      iii. Weakness of isometric internal rotation (if tear involves the subscapularis)
   b. Significant atrophy of supraspinatus and infraspinatus
   c. Often has abrasion sign
3. Neurologic causes of weakness
   a. Brachial neuritis: weakness confined to distribution of peripheral nerve affected (suprascapular nerve involvement produces a pattern of weakness similar to that of a rotator cuff tear)
   b. Cervical radiculopathy
      i. Weakness and sensory loss confined to distribution of nerve roots involved (C5–6 radiculopathy produces a pattern of weakness that includes the cuff and deltoid muscles along with the elbow flexors and supinators)
      ii. Aggravation of symptoms on turning chin toward the affected side
C. Radiographs: an anteroposterior view in plane of scapula and proper axillary view
   1. Incomplete thickness rotator cuff lesion: radiographs usually normal; may show sclerosis of acromial undersurface
   2. Complete thickness rotator cuff tear
      a. Radiographs may show superior displacement of the humeral head in relation to acromion and traction spur formation in the coracoacromial ligament
      b. Radiographs may show cystic changes in the greater tuberosity

IV. Roughness

The basic evaluation seeks to localize the site of roughness and determine the pres-

ence of treatable pathologic changes (see Chapter 5).
A. History
   1. Subacromial abrasion
      a. Compromised function with arms in intermediate positions of elevation
      b. "Catching" of shoulder in mid elevation localized to acromial area
   2. Snapping scapula
      a. Catching or grating of shoulder with movement of the shoulder girdle
      b. Symptoms localized to the posterior medial corner of the scapula
   3. Glenohumeral roughness
      a. Primary degenerative joint disease
         i. Age typically 50 to 75 years at presentation
         ii. Onset without major joint trauma or surgery
         iii. Limited motion and function
         iv. Functional problems often include difficulty sleeping, difficulty tucking in a shirt, difficulty placing the hand behind the head with the arm out to the side, difficulty lifting 8 lb to the level of the shoulder, and difficulty washing the back of the opposite shoulder
      b. Secondary degenerative joint disease
         i. Major shoulder joint injury or disease
         ii. Limited motion and function
      c. Rheumatoid arthritis
         i. Age typically 40 to 65 years at presentation for shoulder problem
         ii. Systemic manifestations of rheumatoid arthritis
         iii. Limited motion and difficulties performing virtually all of the Simple Shoulder Test functions.
      d. Avascular necrosis
         i. Age typically 25 to 50 years at presentation
         ii. Risk factors, such as steroid use
         iii. Limited function, particularly in the ability to allow the arm

to hang comfortably at the side or to sleep on the affected side
   e. Capsulorrhaphy arthropathy
      i. Age ranges from 25 to 60 years at presentation
      ii. Previous repair for glenohumeral instability
      iii. Limited function, especially difficulty sleeping, and limited motion, particularly external rotation
   f. Cuff tear arthropathy
      i. Age typically 60 to 80 years at presentation
      ii. Limited motion, particularly in elevation of the arm
      iii. Limited function in almost all of the activities of the Simple Shoulder Test
      iv. Previously documented cuff tear
B. Physical Examination
   1. Subacromial abrasion
      a. Abrasion sign: crepitance on isolated humeroscapular rotation when humerus is elevated to 90 degrees. Patients should recognize this crepitance as the cause of their functional limitation
      b. May also have tendon signs (weakness or pain on isometric challenge of cuff muscles)
      c. May have associated stiffness, especially of the posterior capsule, manifesting as limited cross-body adduction and internal rotation
   2. Snapping scapula
      a. No symptomatic crepitance on isolated humeroscapular motion
      b. Crepitance on active or passive isolated scapulothoracic motion, often with contortive movements
      c. May have slumping shoulder posture
   3. Glenohumeral roughness
      a. Degenerative joint disease (primary or secondary)
         i. Limited motion, especially in external rotation
         ii. Dry glenohumeral crepitance on isolated humeroscapular motion
      b. Rheumatoid arthritis

         i. Limited motion
         ii. Weakness and muscle atrophy
         iii. May have joint effusion or synovitis
         iv. Dry glenohumeral crepitance on isolated humeroscapular motion
         v. Other manifestations of rheumatoid arthritis
      c. Avascular necrosis
         i. Range of motion often not severely limited
         ii. May have glenohumeral "clunk" or catch on isolated humeroscapular motion
      d. Capsulorrhaphy arthropathy
         i. Evidence of previous surgery
         ii. Limited motion, especially in external rotation
         iii. Dry glenohumeral crepitance on isolated humeroscapular motion
      e. Cuff tear arthropathy
         i. Limited humeroscapular elevation
         ii. Dry glenohumeral and subacromial crepitance on isolated humeroscapular motion
         iii. Severe supraspinatus and infraspinatus atrophy
         iv. Weakness of isometric elevation and external rotation
         v. Palpable defect in rotator cuff near greater tuberosity
         vi. Superior displacement of humeral head relative to scapula
C. Radiographs: an anteroposterior view in plane of scapula and proper axillary view.
   1. Subacromial abrasion: may have primary or secondary changes of the undersurface of the coracoacromial arch, such as sclerosis or traction spurs in the coracoacromial ligament
   2. Snapping scapula: rarely, the lateral view of the scapula may reveal an osteochondroma on the costal aspect
   3. Glenohumeral roughness
      a. Degenerative joint disease (primary or secondary)
         i. Joint space narrowing (typically, axillary view shows posterior glenoid erosion with

posterior subluxation of humeral head). This joint space narrowing may be particularly evident on the anteroposterior view in the plane of the scapula if the arm is placed in the centering position of 45 degrees of abduction and neutral rotation with respect to the thorax
 ii. Periarticular sclerosis
 iii. Periarticular osteophytes
b. Rheumatoid arthritis
 i. Joint space narrowing
 ii. Osteopenia
 iii. Periarticular erosions
 iv. Medial erosion of glenoid
 v. Minimal or absent sclerosis and osteophytes
c. Avascular necrosis
 i. Joint space often not narrowed until late phases of disease process
 ii. Sclerosis within humeral head
 iii. Collapse of subchondral bone of humeral head
d. Capsulorrhaphy arthropathy
 i. Joint space narrowing
 ii. Periarticular sclerosis and osteophytes
 iii. Posterior glenoid erosion with posterior subluxation of humeral head
 iv. May reveal evidence of previous surgical capsulorrhaphy
e. Cuff tear arthropathy
 i. Contact between humeral head and acromion
 ii. Joint space narrowing
 iii. Periarticular sclerosis and osteophytes
 iv. Femoralization of proximal humerus
 v. Acetabularization of glenocoracoacromial arch

INITIAL MANAGEMENT: PATIENT EDUCATION AND PATIENT-CONDUCTED HOME PROGRAMS

For chronic mechanical problems of stiffness, instability, weakness, and roughness, the initial management usually can be determined by the basic evaluation described in the previous section. Patients are informed about the probable nature of their condition as well as the options for management. Unless the basic evaluation suggests otherwise, patients are encouraged to participate in the appropriate self-help program, as follows:

1. Home Exercise Program for the Stiff Shoulder (see Chapter 2)
2. Home Exercise Program for Atraumatic Instability (see Chapter 3)
3. Home Exercise Program for the Weak Shoulder (see Chapter 4)
4. Home Exercise Program for the Rough Shoulder (see Chapter 5).

Because the conditions being managed are chronic, there is adequate time to evaluate the results of simple, patient-conducted programs and to observe the change of symptoms and function over several weeks or months. Patients are reminded that chronic conditions do not resolve overnight. Reevaluation of the patient at 6 to 12 weeks provides an opportunity to confirm the history and physical findings, to determine the benefit of their home program, and to consider alternative diagnoses and management plans.

FURTHER EVALUATION

Most chronic mechanical problems of the shoulder can be evaluated with the basic clinical examination. Expensive tests are reserved for when they will have an important effect on the patient's management. The need for surgery or other forms of advanced management is determined not by additional tests but by factors such as the functional deficit produced by the problem, the diligence of and the response to exercises, and the opportunity for improvement with a more aggressive approach.

Stiffness. Additional tests or consultation may be indicated if the basic evaluation and observation suggest that other factors may be contributing to refractory shoulder stiffness, such as cervical radiculopathy, tumor, diabetes, cardiac pathology, and motivational problems.

Instability. Additional tests are usually not indicated in that they rarely change the treatment of instability.

Weakness. Electromyography and nerve conduction tests may be needed to differentiate neurologic causes of weakness (e.g., cervical radiculopathy and brachial neuritis) from musculotendinous causes of weakness (e.g., rotator cuff tear). Rotator cuff imaging (e.g., arthrography, ultrasonography, and arthroscopy) is indicated only if it has the po-

tential to change the management (not just to "confirm" the diagnosis). For example, cuff imaging may be necessary to evaluate the presence, location, and extent of a suspected incomplete thickness cuff lesion that has not responded to a course of non-operative management and for which surgery is being contemplated.

Roughness. Additional tests to evaluate shoulder roughness usually do not change the management of the patient. The thera-

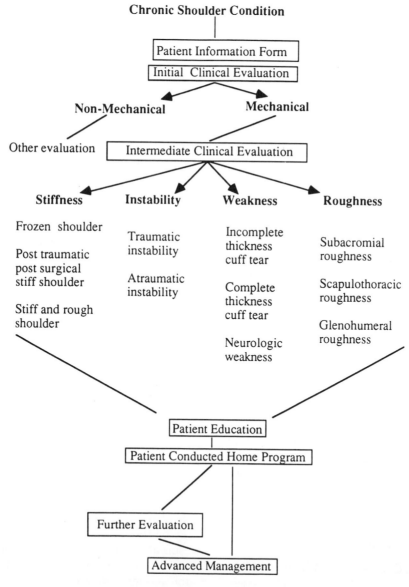

FIGURE 6–1.

Schematic for evaluation and management of chronic shoulder problems.

peutic options are usually evident from the history, physical examination, and plain radiographs.

ADVANCED MANAGEMENT

Stiffness. Isolated glenohumeral stiffness almost always responds to a persistent patient-conducted mobilization program. In selected refractory cases, examination under anesthesia or surgical release, or both, are considered.

Instability. Recurrent *traumatic* instability often requires surgical repair of the traumatic lesion. *Atraumatic* instability is usually managed non-operatively. Global capsular tightening may be used for selected patients with atraumatic instability that is refractory to a concerted effort at non-operative management.

Weakness. Strength lost through disuse can often be improved with a patient-conducted strengthening program. Surgical repair of a rotator cuff defect can restore strength provided the muscle is functional and the cuff tissue is of sufficient quantity and quality to enable a durable surgical repair. It is appropriate to obtain imaging studies prior to cuff repair surgery if the diagnosis is uncertain. However, the predictive factors listed in Table 4–2 appear to be more closely associated with the reparability of the cuff defect than the appearance on cuff imaging.

Roughness. Functionally significant subacromial roughness that has been refractory to a good persistent effort at the home program may be considered for surgery as long as stiffness has been resolved preoperatively. A conventional acromioplasty is performed if the cuff is intact or reparable. A conservative subacromial smoothing is considered if the cuff is irreparable.

Scapulothoracic roughness is a highly variable syndrome. Shoulders suspicious for anterior scapular osteochondromata should be investigated by CT scan with surgical excision if the diagnosis is confirmed. Postural snapping scapulae need persistent postural strengthening exercises. Surgery for postural snapping is limited in its effectiveness and is reserved for highly selected situations.

Functionally significant glenohumeral roughness that is refractory to non-operative management can often be treated by glenohumeral arthroplasty, provided there is sufficient muscle function, glenohumeral bone stock, patient cooperation, and absence of contraindications.

Figure 6–1 indicates in summary form how the initial clinical evaluation selects out the mechanical problems; how the intermediate clinical evaluation separates out the different types of mechanical problems; and how the initial treatment provides home programs for the different mechanical problems. Further evaluation is used when it will affect the treatment, and advanced management is reserved for those patients most likely to benefit from it.

Bibliography

1. Arntz, C.A.; Jackins, S.E.; and Matsen, F.A. III: Prosthetic replacement of the shoulder for the treatment of defects in the rotator cuff and the surface of the glenohumeral joint. *J. Bone Joint Surg.*, 75-A(4):485–491, 1993.
2. Barrett, W.P.; Franklin, J.L.; Jackins, S.E.; Wyss, C.R.; and Matsen, F.A. III: Total shoulder arthroplasty. *J. Bone Joint Surg.*, 69-A:865–872, 1987.
3. Clark, J.M.; and Harryman, D.T. II: The rotator cuff: Gross and microscopic anatomy of the tendons, ligaments, and capsule. *J. Bone Joint Surg.*, 74-A(5):713–725, 1992.
4. Clark, J.M.; Sidles, J.A.; and Matsen, F.A. III: The relationship of the glenohumeral joint capsule to the rotator cuff. *Clin. Orthop.*, 254:29–34, 1990.
5. Collins, D.N.; Harryman, D.T. II; Lippitt, S.B.; Jackins, S.E.; and Matsen, F.A. III: The technique of glenohumeral arthroplasty. *Techniques Orthop.*, 6(1):43–59, 1991.
6. Collins, D.N.; Tencer A.; Sidles, J.A.; and Matsen, F.A. III: Edge displacement and deformation of glenoid components in response to eccentric loading: The effect of preparation of the glenoid bone. *J. Bone Joint Surg.*, 74A(4):501–507, 1992.
7. Franklin, J.L.; Barrett, W.P.; Jackins, S.E.; and Matsen, F.A. III: Glenoid loosening in total shoulder arthroplasty: Association with rotator cuff deficiency. *J. Arthroplasty*, 3(1):1–8, 1988.
8. Gibb, T.D.; Sidles, J.A.; Harryman, D.T. II; McQuade, K.J.; and Matsen, F.A. III: The effect of capsular venting on glenohumeral laxity. *Clin. Orthop.*, 268:120–127, 1991.
9. Harryman, D.T. II: Common surgical approaches to the shoulder. In *Instructional Course Lectures*, Eilert, R.E. (ed.). American Academy of Orthopaedic Surgeons, Park Ridge, IL, Vol. 41, 1992.
10. Harryman, D. T. II: Shoulders: Frozen and stiff. In *Instructional Course Lectures*, Heckman, J. D. (ed.). American Academy of Orthopaedic Surgeons, Park Ridge, IL, Vol. 42, 1992.
11. Harryman, D.T. II; Mack, L.A.; Wang, K.Y.; Jackins, S.E.; Richardson, M.L.; and Matsen, F.A. III: Repairs of the rotator cuff: Correlation of functional results with integrity of the cuff. *J. Bone Joint Surg.*, 73-A(8):982–989, 1991.
12. Harryman, D.T. II; Sidles, J.A.; Clark, J.M.; McQuade, K.J.; Gibb, T.D.; and Matsen, F.A. III: Translation of the humeral head on the glenoid with passive glenohumeral motions. *J. Bone Joint Surg.*, 72-A:1334–1343, 1990.
13. Harryman, D.T. II; Sidles, J.A.; Harris, S.L.; and Matsen, F.A. III: Laxity of the normal glenohumeral joint: A quantitative in vivo assessment. *J. Shoulder Elbow Surg.*, 1:113–118, 1992.
14. Harryman, D.T. II; Sidles J.A.; Lippitt, S.B.; Harris, S.L.; and Matsen, F.A. III: The effect of glenohumeral conformity and humeral neck length on the motion and stability in glenohumeral arthroplasty. *J. Bone Joint Surg.*, In review.
15. Harryman, D.T. II; Sidles, J.A.; and Matsen, F.A. III: The humeral head translates on the glenoid with passive motion. In *Surgery of the Shoulder*, Hawkins, R.J.; Morrey, B.F.; and Post, M. (eds.). Mosby-Year Book, St. Louis, pp. 186–190, 1990.
16. Harryman, D.T. II; Sidles, J.A.; and Matsen, F.A. III: The role of the rotator interval capsule in passive motion and stability of the shoulder. *J. Bone Joint Surg.*, 74-A(1):53–66, 1992.
17. Kilcoyne, R.F.; Shuman, W.P.; Matsen, F.A. III; Morris, M.; and Rockwood, C.A.: The Neer classification of displaced proximal humeral fractures: Spectrum of findings on plain radiographs and CT scans [Pictorial Essay]. *AJR*, 154:1029–1033, 1990.
18. Lippitt, S.B.; Harryman, D.T. II; and Matsen, F.A. III: A practical tool for evaluating function: The Simple Shoulder Test. In *The Shoulder: A Balance of Mobility and Stability*, Matsen, F.A. III; Fu, F.H.; and Hawkins, R.J. (eds.). American Academy of Orthopaedic Surgeons, Rosemont, IL, pp. 501–518, September, 1993.
19. Lippitt, S.B.; Harryman, D.T. II; Sidles, J.A.; and Matsen, F.A. III: Diagnosis and management of AMBRI syndrome. *Techniques Orthop.*, 10(1):61–73, 1991.

20. Lippitt, S.B.; and Matsen, F.A. III: Mechanisms of glenohumeral joint stability. *Clin. Orthop.*, 291:20–28, 1993.

20a. Lippett, S.B.; Vanderhooft, E.; Harris, S.L.; Sidles, J.A.; Harryman, D.R.; and Matsen, F.A. III: Glenohumeral stability from concavity compression: A quantitative analysis. *J. Shoulder Elbow Surg.*, 2(1):27–35, 1993.

21. Mack, L.A.; Gannon, M.K.; Kilcoyne, R.F.; and Matsen, F.A. III: Sonographic evaluation of the rotator cuff: Accuracy in patients without prior surgery. *Clin. Orthop.*, 234:21–28, 1988.

22. Mack, L.A.; Matsen, F.A. III; Kilcoyne, R.F.; Davies, P.K.; and Sickler, M.A.: Ultrasound: US evaluation of the rotator cuff. *Radiology*, 157:205–209, 1985.

23. Mack, L.A.; Nyberg, D.A.; Kilcoyne, R.F.; Harvey, D.; and Matsen, F.A. III: Sonography of the postoperative shoulder. *AJR*, 150:1089–1094, 1988.

24. Mack, L.A.; Nyberg, D.A.; and Matsen, F.A. III: Sonographic evaluation of the rotator cuff. *Radiol Clin. North Am.*, 26(1):161–177, 1988.

25. Mack, L.A.; Rogers, J.V.; Winter, T.C.; and Matsen, F.A. III: Ultrasound of the rotator cuff. In *Diagnostic Imaging of the Shoulder,* Seeger, L.L. (ed.). Williams & Wilkins, Baltimore, pp. 96–139, 1992.

26. Matsen, F.A. III; and Arntz, C.T.: Rotator cuff tendon failure. In *The Shoulder.* Rockwood, C.A. and Matsen, F.A. (eds.). WB Saunders, Philadelphia, Vol. 2, pp. 647–665, 1990.

27. Matsen, F.A. III; and Arntz, C.T.: Subacromial impingement. In *The Shoulder.* Rockwood, C.A.; and Matsen, F.A. (eds.). WB Saunders, Philadelphia, Vol. 2, pp. 623–636, 1990.

28. Matsen, F.A. III; Bonica, J.J.; and Franklin, J.L.: Pain in the shoulder, arm, and elbow. In *The Management of Pain.* Bonica, J.J. (ed.). Lea & Febiger, Philadelphia, 2nd Edition, Vol. 1, pp. 906–923, 1990.

29. Matsen, F.A. III; Harryman, D.T. II; and Sidles, J.A.: Mechanics of glenohumeral instability. *Clin. Sports Med.*, 10(4):783–788, 1991.

30. Matsen, F.A. III; and Thomas, S.T.: Glenohumeral instability. In *Surgery of the Musculoskeletal System.* Evarts, C.M. (ed.). Churchill Livingstone, New York, 2nd Edition, Vol. 2, pp. 1439–1469, 1990.

31. Matsen, F.A. III; Thomas, S.C.; and Rockwood, C.A.: Glenohumeral instability. In *The Shoulder.* Rockwood, C.A.; and Matsen, F.A. III (eds.). WB Saunders, Philadelphia, Vol. 1, pp. 526–569, 1990.

32. Matsen, F.A. III; and Zuckerman, J.D.: Anterior glenohumeral instability. *Clin. Sports Med.*, 2:319–328, 1983.

33. Pearl, M.L.; Harris, S.L.; Lippitt, S.B.; Sidles, J.A.; Harryman, D.T. II; and Matsen, F.A. III: A system for describing positions of the humerus relative to the thorax and its use in the presentation of several functionally important arm positions. *J. Shoulder Elbow Surg.*, 1:113–118, 1992.

34. Pearl, M.L.; Jackins, S.E.; Lippitt, S.B.; Sidles, J.A.; and Matsen, F.A. III: Humero-scapular positions in a shoulder range of motion examination. *J. Shoulder Elbow Surg.*, 1(6):296–305, 1993.

35. Pearl, M.L.; Sidles, J.A.; Lippitt, S.B.; Harryman, D.T.; and Matsen, F.A. III: Codman's paradox: 60 years later. *J. Shoulder Elbow Surg.*, 1:219–225, 1992.

36. Rockwood, C.A.; and Matsen, F.A. III (eds.): *The Shoulder.* WB Saunders, Philadelphia, 1990.

37. Rockwood, C.A.; Thomas, S.C.; and Matsen, F.A. III: Subluxation and dislocations about the glenohumeral joint. In *Rockwood and Green's Fractures in Adults.* Rockwood, C.A.; and Green, D. (eds.). JB Lippincott, Philadelphia, 3rd Edition, 1991.

38. Sidles, J.A.; Harryman, D.T. II; Harris, S.L.; and Matsen, F.A. III: The functional effects of fusion position in glenohumeral arthrodesis. *J. Bone Joint Surg.*, In review.

39. Sidles, J.A.; and Pearl, M.L.: Description and measurement of shoulder motion. In *The Shoulder: A Balance of Mobility and Stability,* Matsen, F.A. III; Fu, F.H.; and Hawkins, R.J. (eds.). American Academy of Orthopaedic Surgeons, Rosemont, IL, pp. 129–140, September, 1993.

40. Thomas, S.C.; and Matsen, F.A. III: An approach to the repair of glenohumeral ligament avulsion in the management of traumatic anterior glenohumeral instability. *J. Bone Joint Surg.*, 71-A(4):506–513, 1989.

41. Zuckerman, J.E.; and Matsen, F.A. III: Complications about the glenohumeral joint related to the use of screws and staples. *J. Bone Joint Surg.*, 66-A:175–180, 1984.

Appendix

Equipment Manufacturers

Item	Company	Address and Phone No.	Part Description
1. Global System	DePuy	700 Orthopaedic Drive US Highway 30, East Warsaw, IN 46580 1-800-366-8143	No catalog number
2. Darrach Retractors	George Tiemann & Co.	25 Plant Avenue Hauppaugh, NJ 11788 1-800-843-6266	Medium (No. 80–201) Large (No. 80–202) X-Large (No. 80–203)
3. AO Osteotomes	Synthes	1690 Russell Road Paoli, PA 19301 1-800-523-0322	Handle: No. 399.54 4 Blades: Nos. 399.58, 399.57, 399.56, and 399.55
4. Balfour Retractors	Sklar	889 S. Matlock West Chester, PA 19380 1-800-221-0202	No. 60–6670—Non-slip retaining (removing the center blade)
5. Fukuda Retractors	George Tiemann & Co.	25 Plant Avenue Hauppaugh, NJ 11788 1-800-843-6266	No. 1869L-99
6. 000 Angled Curette	Codman	Johnson & Johnson PO Box 4000 New Brunswick, NJ 08903 1-800-255-2500	No. 23–1041
7. Hohmann Retractors	Synthes	1690 Russell Road Paoli, PA 19301 1-800-523-0322	Narrow (No. 399.27): 18 mm width, 235 mm length Wide (No. 399.22): 43 mm width, 240 mm length
8. Pine Cone/Wire Passer	3M	3M Surgical Products 17132 Pullman Street Irvine, CA 92714 1-800-221-0202	Pine Cone (No. L40B Burr): 4.0 mm cut head Wire passer (No. M15W Burr): 1.5 mm cut head
9. Angled Needle Holder	Sklar	889 S. Matlock West Chester, PA 19380 1-800-221-0202	Heaney (No. 20–4682)
10. Sofield Retractors	Zimmer	PO Box 708 Warsaw, IN 46581 1-800-348-2759	The set: No. 233-01, 233-02, 233-03, 233-04, 233-05, 233-06. The clip: 233-07
11. Carbojet	ISD (Innovative Surgical Devices, Inc.—Karen Roche)	413 South Martha Street Stillwater, MN 55082 612-430-3940	No catalog number Currently using "glenoid tip" for shoulder procedures
12. Neer System	Kirschner Medical Corp.	9690 Deerco Road Timonium, MD 21093 1-800-374-7557	No catalog number

Index

Note: Page numbers in *italics* refer to illustrations; page numbers followed by t refer to tables.

Abrasion, 151–154
  rotator cuff, *117*, 123, *123*, 126, *126*
  subacromial, diagnostic criteria for, 4t, 155t
    evaluation of, history in, 154, 225
      physical examination in, *126*, 226
      radiography in, 161, 226
    treatment of, 176–178
Abrasion sign, 126, *126*, 176, 224
Acomial shape, 161
Acromion, as scapular landmark, 29–30, *29*, *30*
Acromioplasty, 137, *137*
  contraindications to, 136, 176
  failed, 178
  for rough shoulder, 176–178
Adduction, cross-body, 20, *21*
    exercise for, 47, *49*, 170, *171*, 216
    normal values for, 22t
Adhesion-cohesion, stability and, 71–72
Aerobic exercise, after arthroplasty, 216
  for rough shoulder, 174–175
  for stiff or frozen shoulder, 49
Age. See also specific disorder.
  diagnosis and, 5–6, 6t, *7–9*
AMBRII, 81. See also *Atraumatic instability.*
Analgesics, for rough shoulder, 175
  for stiff or frozen shoulder, 49
Angle of humeroscapular elevation, 29, *30*. See also
    Humeroscapular positions.
Angle of humerothoracic elevation, 20, *22*. See also
    Humerothoracic positions.
Angles of balance stability, 63, 63t
Anterior glenohumeral instability, traumatic. See
    Traumatic anterior glenohumeral instability.
Apprehension, glenohumeral, 61
Apprehension test, 80t, 101, 223
Arthritis. See also *Degenerative joint disease;*
    Rheumatoid arthritis.
  inflammatory, 152

Arthritis *(Continued)*
  post-traumatic, arthroplasty for, 200, 214, 219
Arthrodesis, 148–149, *149*, 179
Arthrography, in rotator cuff lesions, 128–129
Arthropathy, capsulorrhaphy and, 152
  age and, 5–6, 6t, *7–9*, *157*
  arthroplasty for, 198, 200, *200*
  diagnostic criteria for, 5t, 156t
  evaluation of, history in, 226
    physical examination in, 226
    radiography in, 227
  obligate translation and, 40
  Simple Shoulder Test responses in, *164*
  cuff tear, 122–123, *123*, 152
    age and, *158*
    arthroplasty and, 219
      results of, 219t
      smoothness of, 197–198
      stability of, 191, 193
    diagnostic criteria for, 5t, 156t
    evaluation of, history in, 226
      physical examination in, 226
      radiography in, 128, *128*, 227
    Simple Shoulder Test responses in, *166*
  neurotrophic, 152
Arthroplasty, 179–219
  concavity compression and, 71, 192–193, *193*
  contraindications to, 179
  glenoid orientation in, 192, *192*, 210–211, *210*, *211*
  hemiarthroplasty, 179
  motion and, 181–182, *181–183*, 184, *185–188*, 186t,
    187
  joint stuffing and, 181–182, *182–183*, 184, *185*
  non-prosthetic, 179
  procedure for, 198–213
    care after, 213, 215–218
    component selection in, 200–201, *201*
    glenoid preparation in, 209–212, *210*, *211*

235

Arthroplasty *(Continued)*
    contraindications to, 212
   humeral body insertion in, 212
   humeral preparation in, 205, *206–209*, 207–209
    osteotomy planes in, 205, 207, *207*
   pathological determinants of, 198, *199*, 200, *200*
   positioning for, 202
   radiography before, 200
   skin incision in, 202, *202–205*, 204–205
   soft tissue balance in, 212–213
  results of, 213–214, *214*, 219, 219t
  shock absorption and, 193–194, *193*, *194*
  smoothness of, 197–198
  stability of, 187–189, 189t, *189–194*, 191–195
   glenoid bone preparation and, 194–195, *196*
   joint stuffing and, 188–189, *189*, 189t
  strength of, 195, 197, *197*, *198*
Atraumatic instability, 80–96
  advanced management of, 229
  age and, 5–6, 6t, *7–9*, 81, *82*
  capsular laxity and, *79*
  defined, 61
  diagnostic criteria for, 3t, 80t
  evaluation of, 80–84, 80t, 223–224
   history in, 81–82, 223–224
   physical examination in, 82, 84, 224
   radiography in, 84, 224
   Simple Shoulder Test responses in, 82, *83*
  treatment of, 84–97
   exercise, 84–86, *86–88*, 88
   surgical, 89–92, *90*, *92–95*, 95–96
    care after, 90–91, 95–96
Avascular necrosis, age and, 5–6, 6t, *7–9*, 158
  diagnostic criteria for, 4t, 155t
  evaluation of, history in, 154, 225–226
   physical examination in, 226
   radiography in, 160, 227
  hemiarthroplasty for, 198
  Simple Shoulder Test responses in, *166*
Avulsion, bone, with rotator cuff lesion, 118, *119*
  instability and. See *Traumatic anterior glenohumeral*
   instability.
Axillary nerve, arthroplasty and, 204, *205*
  examination of, 127–128
  open release surgery and, 52, *52*

Balance, glenohumeral, 61–65, *62–65*, 63t
  angles of stability and, 63, 63t
  arc of stability from, 61–62, *62*
  humeroscapular positions and, 63–65, *64*
  muscles and, 64–65, *64*, *65*
  muscular, 114–115, *115*
  rotator cuff and, 116, *116*
  soft tissue, in arthroplasty, 212–213
Bankart lesion, balance and, 62, *63*
  repair of, 68, *70*, *103*. See also *Traumatic anterior*
   glenohumeral instability.
Bone graft, glenoid, 211, *211*
Boutonnière deformity, 122, *122*
Brace, neutral rotation, *90*
  after atraumatic instability surgery, 95
Brachial neuritis, 224, 225
Bursitis, rotator cuff lesion progression as, 123

Canal-fitting humeral prosthesis, 184, *186*, 187, *187*,
  188

Capsular shift, 89–96
Capsule, glenohumeral, capsuloligamentous constraint
  and, 74–76, *75*, *76*
  contracture of, 39–40, 39t
   obligate translation and, 39–41, *39*, *40*
   surgical release of, 53, *55*
   humeroscapular motion limitation and, 37, *37*, 38t,
    39–40, 39t
  laxity of, normal, 78, 78t, *79*
   stability and, 76, *77*, 78, 78t, *79*, 80
Capsuloligamentous constraint, stability and, 74–76,
  75, *76*
Capsulorrhaphy arthropathy, 152
  age and, 5–6, 6t, *7–9*, 157
  arthroplasty for, 198, 200, *200*
  diagnostic criteria for, 5t, 156t
  evaluation of, history in, 226
   physical examination in, 226
   radiography in, 227
  obligate translation and, 40
  Simple Shoulder Test responses in, *164*
Carbojet, 232
Cement, in arthroplasty, 211, 212
Centering point, for arthroplasty glenoid orientation,
  192, *192*, 210–211, *210*
Cervical radiculopathy, weakness and, 124, 224, 225
  physical examination in, 126
Codman's paradox, 24, 27, *28*
Cohesion, stability and, 71–72
Computed tomography (CT), in roughness, 159
  in traumatic anterior glenohumeral instability, 102
Concavity compression, 65–68, *66–70*, 68t, 69t
  arthroplasty stability and, 192–193, *193*
  labrum and, 68, *69*, 69t, *70*
  rotator cuff lesions and, 122, *122*
  superior stability and, 68, 70–71, *70*, *71*
Continuous passive motion, after open shoulder
  release, 53, 58
  after rotator cuff surgery, 136–137, 140
  after stiff shoulder manipulation, 50, *50*
Coracoacromial arch, cuff abrasion by, *117*, 123, *123*,
  126, *126*
Coracoid process, as scapular landmark, 29–30, *29*, *30*
Criteria, diagnostic, for chronic shoulder conditions, 2,
  3t–5t, 5
Cross-body adduction, 20, *21*
  exercise for, 47, *49*, 170, *171*, 216
  normal values for, 22t
CT. See *Computed tomography (CT).*
Cuff. See *Rotator cuff.*
Cuff tear arthropathy. See *Arthropathy.*
Curette, manufacturer of, 232

Degenerative joint disease, 152
  age and, 5–6, 6t, *7–9*, 157
  arthroplasty for, 198, *199*. See also *Arthroplasty.*
   glenoid preparation in, 209–210
   results of, 213, *214*
  evaluation of, 225–226
   history in, 154, 225
   physical examination in, 154–160, 226
   radiography in, 160, 226–227
  primary, diagnostic criteria for, 4t, 155t
  secondary, arthroplasty for, 200, 214, 219
   diagnostic criteria for, 4t, 155t
  Simple Shoulder Test responses in, *162*
   after arthroplasty, 213, *214*
Deltoid muscles, arthroplasty and, 195

Deltoid muscles *(Continued)*
  balance and, 114–115, *115*
    rotator cuff lesion repair and, 135–136, *135*, *136*
    surgical compromise of, 130, 135
Diagnosis, age at presentation and, 5–6, 6t, *7–9*
  criteria for, of chronic shoulder conditions, 2, 3t–5t, 5
  Simple Shoulder Test in, 6, 10–17
  unknown, 2, 5
Dislocation, traumatic. See *Traumatic anterior glenohumeral instability.*
Driving, after arthroplasty, 217

Education, patient, 227. See also *Patient information forms.*
Electromyography, in rotator cuff lesions, 129
  in traumatic anterior glenohumeral instability, 102
Elevation, 20, *20*
  after open shoulder release, 53, *56–57*, 58
  exercise for, 45–46, *46*, 167, *168*, 215–216
  humeroscapular. See *Humeroscapular positions.*
  humerothoracic. See *Humerothoracic positions.*
  joint stuffing and, *182*, *183*
  muscular balance and, 114–115, *115*
  normal values for, 22t
Equipment manufacturers, 232
Evaluation of shoulder, 1–17. See also specific disorder.
  additional, 227–229
  basic, 2, 5
  diagnostic criteria in, 2, 3t–5t, 5
  for instability, 223–224
  for motion, 20, *20*, *21*. See also *Motion.*
  for roughness, 225–227
  for stiffness, 222–223
  for treatment, 10, *13*, 17
  for weakness, 224–225
  initial, 222
    mechanical vs. non-mechanical problems in, 222
  intermediate, 222
  schematic for, *228*
  Simple Shoulder Test in, 6, 10–17. See also *Simple Shoulder Test (SST).*
Exercise, after arthroplasty, 213, 215–218
  continuous passive, after open shoulder release, 53, 58
    after rotator cuff surgery, 136–137, 140
    after stiff shoulder manipulation, 50, *50*
  for atraumatic instability, 84–86, *86–88*, 88
    postoperative, 90–91, 95–96
  for rotator cuff deficiency, 130, 131–132, *131*
    postoperative, 137, 140, 141
  for rough shoulder, 161, 167, *168–174*, 170–171, 174–175, 176
  for stiff or frozen shoulder, 43, 45–47, *46–49*
  for traumatic anterior glenohumeral instability, post-operative, 107, 108
External rotation, 20, *21*. See also *Rotation.*
  normal values for, 22t

Facioscapulohumeral muscular dystrophy, weakness and, 125
Force, muscle, 112, *112–115*, 114–115
Fracture, glenoid rim. See also *Traumatic anterior glenohumeral instability.*
  balance and, 62, *63*

Fracture *(Continued)*
  repair of, 68, *70*
  humeral head, hemiarthroplasty for, 198
Frozen shoulder, 39
  advanced management of, 229
  age and, 5–6, 6t, *7–9*, 42
  diagnostic criteria for, 3t, 41t
  evaluation of, 41, *42*, 43, 222–223
    additional, 227
    history in, 41, 223
    physical examination in, 41, 43, 223
    radiography in, 43, *44*, 223
    Simple Shoulder Test responses in, *42*
  treatment of, 43, 45–58
    exercise, 43, 45–47, *46–49*
    manipulative, 43, 50, *50*
    surgical, 50–53, *52–57*, 58
      adequacy of, 53
      capsule release in, 53, *55*
      care after, 53, *56–57*, 58
      motion interface reestablishment in, 52, *52*
      rotator interval opening in, 52
      subscapularis lengthening in, 52–53, *53*, *54*
Full thickness rotator cuff tear. See also *Rotator cuff.*
  age and, 5–6, 6t, *7–9*, 118, *118*
  diagnostic criteria for, 3t, 124t
  evaluation of, 124–129, 224–225
    history in, 124–129
    physical examination in, 126–128
    radiography in, 128–129
  Simple Shoulder Test responses in, 125, *125*
  treatment of, 129–140

Glenohumeral apprehension, 61
Glenohumeral arthrodesis, 148–149, *149*, 179
Glenohumeral arthroplasty. See *Arthroplasty.*
Glenohumeral balance, 61–65, *62–65*, 63t
  angles of stability and, 63, 63t
  arc of stability from, 61–62, *62*
  humeroscapular positions and, 63–65, *64*
  muscles and, 64–65, *64–65*
Glenohumeral capsule, capsuloligamentous constraint and, 74–76, *75*, *76*
  contracture of, 39–40, 39t
    obligate translation and, 39–41, *39*, *40*
    surgical release of, 53, *55*
  humeroscapular motion limitation and, 37, *37*, 38t, 39t, 39–40
  laxity of, as contrasted with stability, 78
  normal, 78, 78t, *79*
Glenohumeral ligament, inferior, avulsion of, 97–99, *98*. See also *Traumatic anterior glenohumeral instability.*
  throwing and, 76, *76*
Glenohumeral suction cup, stability and, 72–73, *72*
Glenohumeral translation, definition of, 60, *60*
Glenoid bone, preparation of, for arthroplasty, 209–212, *210*, *211*
  bone graft with, 211, *211*
Glenoid center line, 60, *60*
  in arthroplasty, 192, 210, *211*
Glenoid concavity, compression of, 65–68, *66–70*, 68t, 69t
  arthroplasty stability and, 192–193, *193*
  labrum and, 68, *69*, 69t, *70*
  rotator cuff lesions and, 122, *122*
  superior stability and, 68, 70–71, *70*, *71*
  depth of, 66, *66*

Glenoid concavity *(Continued)*
    rotator cuff lesions and, 122
    stability and, 65–68, *66–70*, 68t
Glenoid fossa, balance and, 61, *62*
    depth of, 66, *66*
Glenoid prosthesis. See *Prosthesis.*
Glenoid rim fracture, balance and, 62, *63*
    repair of, 68, *70*. See also *Traumatic anterior gleno-humeral instability.*
Glenoidplasty, non-prosthetic, 212
Global diagrams, of capsuloligamentous constraint, *75*
    of humeroscapular positions, 31, *32–33*, 34
    of humerothoracic positions, 22, 24, *25–27*
        Codman's paradox and, 24, 27, *28*
Global System, 232
Goat's beard osteophyte, 198, *199*
Guidelines. See *Practice guidelines.*

Hemiarthroplasty, humeral, 179. See also *Arthroplasty.*
    indications for, 179, 198
    smoothness of, 197–198
    stability of, 193
    special, in cuff tear arthropathy, 219
        results of, 219t
Hip, stabilizing mechanisms of, 61, *61*
History. See *Medical history.*
Home exercise. See *Patient information forms.*
Humeral hemiarthroplasty, 179. See also *Arthroplasty.*
    indications for, 179, 198
    smoothness of, 197–198
    stability of, 193
Humeroscapular motion interface, 34, *34–36*, 152–153
    postoperative scarring in, 135
    reestablishment of, 52
    roughness at, 176
        surgery for, 176, 178, 198
Humeroscapular positions, 29–37
    balance and, 63–65, *64*
    global diagrams of, 31, *32–33*, 34
    limitation of, 34, 37, *37*, *38*, 38t, 39–41, *39*, *40*
        by abutment against glenoid, 37, *38*, *117*
        by bony contact, 37
        by capsule and ligaments, 34, 37, *37*, 38t
        by soft tissue causes, 39–41, *39*, *40*
    maximum elevation in, 30–31, 31t
    motion interface for, 34, *34–36*, 152–153
        postoperative scarring in, 135
        reestablishment of, 52
    scapular landmarks for, 29–30, *29*, *30*
Humerothoracic positions, 20, 22–29
    balance and, 63–65, *64*
    Codman's paradox and, 24, 27, *28*
    global diagrams of, 22, 24, *25–27*
    limitation of, 27, 29
    normal values for, 22, 23t, 24t
Humerus, geometry of, 186t
    orthopaedic axis of, 184, *186*
    preparation of, for arthroplasty, 205, *206–209*, 207–209
        osteotomy planes in, 205, 207, *207*
    prosthetic. See *Prosthesis.*

Impingement syndrome, 123
Incomplete rotator cuff lesion. See also *Rotator cuff.*
    age and, 5–6, 6t, *7–9*, 118
    bone avulsion with, 118, *119*

Incomplete rotator cuff lesion *(Continued)*
    diagnostic criteria for, 3t–4t, 124t
    evaluation of, 224–225
    repair of, 140, 142, *142*
Inferior glenohumeral ligament, avulsion of, 97–99, *98*.
        See also *Traumatic anterior glenohumeral instability.*
    throwing and, 76, *76*
Inflammatory arthritis, 152
Information forms. See *Patient information forms.*
Infraspinatus muscle, stability and, 70, *71*
Infraspinatus tendon, rotator cuff lesions and, 122, *122*
    testing of, 126, *127*
Innervation, deltoid, 130
    joint motion and, 126–127
    open release surgery and, 52, *52*
Instability. See also *Atraumatic instability*; *Stability*;
        Traumatic anterior glenohumeral instability.
    evaluation of, 223–224
        additional, 228
    glenohumeral, 60, 80
        intermediate forms of, 107, 109
Internal rotation, 20, *21*. See also *Rotation.*
    normal values for, 22t
Ivory Soap sign, 211

Joint disease, degenerative. See *Degenerative joint disease.*
Joint stuffing, by prosthesis, 181–182, *182–183*, 184, *185*
    stability and, 188–189, *189*, 189t
    strength and, 195, *198*
Juvenile rheumatoid arthritis, arthroplasty for, 214

Knee, muscular balance of, 114
    stabilizing mechanisms of, 61, *62*

Labrum, avulsion of, 97–99, *98*. See also *Traumatic anterior glenohumeral instability.*
    stability and, 68, *69*, 69t, *70*
Laxity, arthroplasty and, 188–189, *189–191*
    capsular, as contrasted with stability, 78
    normal, 78, 78t, *79*
    evaluation of, during arthroplasty, 207, *208*
        in atraumatic instability, 84
    glenohumeral translational, definition of, 60, *60*
    traumatic anterior glenohumeral instability and, 101–102
Ligament(s). See also specific ligament.
    as stabilizers, 61, *62*
    capsuloligamentous constraint and, 74–76, *75*, *76*
Limited joint volume, stability and, 73–74, *74*
Loose shoulder. See *Atraumatic instability.*

Magnetic resonance imaging (MRI), in rotator cuff lesions, 128–129
Manipulation, for stiff or frozen shoulder, 43, 50, *50*
Median nerve, examination of, 128
Medical history, in atraumatic instability, 81–82, 223–224
    in intermediate instability, 107, 109
    in roughness, 154, *157–158*, 225–226
    in stiff or frozen shoulder, 41, 223

Medical history *(Continued)*
  in traumatic anterior glenohumeral instability, 99–100, 223
  in weakness, 124–126, 224
Medication, for rough shoulder, 175
  for stiff or frozen shoulder, 49
Moment arm, 112, *112*
Motion, 19–58. See also *Frozen shoulder; Stiff shoulder.*
  after rotator cuff surgery, 145t, 146t, *147, 148*
  arthroplasty and, 181–182, *181–183,* 184, *185–188,* 186t, 187
    joint stuffing and, 181–182, *182–183,* 184, *185*
  continuous passive, after open shoulder release, 53, 58
    after rotator cuff surgery, 136–137, 140
    after stiff shoulder manipulation, 50, *50*
  humeroscapular positions and, 29–37
    global diagrams of, 31, *32–33,* 34
    limitation of, by abutment against glenoid, 37, *38, 117*
      by bony contact, 37
      by capsule and ligaments, 34, 37, *37,* 38t
      by soft tissue causes, 39–41, *39, 40*
    maximum elevation in, 30–31, 31t
    motion interface for, 34, *34–36*
      postoperative scarring in, 135
      reestablishment of, 52
    scapular landmarks for, 29–30, *29, 30*
  humerothoracic positions and, 20, 22–29
    Codman's paradox and, 24, 27, *28*
    global diagrams for, 22, 24, *25–27*
    limitation of, 27, 29
    normal values for, 22, 23t, 24t
  quick assessment of, 20, *20, 21*
  scapulothoracic positions and, 37–38
    limitation of, 38, 39
  smoothness and, 152–154, *153*
MRI (magnetic resonance imaging), in rotator cuff lesions, 128–129
Muscle(s), 112, *112–115,* 114–115. See also *Rotator cuff;* and specific muscle.
  balance of, 114–115, *115*
    rotator cuff and, 116, *116*
  glenohumeral balance and, 64–65, *64, 65*
  prosthesis stability and, 189, 191
  superior stability and, 70, *70, 71*
Muscular dystrophy, facioscapulohumeral, weakness and, 125
Musculocutaneous nerve, examination of, 128

Necrosis, avascular. See *Avascular necrosis.*
Needle holder, manufacturer of, 232
Neer System, 232
Nerve(s). See *Innervation;* and specific nerve.
Net humeral joint reaction force, 60, *60*
  arthroplasty and, 189, 191–192
  balance and, 61–65, *62, 64, 65*
Neuritis, brachial, 224, 225
Neuropathy, weakness and, 124–126, 224, 225
  physical examination in, 126–128, 225
Neurotrophic arthropathy, 152
Non-articular humeroscapular motion interface. See *Humeroscapular motion interface.*
Non-mechanical problems, 222
Non-prosthetic arthroplasty, 179
Non-prosthetic glenoplasty, 212
Notch phenomenon, 120, *121*

Obligate translation, 39–41, *39, 40*
  arthroplasty and, 189, 189t
Open shoulder release, 50–53, *52–57,* 58
  adequate, 53
  capsule release in, 53, *55*
  care after, 53, *56–57,* 58
  motion interface reestablishment in, 52, *52*
  rotator interval opening in, 52
  subscapularis lengthening in, 52–53, *53, 54*
Orthopaedic axis of humerus, 184, *186*
Osteoarthritis. See *Degenerative joint disease.*
Osteophytes, arthroplasty and, 205, *206*
  excision of, 208, *208*
  goat's beard, 198, *199*
Osteotomes, manufacturers of, 232
Osteotomy, humeral, 205, 207, *207*

Pain, 2, 222
  traumatic anterior glenohumeral instability and, 102
Patient education, 227
Patient information forms, for arthroplasty rehabilitation, 215–218
  for initial evaluation, 13t–16t, 222
  in atraumatic instability, for exercise, 85 86, *86 88,* 88
    postoperative, 96
    for surgical repair, 90–91, *90*
  in rotator cuff lesions, for exercise, 131–132, *131*
    postoperative, 141
    for surgery, 133–134
  in roughness, for exercise, 167, *168–174,* 170–171, 174–175
    for prosthetic arthroplasty, 180
    for subacromial surgery, 177
  in stiff or frozen shoulder, for exercise, 45–49
    for open surgical release, 51
  in traumatic anterior glenohumeral instability, for rehabilitation, 108
    for surgery, 104
Physical examination, in atraumatic instability, 82, 84, 224
  in intermediate instability, 107, 109
  in rotator cuff lesions, 126–128, *126, 127,* 224–225
  in roughness, 154, 156, 159
  in stiff or frozen shoulder, 41, 43, 223
  in traumatic anterior glenohumeral instability, 100–102, 224
  in weakness, 224–225
Plane of humeroscapular elevation, 29, *30.* See also *Humeroscapular positions.*
Plane of humerothoracic elevation, 20, 22, *23.* See also *Humerothoracic positions.*
Plane of scapula, 29–30, *30*
Polyethylene, shock absorption and, 193–194, *193, 194*
Posteroinferior recess, reduction of, 89–92, *90, 92–95,* 95–96
Postoperative care, after arthroplasty, 213, 215–218
  after atraumatic instability surgery, 90–91, 95–96
  after open shoulder release, 53, *56–57,* 58
  after rotator cuff surgery, 137, 140, 141
  after traumatic anterior glenohumeral instability surgery, 107, 108
Practice guidelines, 222–229
  for advanced management, 229
  for further evaluation, 227–229
  for glenohumeral instability, 223–224
  for initial evaluation, 222
  for initial management, 227

Practice guidelines *(Continued)*
  for roughness, 225–227
  for stiff shoulder, 222–223
  for weakness, 224–225
  schematic for, *228*
Press plus exercise, 85, *87*, 132, 171, *174*
Primary degenerative joint disease. See *Degenerative joint disease.*
Progressive supine press, 131–132, *131*, 137, 217
Prosthesis, glenoid component of, 211–212
    bone preparation for, 194–195, *196*
    contraindications to, 212
    rim destruction in, 189, *190, 191*
    selection of, 200–201
    thickness of, 184
   humeral component of, arc of motion and, 181, *181*
    canal-fitting, 184, *186*, 187, *187, 188*
    insertion of, 212
    positioning of, 184, *185*
    selection of, 201, *201*
   joint stuffing by, 181–182, *182–183*, 184, *185*
    stability and, 188–189, *189*, 189t
    strength and, 195, *198*
   motion and, 181–182, *181–183*, 184, *185–186*, 186
   selection of, 200–201, *201*
   shock absorption and, 193–194, *193, 194*
   soft tissue balance and, 212–213
   stability of, 187–189, *189–194*, 191–195
   strength of, 195, 197, *197, 198*
   trial, 207–208, *208*

Radial nerve, examination of, 128
Radiculopathy, cervical, weakness and, 124, 224, 225
Radiography, before arthroplasty, 200
  in atraumatic instability, 84, 224
  in roughness, 159–161, *159, 160*, 226–227
  in stiff or frozen shoulder, 43, *44*, 223
  in traumatic anterior glenohumeral instability, 102, 224
  in weakness, 128, 225
Range of motion. See *Motion.*
Rehabilitation. See *Exercise; Postoperative care.*
Retractors, manufacturers of, 232
Rheumatoid arthritis, age and, 5–6, 6t, *7–9, 157*
  arthroplasty for, 198, *199*, 213–214. See also *Arthroplasty.*
    glenoid reaming in, 211
  diagnostic criteria for, 4t, 155t
  evaluation of, history in, 225
    physical examination in, 226
    radiography in, 227
  Simple Shoulder Test responses in, *163*
Rocking horse mechanism, 189, *190*
Rotation, after open shoulder release, 53, *56–57*, 58
  Codman's paradox and, 24, 27, *28*
  exercise for, 46–47, *47*, *48*, 85, *86*, 167, *169, 170, 171, 172, 173*, 216
  external, 20, *21*
  humeroscapular positions and, global diagrams for, *33*
    motion interface for, 34, *34–36*
      postoperative scarring in, 135
      reestablishment of, 52
  humerothoracic positions and, global diagrams for, 24, *26*
  internal, 20, *21*
  joint stuffing and, *182*
  muscular balance and, 114–115, *115*

Rotation *(Continued)*
  normal values for, 22t
  rotator cuff and, 116, *116–118*, 118
Rotator cuff, 115–124
  abutment against glenoid, 37, *38, 117*
  age and, 118, *118*
  arthroplasty and, 195, 197, *197*, 208–209, *209*
  balance and, 116, *116*
  lesions of, 118–149
    advanced management of, 229
    arthrodesis for, 148–149, *149*
    cuff tear arthropathy, 122–123, *123*, 152
      age and, *158*
      arthroplasty and, 191, 193, 197–198, 219, 219t
      diagnostic criteria for, 5t, 156t
      evaluation of, 226, 227
      radiography in, 128, *128*
      Simple Shoulder Test responses in, *166*
    electromyography in, 129
    evaluation of, 224–225
    exercise treatment of, 130, 131–132, *131*
      postoperative, 137, 140, 141, 216–217
    full thickness, age and, 5–6, 6t, *7–9*, 118, *118*
      diagnostic criteria for, 3t, 124t
      Simple Shoulder Test responses in, 125, *125*
    history in, 124–126, 224
    incomplete, age and, 5–6, 6t, *7–9*, 118
      bone avulsion with, 118, *119*
      diagnostic criteria for, 3t–4t, 124t
      repair of, 140, 142, *142*
    physical examination in, 126–128, *126, 127*, 224–225
    progression of, 118, *119–123*, 120, 122–124
    radiography in, 128–129, *128*, 225
    repair of, 129–149
      arthroplasty with, 195, 197, 208–209, *209*
      care after, 137, 140, 141
      complications of, 130, 135
      feasability of, 125–126, 129–130, 129t
      insufficient tissue for, 136–137, *136*
      results of, 142–143, 144–146t, *147, 148*
      technique for, 135–140, *135–139*, 142, *142*
    tendon failure in, 118, *119–122*, 120, 122
  Rotator interval, release of, 52
Rotator-interval capsule/coracohumeral ligament complex, humeroscapular motion limitation and, 37, *37*, 38t
  reconstruction of, 89–92, *90*, *92–95*, 95–96
Roughness, 151–219
  advanced management of, 229
  causes of, 152–154, *153*
  evaluation of, 154, 155t–156t, 156, *157–160*, 159–161, 225–227
    additional tests in, 228–229
    age at presentation and, *157–158*
    diagnostic criteria in, 155t–156t
    history in, 154, *157–158*, 225–226
    physical examination in, 154, 156, 159, 226
    radiography in, 159–161, *159, 160*, 226–227
    Simple Shoulder Test responses in, *162–166*
  treatment of, exercise, 161, 167, *168–174*, 170–171, 174–175, 176
    surgical, 161, 176, 178–219
      for glenohumeral roughness. See *Arthroplasty.*
      for humeroscapular roughness, 176–178
      for scapulothoracic roughness, 161

Scapula. See also *Humeroscapular positions.*

Scapula *(Continued)*
 landmarks of, 29–30, *29*, *30*
 plane of, 29–30, *30*
 roughness and, 152, *153*
  evaluation of, 156, 159, 225, 226
   history in, 226
   physical examination in, 156, 226
   radiography in, 159, *159*, 226
  treatment of, 161
Scapulothoracic motion interface, roughness at, 152, *153*
  evaluation of, 156, 159
  treatment of, 161
Scapulothoracic positions, 37–38
  limitation of, 38, 39
Secondary degenerative joint disease. See also
  Degenerative joint disease.
  arthroplasty for, 200, 214, 219. See also *Arthroplasty.*
  diagnostic criteria for, 4t, 155t
  evaluation of, 225–227
Self-help programs. See *Patient information forms.*
Shoulder. See also specific parts.
  chronic conditions of, diagnostic criteria for, 3t–5t
  evaluation of. See *Evaluation of shoulder.*
  frozen. See *Frozen shoulder.*
  loose. See *Atraumatic instability.*
  rough, 152–154, *153*. See also *Roughness.*
  stiff. See *Stiff shoulder.*
  treatable, 2
  undiagnosable, 2, 3
  untreatable, 2
  weak, 124. See also *Rotator cuff.*
Shoulder Information Form, 13–16t, 222
Shoulder shrug exercise, 86, *87*, 88, 171, 174, *174*
Simple Shoulder Test (SST), 6, 10–17
  humeroscapular positions in, 30, 31t
   global diagrams of, *32*, *33*
  humerothoracic positions in, 22, 24t
   global diagrams of, *25*, *26*
  in atraumatic instability, 82, *83*
  in frozen shoulder, *42*
  in full thickness rotator cuff tear, 125, *125*
  in rough shoulder, *162–166*
   from avascular necrosis, *165*
   from capsulorrhaphy arthropathy, *164*
   from cuff tear arthropathy, *166*
   from degenerative joint disease, *162*
   from rheumatoid arthritis, *163*
  in traumatic anterior glenohumeral instability, 100, *101*
  normal performance on, 10, *11*
  reproducibility of, 10, *12*
  Shoulder Information Form with, 13–16t
  treatment evaluation by, 10, *13*
Smoothness, 152–154, *153*. See also *Roughness.*
  of arthroplasty, 197–198
Soft tissue balance, in arthroplasty, 212–213
Special hemiarthroplasty, in cuff tear arthropathy, 219
  results of, 219t
SST. See *Simple Shoulder Test (SST).*
Stability, 59–109. See also *Atraumatic instability;*
  Traumatic anterior glenohumeral instability.
  arthroplasty and, 187–189, 189t, *189–194*, 191–195
   joint stuffing and, 188–189, *189*, 189t
  capsular laxity and, 76, *77*, 78, 78t, *79*, 80
  definitions concerning, 60–61, *60*
  glenohumeral, 60
  intermediate, 107, 109
  mechanism(s) for, 61, *61*, *62*
   adhesion-cohesion as, 71–72

Stability *(Continued)*
  balance as, 61–65, *62–65*, 63t
   angles of stability and, 63, 63t
   arc of stability from, 61–62, *62*
   humeroscapular positions and, 63–65, *64*
   muscles and, 64–65, *64*, *65*
  capsuloligamentous constraint as, 74–76, *75*, *76*
  concavity compression as, 65–68, *66–70*, 68t, 69t
   in arthroplasty, 192–193, *193*
   labrum and, 68, *69*, 69t, *70*
   rotator cuff lesions and, 122, *122*
   superior stability and, 68, 70–71, *70*, *71*
  glenohumeral suction cup as, 72–73, *72*
  limited joint volume as, 73–74, *74*
  superior, mechanisms for, 68, 70–71, *70*, *71*
  postoperative loss of, 135
Stiff shoulder, 39
  advanced management of, 229
  diagnostic criteria for, 3t, 41t
  evaluation of, 41, *42*, 43, 222–223
   additional, 227
   history in, 41, 223
   physical examination in, 41, 43, 223
   radiography in, 43, *44*, 223
  treatment of, 43, 45–58
   exercise, 43, 45–47, *46–49*
   manipulative, 43, 50, *50*
   surgical, 50–53, *52–57*, 58
    adequacy of, 53
    capsule release in, 53, *55*
    care after, 53, *56–57*, 58
    motion interface reestablishment in, 52, *52*
    rotator interval opening in, 52
    subscapularis lengthening in, 52–53, *53*, *54*
Strength, 111–149. See also *Rotator cuff.*
  arthroplasty and, 195, 197, *197*, *198*
  muscles and, 112, *112–115*, 114–115
Stretching exercises, 45–47, *46–49*, 49, 167, *168–171*, 170
Stuffing, by prosthesis, 181–182, *182–183*, 184, *185*
  stability and, 188–189, *189*, 189t
  strength and, 195, *198*
Subacromial abrasion, diagnostic criteria for, 4t, 155t
  evaluation of, history in, 154, 225
   physical examination in, *126*, 226
   radiography in, 161, 226
  treatment of, 176–178
Subacromial space, 153
Subluxation, rotator cuff lesion progression and, 123–124
Subscapularis tendon, arthroplasty and, 202, *203*, 204, *204*
  lengthening of, 52–53, *53*, *54*, 202, *203*, 204, *204*
  Z-plasty for, 204, *204*
  testing of, 126, *127*
Suction cup, glenohumeral, stability and, 72–73, *72*
Supine press exercise, 131–132, *131*, 137, 217
Suprascapular nerve, examination of, 128
Suprascapular neuropathy, weakness and, 125
Supraspinatus muscle, stability and, 70, *70*, 71
Supraspinatus tendon, in open shoulder release, 52
  rotator cuff lesions and, 118, *119–122*, 120, 122
  testing of, 126, *127*
Surgeon, treatment evaluation by, 10, 17
Surgery, equipment manufacturers for, 232
  for atraumatic instability, 89–92, *90*, *92–95*, 95–96
   care after, 90–91, 95–96
  for rotator cuff lesions, 129–149
   arthrodesis, 148–149, *149*
   care after, 137, 140, 141

Surgery *(Continued)*
  complications of, 130, 135
    feasability of, 125–126, 129–130, 129t
    insufficient tissue for, 136–137, *136*
    partial thickness defects and, 140, 142, *142*
    results of, 142–143, 144t–146t, *147, 148*
    technique for, 135–140, *135–139*, 142, *142*
  for rough shoulder, glenohumeral. See *Arthroplasty.*
    humeroscapular, 176–178
    scapulothoracic, 161
  for stiff or frozen shoulder, 50–53, *52–57*, 58
    adequacy of, 53
    capsule release in, 53, *55*
    care after, 53, *56–57*, 58
    motion interface reestablishment in, 52, *52*
    rotator interval opening in, 52
    subscapularis lengthening in, 52–53, *53, 54*
  for traumatic anterior glenohumeral instability, 102–
    109
    care after, 107, 108
    indications for, 103
    technique for, 103, 105–107, *105, 106*
  stiff shoulder after. See *Stiff shoulder.*
Synovial fluid, stability and, 71–72

Tendinitis, rotator cuff lesion progression as, 123
Tendon(s). See also specific tendons.
  rotator cuff lesions and, 118, *119–122*, 120, 122, 136,
    143
    postoperative evaluation of, 143, 144t–146t
Tendon signs, 126, *127*, 224, 225
Thoracic nerve, examination of, 128
Thoracic nerve palsy, weakness and, 124
Throwing, global diagram of, *27*
  inferior glenohumeral ligament and, 76, *76*
Torque, 112, *112*
Translation. See also *Laxity.*
  arthroplasty and, 188–189, *189–191*
  glenohumeral, 60, *60*
  obligate, 39–41, *39, 40*
Trauma, anterior glenohumeral instability after. See
    Traumatic anterior glenohumeral instability.
  degenerative joint disease after. See *Secondary de-
    generative joint disease.*
  stiff shoulder after. See *Stiff shoulder.*
Traumatic anterior glenohumeral instability, 97–109

Traumatic anterior glenohumeral instability *(Continued)*
  advanced management of, 229
  age and, 5–6, 6t, *7–9*, 99, *99*
  capsular laxity and, *79*
  cause of, 97–99, *97, 98*
  defined, 61
  diagnostic criteria for, 3t, 80t
  evaluation of, 99–102, 223
    history in, 99–100, 223
    physical examination in, 100–102, 224
    radiography in, 102, 224
    Simple Shoulder Test responses in, 100, *101*
  treatment of, 102–109
    surgical, 103–109
      care after, 107, 108
      indications for, 103
      technique for, 103, 105–107, *105, 106*
Tuberosity union, 209
TUBS syndrome, 99. See also *Traumatic anterior
    glenohumeral instability.*

Ulnar nerve, examination of, 128
Ultrasonography, in rotator cuff lesions, 128–129

Volume, joint, stability and, 73–74, *74*

Water exercises, after arthroplasty, 217
Weakness, 124
  advanced management of, 229
  evaluation of, 224–225
    additional, 228
    history in, 124–126, 224
    physical examination in, 126–128, 224–225
    radiography in, 128, 225
  exercise treatment of, 130, 131–132, *131*
Wire passer, manufacturer of, 232

Zipper phenomenon, 118, 120
Z-plasty, for subscapularis tendon lengthening, 204,
    204